# ARCHITECTURAL DESIGN AND INDOOR MICROBIAL POLLUTION

# ARCHITECTURAL DESIGN AND INDOOR MICROBIAL POLLUTION

*Edited by*

**RUTH B. KUNDSIN**

Department of Microbiology and Molecular Genetics

Harvard Medical School

Brigham and Women's Hospital



New York Oxford

OXFORD UNIVERSITY PRESS

1988

Oxford University Press

Oxford New York Toronto
Delhi Bombay Calcutta Madras Karachi
Petaling Jaya Singapore Hong Kong Tokyo
Nairobi Dar es Salaam Cape Town
Melbourne Auckland

and associated companies in
Berlin Ibadan



Published by Oxford University Press, Inc.,
200 Madison Avenue, New York, New York 10016



**Library of Congress Cataloging-in-Publication Data**

Architectural design and indoor microbial pollution.

Based on seminar held at the annual Meeting of the American Society for Microbiology, March 1986, in Washington, D.C.
Includes bibliographies and index.
1. Buildings--Environmental engineering--Congresses.
2. Air--Pollution, Indoor--Health aspects--Congresses.
3. Air--Microbiology--Congresses. I. Kundsin, Ruth B., 1916– . II. American Society for Microbiology. Meeting (86th : 1986 : Washington, D.C.) [DNLM:
1. Air Microbiology--congresses. 2. Air Pollution--adverse effects--congresses. 3. Climate--congresses.
4. Facility Design and Construction--congresses.

WA 750 A673 1986]
TH6014.A73 1988 628.5′36 88–12626
ISBN 0–19–504436–3

10 9 8 7 6 5 4 3 2 1

Printed in the United States of America

# Preface

Architecture is an art form. However unlike other art forms such as painting, sculpture, dance, theatre, and music which one can enjoy without physical involvement, architecture defines space, space which has occupants. Because of this difference, architects may be designing a monument but they are also defining a habitation.

Recent evidence of serious disease resulting from the design of heating, ventilating and air conditioning systems has resulted in concern for the type of construction that creates such health problems.

In order to address the problems of construction and its relation to indoor microbial pollution, a seminar was held at the annual meeting of the American Society of Microbiology in March 1986, in Washington, DC. The seminar, entitled *Impact of Architectural Design on Microbial Pollution*, was convened together with Anita K. Highsmith of the Centers for Disease Control, Atlanta, GA. Participants were Peter S. Hockaday, MBT Associates of San Francisco, CA; Philip Morey, at the time with the National Institute for Occupational Safety and Health, Morgantown, WV; James E. Woods, Jr., Honeywell, Bloomington, MN; Carl W. Walter, the Harvard Medical School, Boston, MA; Anita K. Highsmith of CDC, Atlanta; and myself, Ruth B. Kundsin, of the Brigham and Women's Hospital, Boston, MA.

The seminar served as the inspiration for this book. It became apparent that many disciplines were involved in ascertaining that buildings were safe. Other knowledgeable contributors were solicited and invited to present their findings, so that in addition to our original six participants we now have twelve.

To-date the emphasis has been on chemical contaminants. The NIOSH/OSHA *Pocket Guide to Chemical Hazards* published by the U.S. Department of Health, Education, and Welfare lists 370 chemicals which are considered hazardous. No similar list exists for microbial contaminants.

The microbiological hazard of enclosed space is increased wherever people congregate. The method of handling the air supply and the microbial quality of the air intake determines the background microbiology, added to that is the microbial contribution of the occupants. Thus the environment reflects the sum of all microorganisms contributed by animate and inanimate sources. It is these sources that are defined in this book.

The authors of the ensuing chapters represent those who design as well as those who inhabit structure-enclosed spaces. Some have particular expertise in evaluating the enclosed spaces. The observations of thoughtful scientists as to the objective determinations and characteristics which comprise a hygienic environment are presented.

*Acknowledgments.* I am deeply indebted to two friends, Carl W. Walter and Anita K. Highsmith, both of whom were participants in the original seminar. They provided the understanding and support that turned an idea into a reality.

*Boston, MA* R. B. K.
*October 1987*

# Contents

# Contributors

James C. Feeley, Ph.D.
Pathogen Control Associates, Inc.
Lilburn, Georgia

Stephen C. Frantz, Ph.D.
Wadsworth Center for Laboratories and Research
New York State Department of Health
Albany, New York

Anita K. Highsmith, M.L.S.
Nosocomial Infections Laboratory Research Branch
Hospital Infections Program
Center for Infectious Diseases
Centers for Disease Control
Atlanta, Georgia

Peter S. Hockaday, AIA
MBT Associates
San Francisco, California

Ruth B. Kundsin, Sc.D.
Department of Microbiology & Molecular Genetics
Harvard Medical School
Brigham & Women's Hospital
Boston, Massachusetts

J. Drennan Lowell, M.D.
Department of Orthopedic Surgery
Brigham and Women's Hospital
Boston, Massachusetts

Philip R. Morey, Ph.D.
Clayton Environmental Consultants
Edison, New Jersey

Edward A. Nardell, M.D.
Tuberculosis Control Officer
Massachusetts Department of Public Health
Department of Pulmonary Medicine
The Cambridge Hospital
Department of Medicine
Harvard Medical School
Formerly, Shelter TB Clinic Physician

Susan H. Pierson, M.D., R.P.T.
Department of Medicine
Mt. Auburn Hospital
Cambridge, Massachusetts

Dean R. Rask, M.S.M.E.
Building Controls Division
Honeywell Indoor Air Quality Diagnostics
Golden Valley, Minnesota

Richard L. Riley, M.D.
Professor Emeritus
The Johns Hopkins Medical Institutions
Baltimore, Maryland

Andrew J. Streifel, M.P.H.
Department of Environmental Health & Safety
University of Minnesota
Minneapolis, Minnesota

Carl W. Walter, M.D.
Department of Surgery
Harvard Medical School
Boston, Massachusetts

James E. Woods, Jr., Ph.D., P.E.
Building Controls Division
Honeywell Indoor Air Quality Diagnostics
Golden Valley, Minnesota

# ARCHITECTURAL DESIGN
# AND INDOOR
# MICROBIAL POLLUTION

# 1
# Ventilation and Disease

CARL W. WALTER

The import of microbiology in the design of heating, ventilating, and air-conditioning systems is only tangentially considered by architects, air-conditioning engineers, and systems engineers. Airborne disease remains but a theory of microbiologists; indeed, most physicians and epidemiologists ignore it, preferring to deal with readily demonstrable vectors—fingers, food, water, insects, and like fomites. This chapter provides selected examples of environments that foster sickness among occupants which should result in a compelling consensus of support for multidisciplinary action aimed at healthy as well as comfortable environments in buildings. It is no longer tenable for architects, engineers, physicians, microbiologists, and epidemiologists to ignore the impact of bioburden spread by ventilation on productivity or incidence of disease due to infection or allergy in hospitals.

## SICK BUILDING SYNDROME

Surprisingly, the American Society of Heating, Refrigeration, and Air Conditioning Engineers (ASHRAE) sets no standard for bioburden (ASHRAE Standard, 1981). Further, the ventilation standards set by the Department of Energy, promulgated to preserve energy, state that airborne organisms are an uncommon vector of nosocomial pathogens (Division of Facilities Utilization, 1978). Greater ventilation is required for beauty parlors and motel rooms than for bedridden hospital patients. The only requirement with putative medical impact relates to increased ventilation to dilute tobacco smoke. Unfortunately, the ventilating air that disperses the smoke can also provide occupants with lethal doses of microorganisms or debilitating allergens. Architects and engineers too often ignore the health of the future occupants of the building they are designing. This is especially the case with airborne viral diseases, such as chickenpox or measles, and nosocomial infections among immunologically compromised patients.

The requirements for hospital facilities of the Department of Health, Education, and Welfare (now the Department of Health and Human Services) describe the mechanical performance of ventilation systems in more hygienically realistic detail than the ASHRAE specifications. However, the specifications for the design of HVAC systems essential to preclude the growth of microbes inside the system are not considered. Duct linings are permitted and terminal filters with 90 percent efficiency are required in aseptic areas (Division of Facilities Utilization, 1978). It is assumed that high-efficiency terminal filters remove microbial contamination entrained elsewhere. This is true only as long as the filter remains dry. Once wetted, fungi and certain bacteria simply grow through the filter and entrain on the downstream side.

The sick building syndrome (Finnegan, Pickering, and Burge, 1984) has emerged from a welter of anecdotal reports to become a documented entity with increasingly clear etiologic factors. Indeed, the demand for correction of the condition has spawned dedicated engineering and commercial enterprises (Baldwin; Foster). Expertise based on field experience is evolving on a national scale (Woods and Morey; Chapters VI, III). Chemical irritants, allergens, insects, and microbes have been defined as the pathogenic messengers of improper design, construction, or maintenance of the ventilation system of the workplace (Spengler and Sexton, 1983).

The prevalence of the sick building syndrome was studied in central England in nine office buildings occupied for more than five years (Finnegan, Pickering, and Burge, 1984). Complaints by workers initiated the study in two buildings—the other seven buildings were selected by the investigators without knowledge of any dissatisfaction among the workers. A physician-conducted questionnaire inquired into work-related symptoms typifying the syndrome either

**Table 1.1** Details of Buildings and Populations Studied in Each

| | Buildings | | | | | | | | |
|---|---|---|---|---|---|---|---|---|---|
| | 1 | 2 | 3 | 4 | 5 | 6 | 7 | 8 | 9 |
| No. of workers in sample | 246 | 65 | 146 | 143 | 272 | 227 | 78 | 88 | 120 |
| Proportion seen (%) | 81.7 | 75.4 | 88.4 | 78.3 | 82.7 | 87.2 | 93.6 | 88.6 | 81.7 |
| Natural ventilation | – | + | – | + | – | – | – | – | + |
| Mechanical ventilation | + | – | + | – | + | + | + | + | – |
| Humidified | + | – | + | – | + | + | – | + | – |
| Air recirculation | + | – | – | – | – | + | + | + | – |

*From* Finnegan, Pickering, and Burge, 1984. By permission of the authors and *British Medical Journal*.
+ = factor present; – = factor absent.

among the entire work force or a random sample. From 75 percent to 93 percent of the workers participated; 1,385 questionnaires were analyzed (Table 1.1). Five of the office buildings were fully air-conditioned; air was recirculated through a mechanical ventilation system in six; three were naturally ventilated (Table 1.2). Comparison between the naturally ventilated buildings and the other buildings at the same location showed a repetitive pattern of nasal, ocular, and mucous membrane symptoms associated with dry skin, lethargy, and headaches among occupants of those buildings with mechanical ventilation. The array of symptoms tended to develop toward the end of the day and abated after leaving the workplace (Table 1.3).

The study concluded that the sick building syndrome is a reaction to the working environment on a scale that merits detailed investigation of etiologic factors by a multidisciplinary group of architects, engineers, and physicians.

The etiology of a clinically defineable entity—hypersensitivity pneumonitis—has been documented as resulting from airborne allergens spread from microbiologic contamination in ventilating, heating, cooling, or humidifying systems in offices, factories, homes, or automobiles (Banaszak, Thiede, and Fink, 1970; Edwards, 1980; Fink, Banaszak, Barboriak et al., 1976; Fink, Banaszak, Thiede, and Barboriak, 1971; Hales, Greene, and Rubin, 1979; Kumar, Marier, and Leech, 1981; Solley and Hyatt, 1980). An exemplary study (Bernstein, Sorenson, Garabant et al., 1983) demonstrated the role

**Table 1.2** Prevalence of Symptoms (%) in Relation to Method of Air Supply: Comparison with Natural Ventilation

| Symptom | Natural Ventilation (n = 259) | Mechanical Ventilation Only (n = 73) | Humidified, No Recirculation (n = 354) | Humidified with Recirculation (n = 477) |
|---|---|---|---|---|
| Nasal | 5.8 | 13.7* | 22.4*** | 17.2*** |
| Eye | 5.8 | 8.2 | 28.3*** | 17.6*** |
| Mucous membrane | 8.1 | 17.8* | 37.9*** | 32.6*** |
| Tight chest | 2.3 | 1.1 | 9.6*** | 7.8** |
| Shortness of breath | 1.6 | | 4.3 | 2.9 |
| Wheeze | 3.1 | | 5.1 | 4.4 |
| Humidifier fever | 1.1 | | 3.4 | 2.1 |
| Current smoker | 28.2 | 30.1 | 29.1 | 26.5 |
| Headache | 15.7 | 37.0*** | 34.7*** | 39.5*** |
| Nosebleed | 0.5 | | 1.4 | 2.2 |
| Dry skin | 5.7 | 5.5 | 16.2*** | 14.9*** |
| Rash | 1.9 | 2.7 | 3.1 | 2.9 |
| Itchy skin | 2.9 | 2.7 | 7.4* | 7.2* |
| Lethargy | 13.8 | 45.2*** | 49.9*** | 52.5*** |

*From* Finnegan, Pickering, and Burge, 1984. By permission of the authors and *British Medical Journal.*

Significance of difference when compared with natural ventilation: $p$* <0.05; **<0.01; ***<0.001.

of *Penicillium* mold from a contaminated office ventilation system in clinical disease in two offices in 1979. The heater-cooler units had not been maintained and their filters had not been changed for two years. The intake was at the bottom of an external shaft covered with rotting leaves (Table 1.4). Two individuals in separate clerical cubicles among fourteen workers in a suite of offices developed hypersensitivity pneumonitis; a third worker was diagnosed as having pulmonary sarcoiditis.

## QUALITY OF VENTILATING AIR

Location of the air intake as the prime consideration in determining the quality of ventilating air is too often disregarded. Fire safety prompts the location of the air intake low in the structure to preclude

**Table 1.3** Prevalence of Symptoms (%) in Each Building Studied

| | Buildings | | | | | | | | |
|---|---|---|---|---|---|---|---|---|---|
| Symptom | 1 | 2 | 3 | 4 | 5* | 6 | 7 | 8* | 9 |
| Nasal | 18.4 | 8.2 | 27.6 | 5.4 | 19.6 | 14.1 | 13.7 | 21.8 | 5.1 |
| Eye | 9.5 | 4.1 | 21.9 | 7.1 | 34.7 | 18.7 | 8.2 | 35.6 | 5.1 |
| Mucous membrane | 24.9 | 8.2 | 34.9 | 9.0 | 39.6 | 32.0 | 17.8 | 55.1 | 7.1 |
| Tight chest | 5.0 | 0 | 7.0 | 3.6 | 11.1 | 6.6 | 1.4 | 17.9 | 2.0 |
| Shortness of breath | 1.0 | 2.0 | 3.2 | 1.8 | 4.9 | 2.0 | 0 | 10.4 | 1.0 |
| Wheeze | 4.0 | 2.0 | 8.6 | 4.5 | 3.1 | 4.0 | 0 | 6.4 | 2.0 |
| Humidifier fever | 2.0 | 0 | 9.3 | 1.8 | 0 | 0.5 | 0 | 0 | 0 |
| Current smoker | 30.8 | 26.5 | 24.0 | 25.0 | 32.0 | 22.2 | 30.1 | 25.6 | 32.7 |
| Headache | NA | NA | 31.0 | 15.2 | 36.4 | 32.3 | 37.0 | 57.7 | 16.3 |
| Nosebleed | NA | NA | | | 2.5 | 1.5 | | 3.9 | 1.0 |
| Dry skin | NA | NA | 5.4 | | 23.1 | 12.6 | 5.5 | 20.5 | 12.2 |
| Rash | NA | NA | 3.9 | 0.9 | 2.7 | 1.5 | 2.7 | 6.4 | 3.1 |
| Itchy skin | NA | NA | 3.9 | 1.8 | 9.3 | 6.1 | 2.7 | 10.4 | 4.1 |
| Lethargy | NA | NA | 36.4 | 13.4 | 56.9 | 42.9 | 45.2 | 76.9 | 14.3 |

*From* Finnegan, Pickering, and Burge, 1984. By permission of the authors and the *British Medical Journal.*

*Building studied at request of management.

NA = not available.

**Table 1.4** Spectrum of Respirable-Size Fungal Organisms Found on Air Sampling in Both Offices in December 1979 Prior to Clean-Up of Ventilation System

| | |
|---|---|
| **Predominant organisms:** | *Penicillium** (over 80 percent of all colonies), *Aspergillus**, *Cladosporium**, *Alternaria**, *Aureobasidium** |
| **Other organisms present:** | *Rhizopus, Mucor, Helminthosporium* |

*From* Bernstein, Sorenson, Garabant, et al., 1983. By permission of *American Industrial Hygiene Association Journal.*

*Organisms that have been implicated in previous case reports of hypersensitivity pneumonitis.

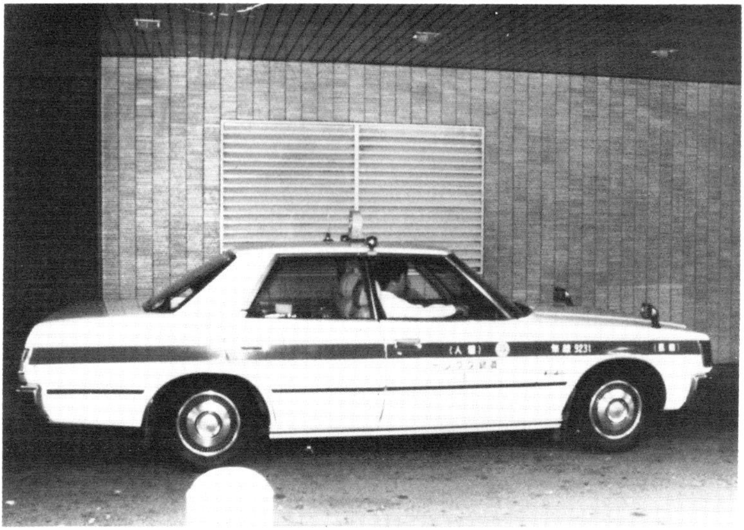

**Figure 1.1.** Air intake shares exhaust of a succession of taxis lined up to serve entrance to hotel.

the aspiration of smoke. Such siting means that exhaust fumes from vehicles at loading docks or parking areas are sucked in (Figure 1.1), as are particles of debris from landscaping. Architectural features that encourage roosting pigeons counterdict the location of an air intake. Exhausts, flat roofs, eaves, vent stacks, chimneys, evaporative coolers, and cooling towers are sources of odors or bioburden that can permeate and foul an entire ventilating system. Pneumonitis due to *Legionella pneumophila* and humidifier fever are examples of diseases caused by the infiltration of the building environment by bacteria. Even rodents and raccoons have colonized hospital air-conditioning systems (Feeley, 1984).

## SELECTED EXAMPLES

### Hospital in Massachusetts

The outdoor environment is seldom suspected as an etiologic factor in overt nosocomial infection. An impressive example is a hospital in Massachusetts that was burdened with serious gram-negative, anaerobic, and fungal wound infections. The inner surfaces of the HVAC system were coated with slime or encrustations of mildew. Recently installed filters had already collected a layer of chaff and bits of feathers. The scrubber contained a slurry of debris and several of the spray nozzles were occluded. The air intake was located behind a simulated doorway opening on a large fourth-floor deck. It faced a neighboring three-story hennery several hundred yards toward the prevailing wind. A series of large vent fans on each floor of the hennery provided comfort for the hens and ensured continuous exposure of the hospital to the airborne by-products of egg production, both gross and microscopic.

*Remedial Action:* Cleaning and upgrading the air-conditioning system would represent a fraction of the cost of relocating the hennery. Had the architect understood and perceived the airborne hazard, he could have located the hospital in favor of patients on the relatively large site abutting the existing hennery.

## Specialty Hospital in Massachusetts

Another example of an architect's ignoring an abutter is a fifteen-story, relatively new specialty hospital in Massachusetts located on the property line of an adjoining hospital. A windowless wall faces a courtyard used by the neighbor as a receiving area for maintenance supplies, contractors' trucks, and trash collection (Figure 1.2). Indeed, the trash compactor obstructs a portion of the ground-level air intake of the specialty hospital.

It is little wonder that the air-conditioning system of the hospital requires frequent maintenance and distributes a variety of odors emanating from the neighbor's trash and the exhaust from trucks. A fire in the compactor would certainly demonstrate the absurdity of the situation.

*Remedial Action:* Awareness of the problem should result in neighborly cooperation.

## Hospital in Florida

A Florida hospital with 310 beds illustrates the impact of an air intake that is defective in design and poorly located. The design of the ventilating system provided for heating, cooling, and humidity

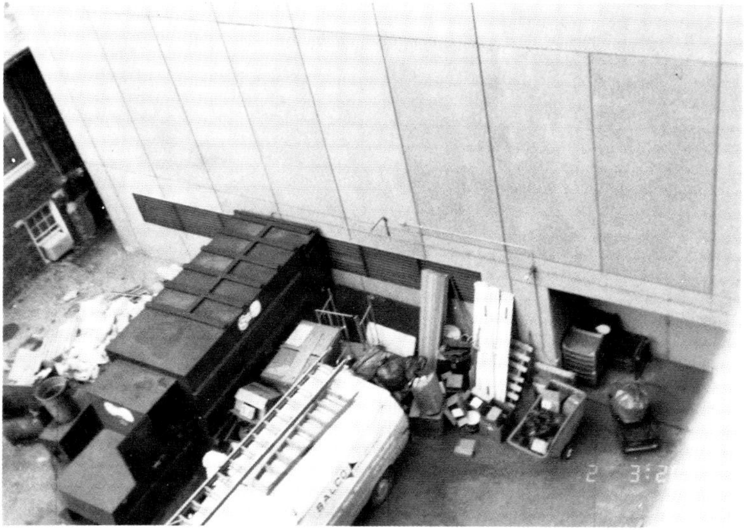

**Figure 1.2.** Careless location of air intake results in ventilation of neighbor's trash processing area. Note also the window air conditioner at the left.

control in the humid Sun Belt. In aseptic areas and nurseries, 100 percent primary air, cleaned by coarse filters and electrostatic precipitators, was used. Clinics and bed areas received 5–15 percent primary air, which was filtered through metal mesh filters and distributed to induction-type air conditioners located above the hung ceiling in each room. Exhaust air was removed through toilets and corridors. The kitchen was supplied with 100 percent primary air filtered through mesh filters. An independent high-rate exhaust system maintained negative pressure in the cooking areas, but the discharge plume coincided with the draft pattern of the air intake for the hospital.

The air intake was through an underground plenum in an 8-foot-deep area-way with the screened intake extending 8 feet above ground. A common intake plenum was used for primary air for the entire hospital including the kitchen; discharge ducts from the hospital were through cupolas on the roof ten stories above ground.

Cross-infection handicapped the operation of the facility almost from the first day. There were several extensive outbreaks of gram-negative postoperative wound infection. Clostridial omphalitis occurred. *Clostridia* were demonstrable in aseptic areas; *Pseudomonas* in clinical areas. The air-conditioning louvers in the nursing units were festooned with green slime. Kitchen and incinerator odors permeated the hospital at night. A severe epidemic of hepatitis occurred.

Inspection of the ventilating system revealed that the screen behind the ground-level intake louvers was choked with trash, leaves, and wood chips from manure that had been spread over the unplanted courtyard. Fragments of similar debris had accumulated on the floor of the intake plenum. There was a high negative pressure in the plenum, enough to cause violent turbulence in the dozen or more blowers that fed from it. The water in the recirculating spray scrubber system was murky and covered with foam and debris. The refrigeration coils were slimy. The fiberglass insulation lining inside the distribution ducts was slimy, as were some of the induction units.

The kitchen opened on a long service corridor that terminated at the receiving platform and, at the other end, at the incinerator and trash collection rooms. The soiled linen room adjoined the room for trash collection. These were located beneath laundry and trash chutes, respectively. A sorting room, contiguous with the linen room, was ventilated by a small exhaust fan mounted in a window opening on an area-way. When turned off, the blades spun in reverse. The door between these rooms had been removed; the door from the sorting room to the corridor was wired open to improve working conditions. An open belt conveyor had been installed in the corridor between the trash room and the incinerator so that carelessly discarded instruments, utensils, and supplies could be scavenged.

Performance of the air-conditioning and ventilating systems was satisfactory when the hospital first opened. However, ventilation soon became ineffective and odor control became a problem. Conditions were much worse at night.

Aside from the faulty maintenance of the screen behind the intake louvers, the intake plenum, and the scrubber which resulted in marginal air flow, no other defects were noted until late in the evening. Then quite suddenly ventilation throughout the hospital improved and concomitantly kitchen and trash odors became offensive. Inspection revealed that the kitchen ventilator and exhaust fan had been shut down. The high negative pressure in the common intake

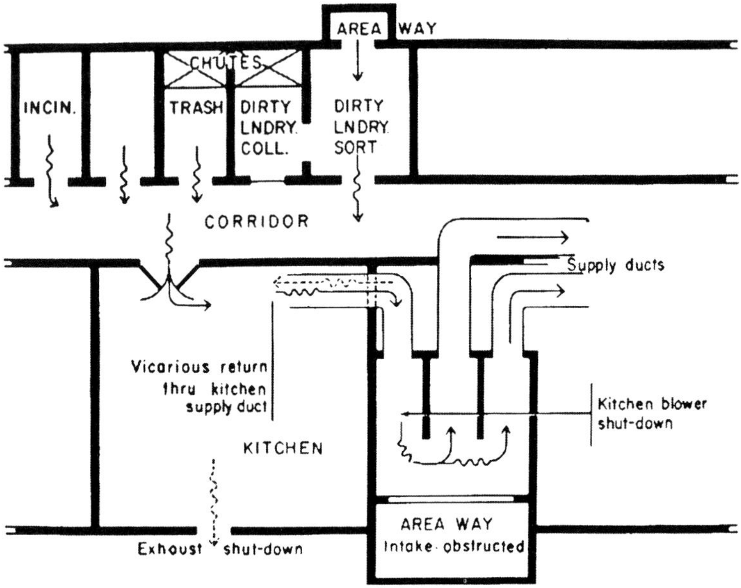


**Figure 1.3.** Diagram of the vicarious airflow when the kitchen blower was stopped. Air was sucked through the kitchen from the corridor and the soiled laundry and trash collection rooms, as well as through the kitchen exhaust fan. (From Walter, 1966. By permission of *ASHRAE Journal*.)

plenum caused reverse flow through the kitchen air ducts. The double-acting doors between the service corridor and the kitchen opened under the pressure gradient to suck in air from the corridor. This air was drawn from the soiled laundry, trash, incinerator, and loading dock areas. The kitchen exhaust system also became an intake.

Several defects in ventilation of epidemiologic significance were demonstrated (Figure 1.3):

1. Reverse flow through the kitchen air-conditioning ducts sucked odors from the kitchen when that system was shut down. The high-rate kitchen exhaust system became an air supply duct.
2. Contamination from soiled linen and trash was sucked into the kitchen from the sorting and scavenging operations to contaminate food and food-processing surfaces.

3. Smoke and odor from the incinerator were drawn from the service corridor through the kitchen air-conditioning duct and distributed throughout the hospital.
4. *Pseudomonas* from soiled linen and trash were carried by the primary air to contaminate the induction-type air conditioners in each hospital room.
5. The exhaust pipe from the standby electric generator located immediately adjacent to the kitchen exhaust blower flooded the kitchen with diesel fumes when the generator was periodically exercised.

*Remedial Action:* The malfunctioning system was partially corrected by elevating the intake louver 10 feet off the ground and quadrupling its capacity to slow the rate of flow. The intake plenum was partitioned to isolate the air supply for each blower. A corrosion-inhibiting germicide dispenser was installed in the recirculating water system for the scrubbers. The fiberglass lining was stripped from the distribution system and a dedicated return air system to the induction units was installed to replace the open space over the suspended ceiling that had been used as the return air plenum.

The *Clostridia* that pervaded the hospital were not eliminated until birds, predominantly pigeons, were prevented from nesting in the exposed trusses supporting the roof of the Sun-Belt-style open-sided laundry on the hospital grounds. Dust, emanating from bird droppings, contaminated the clean laundry to a hazardous degree.

## Buildings in Puerto Rico

"All natural" ventilation has innate problems. This is illustrated by bird colonization of open-sided shelters housing steam sterilizers and packaging operations of two unrelated pharmaceutical operations in Puerto Rico which resulted in shortened shelf life of the sterilized products. Mildewed labels and materials inside the cartons resulted in recalls.

*Remedial Action:* Steam cleaning of the roof trusses, enclosure of the facilities, and ventilation with filtered air corrected the problem.

## Another Hospital in Florida

A faulty air intake was the unrecognized cause of postoperative infections in a Florida hospital that historically experienced mixed clostridial and gram-negative wound infections. These infections were believed to characterize the essentially rural patient population. The causative organisms, plus fungi, were found in environmental cultures, on settle plates, and in dust taken from ventilation diffusors. Inspection revealed pigeons roosting in the large intake plenum of the air-conditioning system. Eight inches of guano and the decomposed carcasses of a half-dozen birds littered the floor. The large, wide-slatted louvers, unprotected by a screen, served as inviting landing strips. The filters, laden with molding dust, had dropped out of their frames and the refrigerating coils were a confluent mass of slime and mold.

*Remedial Action:* The HVAC system and the outside of the building were cleansed. Architectural features were pigeon-proofed and screens replaced the open intake louvers.

## Hospital in Oregon

An example of poor location of an air intake is provided by a hospital in Oregon where miliary abscesses of the lung and fungemia were noted sixteen to eighteen weeks after placement of prosthetic aortic valves. Some patients had noted painful chronic infections in their nail beds. There had been several instances of panophthalmitis due to fungi. Extensive investigation of the operating room and its personnel showed no source for the fungus or the *Staphylococcus epidermidis* that were isolated from blood cultures.

Volumetric air samples from the cardiac catheterization laboratory showed heavy contamination with *Aspergillus* and *S. epidermidis* (Figure 1.4; Walter et al., 1967). The laboratory had been built in the basement as an afterthought in a relatively new hospital. It was air-conditioned by a domestic-type window unit that projected out over a trash compacter. Its filter was moldy. Its refrigeration coils and fan were slimy. Personnel in the laboratory reported little illness—perhaps because they wore masks as part of an elaborate program of asepsis. Fungi were cultured on settle plates exposed on aseptic fields and from angiographic catheters taken from the instrument table after withdrawal from patients.

*Remedial Action:* The trash compactor was relocated and an air conditioner with an adequate bank of filters was installed. All porous materials in the laboratory were replaced and the walls and floor were disinfected.

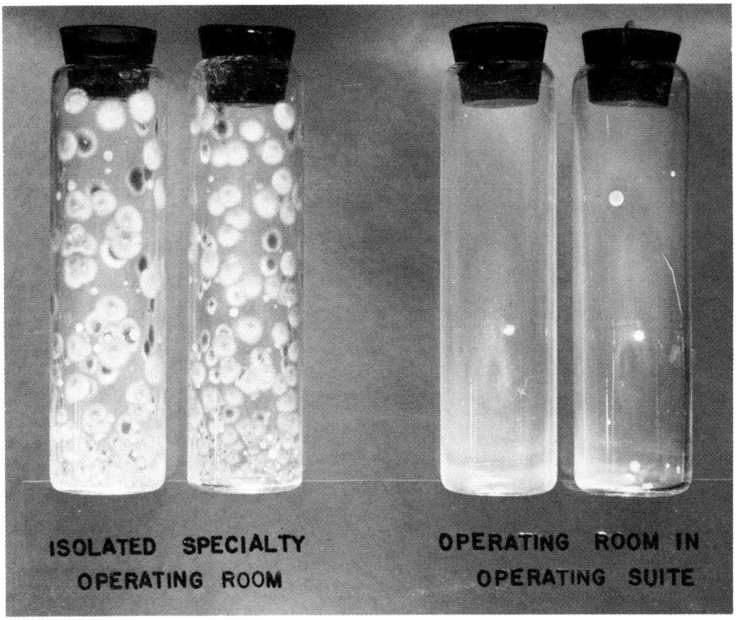


**Figure 1.4.** Well's air centrifuge samples of 5 cu ft of air taken in isolated specialty operating room (left) and operating room (right) demonstrate source of endogenous fungal infections carried to operating room subsequent to cardiac catheterization. (From Walter et al., 1967. By permission of *Clinical Neurosurgery.*)

## Outpatient Clinic, Hospital in Massachusetts

Symptoms of the sick building syndrome allergies among the staff and debilitating respiratory illness in two physicians working in a busy outpatient clinic in a Massachusetts hospital that opened in 1980 prompted an investigation.

A monumental ventilation tower with intake and discharge ports back-to-back is nestled in a corner between a six-slot ambulance dock and a busy driveway where a trash collector is parked (Figure 1.5). With the proper wind, litter from the area between the buildings is wafted above the air intake and gets sucked into the grille. When the winds are less strong, litter rises into the discharge plume and gets sucked into the intake, demonstrating an external shunt between the discharge and the intake which even a passerby on the street can

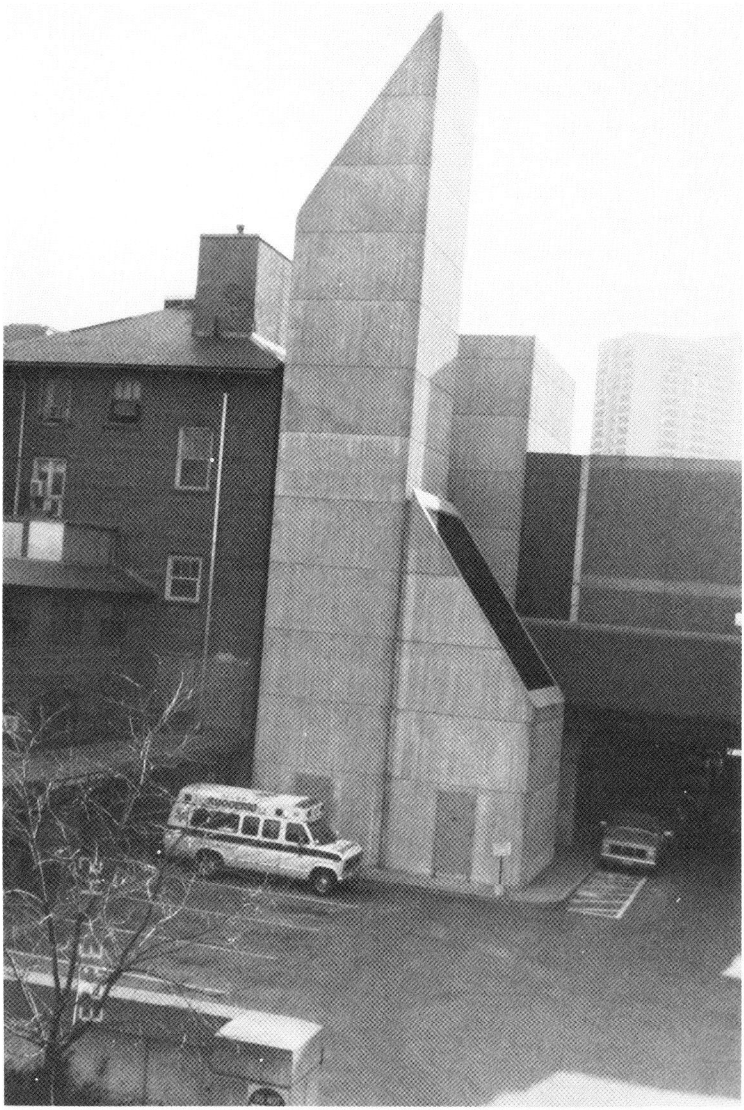

**Figure 1.5.** Ventilation tower with discharge at lower right. Note spawling stucco resulting from condensate of vapor from sanitary vent. Exhaust from rat colony tops elevator shaft that houses colony.

notice. The soaring litter is visual evidence that the parked ambulances are the source of exhaust odors. A view from above (Figure 1.6) shows abutting sources of contamination, such as a small cooling tower and four evaporative condensers. Pools of stagnant water accumulate on an adjoining roof. An exhaust from a laboratory rat colony built in the abandoned elevator shaft discharges into the air intake. The force of the negative pressure is great enough to suck open a trapdoor over a hatch in the mechanical space next to the elevator shaft. The air intake literally sweeps the adjoining roofs. The location of the ventilation tower exposes it to the hazards of fire in the adjoining flammable building complex. The vapors from a sanitary vent have been condensing on the stucco coating the elevator shaft. The inrushing air eroded the stucco and the underlying brick. Looking up seven stories inside the tower at the grille that protects the intake shows that its periphery is open to litter and birds.

The five-story ventilating tower also extends four stories underground to a 20 foot by 60 foot pit extending beneath the driveway, which serves as the intake plenum for HVAC systems for the lower six floors of the hospital. The individual HVAC systems are located on the mechanical floor above the pit that has become a drainage sump. The air intake for each HVAC system draws air from above the sump.

The sump held 12 inches of water that had accumulated from rain and snow, condensate from the cold concrete walls, seepage of groundwater through structural imperfections, as well as sewage dripping from a defective connection in a soil pipe (Figure 1.7). The turbulent, murky water was covered with floating debris, whorls of dead insects, and feathers. No provision had been built to drain the sump other than several abandoned portable household-type sump pumps that discharged water through hoses onto the mechanical floor above, where it spewed out below the intake dampers serving a series of HVAC units, compounding the problem by amplifying the surface of foul water exposed to the inrushing air. Staining of the concrete and residues of debris made it obvious that most of the slurry spilled back into the sump. The intake air is drawn through the plenum rapidly enough to cause white-capped ripples that emit a spray of aerosols.

Samples of the water grew out $>1.5 \times 10^6$ microorganisms/mL. Predominant organisms were *Pseudomonas* sp., *Flavobacterium* sp.,

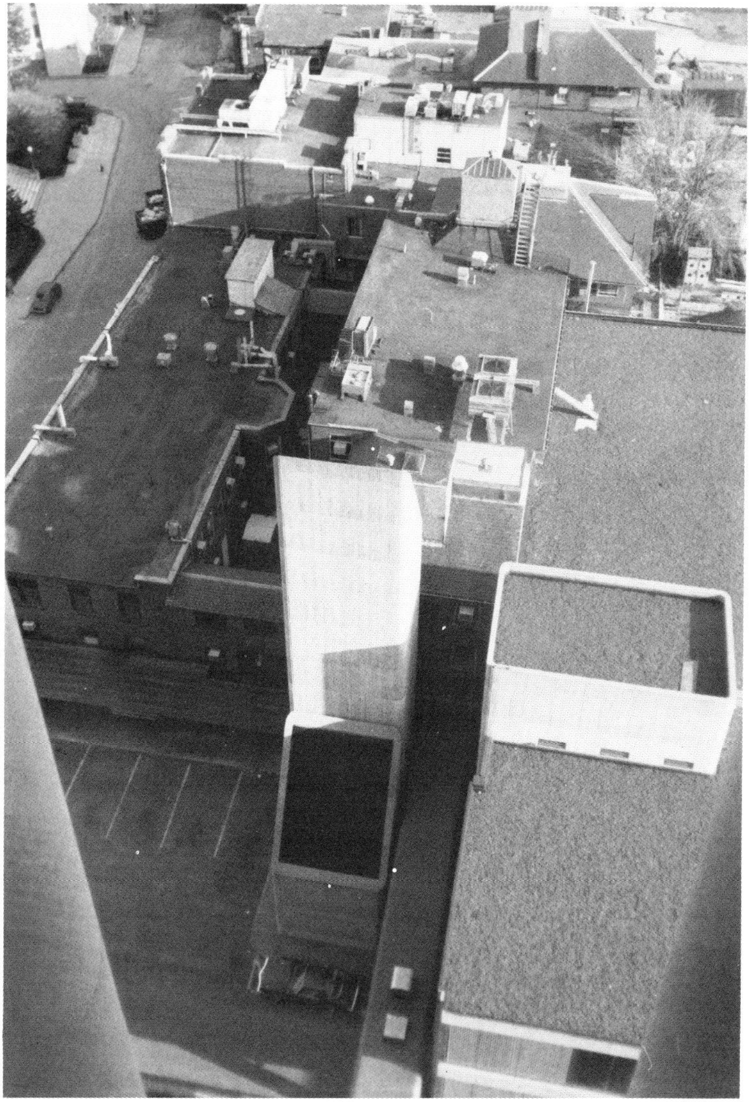

**Figure 1.6.** Sources of contamination abutting the air intake include sanitary vents, an exhaust from a rat colony, and evaporative coolers.

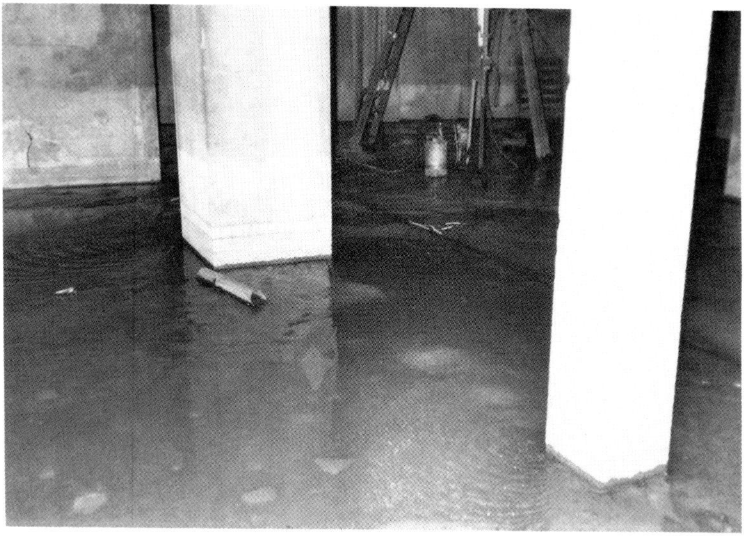

**Figure 1.7.** Undrained sump at bottom of intake plenum that supplies air for lower six floors of hospital, including operating rooms. Note ripples caused by fast stream of air.

*Achromobacter* sp., *Bacillus* sp., and fungi (*Geotrichum* sp. and *Cladosporium* sp.). Gram stain of the water showed protozoa suggestive of *Naegleria.* Wet mounts showed active amoebas, trophozoites as well as cysts, other active protozoa, and myriads of bacteria.

The large exhaust duct, hung from the ceiling, traverses the length of the intake plenum. It is covered with insulation. This insulation is disintegrating and the exposed fiberglass is green and slimy, an obvious source of contamination to be swept up by the inrushing air. The planned role of the insulation in energy conservation is difficult to contemplate.

The components of each air-conditioning system—the HVAC units—were not free-standing. Rather, sheet-metal walls enclosed plenums with one or two concrete walls, floor, or ceiling. The metal walls were lined with deteriorating fiberglass panels. Cracks in the concrete wall of the plenum downstream from the filters of the system in question permitted groundwater three floors underground to leak into the plenum. The cracks were encrusted with salt residue

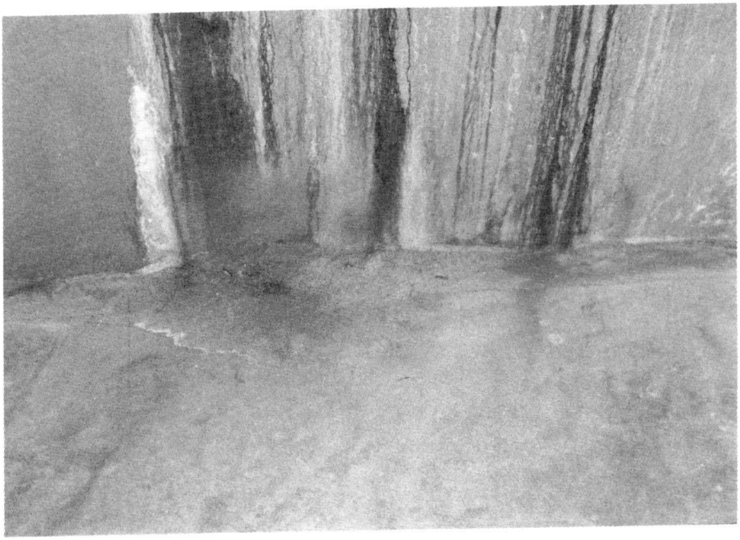

**Figure 1.8.** Groundwater seeping through cracks in the concrete wall of an air-conditioning plenum downstream of filter bank.

and overgrown with mold that spread over the concrete (Figure 1.8). The filters had recently been changed, but the remarkably horizontal drip pan under the chiller coils held an accumulation of grumous slime. Its drain was plugged. The concrete floor was stained and scaly where condensate had overflowed and evaporated. Indeed, the walls and other equipment on the entire mechanical floor showed water marks 8 inches above the floor, evidence of repeated flooding. A putative source of the flooding was an open cess pit located amid several HVAC units where sewage from the underground floors of the hospital accumulates to be pumped up to the sewer under the street.

The metal walls of the HVAC system both proximal and distal to the filter bank and the air-distribution ducts beyond the blower were lined by an inch-thick pad of fiberglass. That affixed to the top of the duct was dry and a dust of mold spores could be shaken from it. The dry fiberglass contained $1.5 \times 10^6$ organisms/g. These were predominantly fungi such as *Penicillium* sp., *Verticillium* sp., *Cladosporium* sp., and micrococci and bacillus species. At the sides the lower portion of the lining and the bottom were wet and slimy. The duct vibrated violently due to turbulence in the blower and the high rate of airflow.

Further investigation of the air distribution system was forbidden by the hospital.

In the offices that were the source of the complaints, the space above the hung ceiling was used as a plenum for return air from several offices. The surfaces of the overhead concrete slab and the concrete beams were spotted with mildew. The slab was stained from unidentified leakage. Functionally, the return plenum with its complex of wires, conduits, pipes, and ducts interconnects the offices. A portion of the return air is mixed with fresh conditioned air and reintroduced into the rooms through the induction unit. The inside walls of flexible plastic terminal ducts distal to the induction unit were dry but dusty. When doors to the corridor are opened or closed, air is pumped from one space to another, belching out of the mildew-stained ceiling-mounted return air grilles.

The entire HVAC system from air intake to induction unit was designed, specified, installed, and operated to distribute pathogens, both microbes and allergens.

Samples trapped on the adhesive surface of clear cellophane tape pressed against the top edge of doors or picture frames in the clinic revealed many particles of fiberglass presumably shed from insulation inside the duct. Incidentally, this cellophane tape technique effectively demonstrates dust mites in an environment. The chitinous shells of the insects are potent allergens.

*Remedial Recommendations:*

1. Slope abutting roofs to ensure prompt drainage.
2. Maintain evaporation coolers to preclude growth of thermophilic bacteria such as *Legionella.*
3. Move sanitary vents and exhausts out of range of intake suction field.
4. Screen intake to exclude gross trash and birds.
5. Slope floor (8 percent) of intake plenum to ensure prompt drainage of condensate, rain, and snow.
6. Provide a sump that is heated above freezing temperature so that water can be pumped to a drain.
7. Seal imperfections in concrete to exclude groundwater that is

potentially contaminated with *Legionella.* Coat concrete walls of HVAC system with mildew-resistant paint such as is used in swimming pools.

8. Strip fiberglass lining from inside HVAC system and duct work.
9. Install dedicated return air ducts from each space to induction units.
10. Organize periodic inspection.

### Animal Facility with Exposed Ductwork

An example of architectural design that fosters the dispersal of bioburden in the occupied space itself is the "organic" treatment of pipes, conduits, cable chases, and ducts suspended in the corridor of a brand-new animal facility (Figure 1.9). Imagine controlling the dust, vermin, pests, and bioburden in this building. The occupants of the building and its research projects will pay dearly for the arrogant vanity of its architect.

*Remedial Action:* A properly installed, hung ceiling would isolate the space and preclude accumulation of dust and vermin.

## LESSONS

### Use Slab-to-Slab Partitions in Hospital Design

Slab-to-slab partitions are imperative in hospitals to preclude cross-infection with viruses, fungal spores, and bacteria such as tubercle bacilli and staphylococci (Smith, 1977; Thacker et al., 1978; Wells, 1933). Such a design also serves to confine smoke to the space of origin and is essential for fire safety. To visualize the impact of this design in terms of contagion, think of aerosols of measles and/or chickenpox viruses as smoke, and one will realize why it is imperative to structurally isolate each patient space in a hospital.

### Provide Access to HVAC Equipment

Ready access to HVAC equipment is an essential specification for its design and installation. Units so crowded that each cannot be

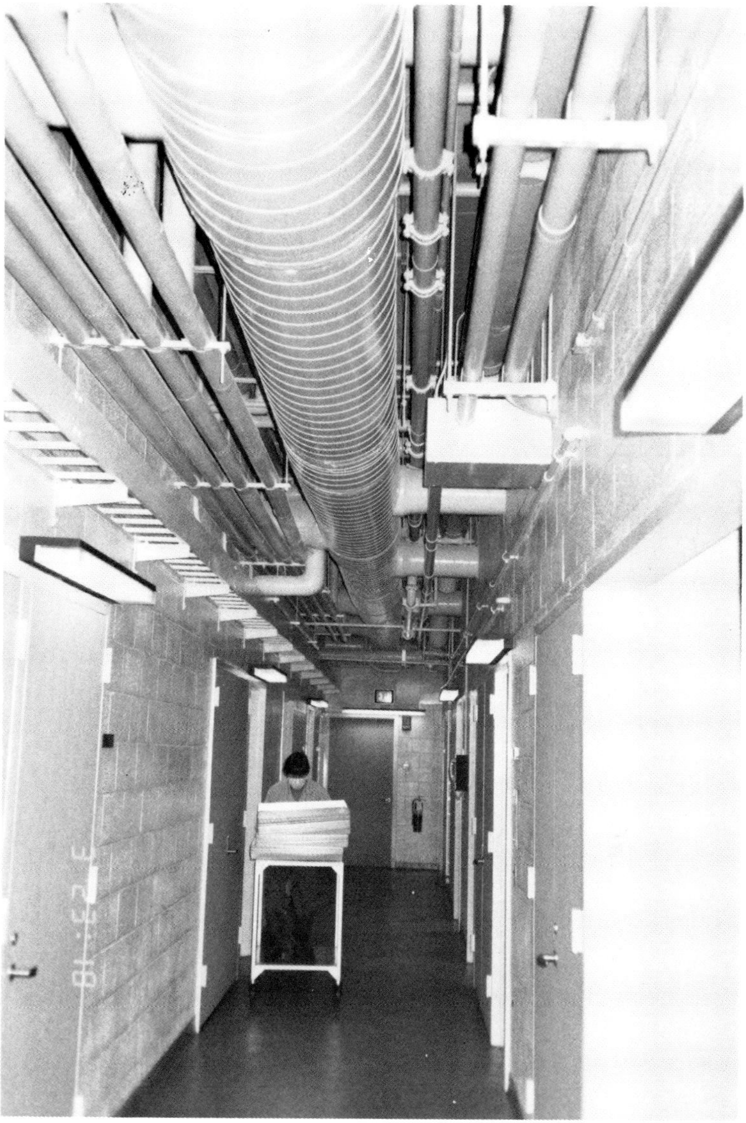

**Figure 1.9.** An unhygienic visceral display of the building services suspended above the corridor of an animal facility.

exposed for cleaning should not be operated. Concealed spaces where water is trapped and stagnates is the nadir of engineering malpractice. A filter that must be bent or cut to permit installation is functionally destroyed before it is installed. Insulation that completely obscures and seals access panels of the HVAC system precludes maintenance, yet that situation has been discovered in several hospitals. These units were choked by years' accumulation of dirt. The accumulation of sludge in scrubbers that cannot be drained or cleaned is another illustration of careless specification and installation.

## Avoid Accumulation of Water

Because it is so difficult to prevent the growth of microbes in water, its accumulation in HVAC systems must be avoided. Humidifying sprays or moist belts are suspect and should not be used. Humidification can safely be accomplished by steam. When a wet system is used, regular cleaning and disinfection must be done.

## Choose Proper Materials for Inner Surface of Distribution Ducts

The inner surface of the distribution ducts must be smooth and moisture-resistant. Absorbent surfaces such as concrete or porous insulation become mildewed and shed spores. The walls should have minimal heat capacity to avoid condensation when the humidity of the circulated air is above the dew point in relation to the temperature of the containing surfaces. Lining ducts with insulation to suppress sound transmission must be prohibited because microbiologic colonization is both predictable and disastrous. The fact that water condenses at the shear interface between a moving stream of air and the duct wall is overlooked. The insulation becomes saturated with water and the binder leached from the fiberglass supports the prodigious growth of fungi and other organisms. Indeed, the lining itself may impinge on the capacity of the duct and causes vibration that shatters the material. Brand-new fiberglass insulation contains $1 \times 10^5$ microorganisms/g; these seed successive crops which entrain to distribute disease.

## Insulate Outside of Ducts

It is important to insulate the outside of ducts to keep the duct at the temperature of the air it transports to prevent condensation. In a dry duct, microbes do not encounter the moisture essential for multiplication.

## Diffuse Air from Ceiling and Exhaust Near Floor

To ensure proper dilution of the microbiologic, allergenic, and chemical contaminants, the air should be diffused from supply fixtures at the ceiling and exhausted near the floor. When both the supply and return fixtures are located in the ceiling, horizontal shunting precludes mixing and dilution at the work level. Comfort and hygiene for the occupants are sacrificed for the additional cost of a properly designed duct system. In many workplaces portable fans are eventually provided to circulate the air in each space—an overt apology for the stupid design criteria of an expensive air-conditioning system.

## Regulate Air Change and Pressure

Rate of air change and maintenance of negative or positive pressure in relation to the corridor is often used to disperse or contain airborne microorganisms. This is effective only in an enclosed space. When the corridor door is open, inversion-convection results in a simultaneous exchange between the interconnected spaces, its rapidity depending on the contrasting temperature of the spaces and in pressure impulses from elevators and stairwells.

## Organize Expert Inspection

Periodic expert inspection is as important to the maintenance of a healthy air-conditioning system as it is to the safety of an airplane. Neglect affects the well-being of occupants of the air-conditioned space less spectacularly than it affects the passengers of an airplane, but continuous exposure to pathogens impairs productivity and destroys morale. Moreover, the neglect affects many more people. Yet, for those who serve as consultants to troubled hospitals, maintenance manuals or inspection schedules are seldom available to demonstrate that management recognizes the performance problems of air-conditioning systems. Biologic problems and hazards are ignored. Indeed, biologic sampling is decried, although it is essential to demonstrate the safety of HVAC systems. The presence of these invisible microbial pathogens demands quality control by professionals instead of the current practice of tallying victims or tracing patterns and rates of airflow in an unoccupied room, while overlooking the hygienic objectives of inspection.

## Protect from Infectious Disease

Consider the active role in infection control that a properly designed isolation unit can play in protecting both patients and staff. Despite the evidence that patients or personnel with infection are the source of bacteria that establish the carrier state, it is difficult to achieve effective isolation in routine hospital practice. Isolation of patients with infection remains a controversial subject and exclusion of bacteria from a susceptible patient is seldom considered. One extreme is conventional isolation by nursing technique, isolation by definition rather than by physical barriers (Centers for Disease Control, 1983a and b). The opposite extreme is the federal requirement of air control in hospital isolation areas (Division of Facilities Utilization, 1978). A basic obstacle is the physician's denial that patients or personnel with overt infection are a hazard.

## Use Appropriate Isolation Techniques

Consider what can be accomplished by the application of bacteriologic principles to aid and abet the care of the critically ill patient who requires protection from nosocomial microorganisms or whose own organisms are a danger to the staff or other patients. Physical barriers are essential to achieve the goal, yet in consideration of psychologic welfare, the patient must be in the open. A successful system of isolation, either exclusion or containment, has evolved after many years of failure to contain sepsis by conventional techniques. It gained acceptance because high levels of cross-infection compelled reform.

Each critically ill patient is housed in a single room that is ventilated with seventeen air changes, with the return air drifting through an ultraviolet curtain at the open doorway to be exhausted from the

**Table 1.5** Results of Ultraviolet Barrier Installation

| Before May 1966 | After May 1966 |
|---|---|
| Crowding—four-bed room | Single room |
| Recirculating air conditioner | Threshold sanitary ventilation |
| | Ultraviolet barrier at doorway |
| | Alcohol hand rinse |
| 42 patients—25 deaths = 60% mortality | 194 patients—58 deaths = 30% mortality |
| 70% deaths due to sepsis | 7% deaths due to sepsis |
| Nurse's nasal carriage of *S. aureus* = 60% | Nurse's nasal carriage of *S. aureus* = 15% |

*From* Walter, C. W. 1980. By permission of the author and the Annals of the New York Academy of Sciences.

corridor near the nurses' station. Eighty-five percent of the air is recirculated; humidity is controlled at 50 percent by a Kathabar lithium chloride scrubber.*

An ultraviolet barrier (energy level 25 $\mu W/cm^2$ at the floor) at each doorway accomplishes two objectives (Walter, 1978). It sterilizes the convection currents through the doorway in either direction—equivalent to ten changes of air per room per minute due to the temperature differential between the room and the corridor—and sterilizes the net volume of ventilating air leaving the room. Die-away studies of an aerosol of *Escherichia coli* in the room demonstrated threshold sanitary ventilation.

A germicide dispenser at each doorway encourages disinfection of the hands of those passing through. The germicide formula (Zephiran at 17 percent, 30 cc; cetyl alcohol, 100 g; isopropanol 99 percent q.s. ad 4,000 mL) forms a sterile chemical glove that persists for hours after rapid drying by evaporation. The cetyl alcohol is deposited as an emollient that prevents chapping.

The clinical results after installation of an ultraviolet barrier in May 1966 are illustrated in Table 1.5.

## SUMMARY

These discussions of selected examples of the ecologic impact of air-conditioning on airborne diseases and nosocomial infections chal-

*Kathabar Systems Division, Sommerset Technologies, Inc., New Brunswick, NJ 08903.

lenge the disciplines involved to develop design, installation, and operational specification criteria for microbiologically safe, environmentally effective, and readily maintained HVAC systems. The control of the multiplication of microorganisms and spread of allergens must be considered crucial to the comfort and hygiene of closed environments. Each of the disciplines involved must contribute expertise to a collaborative effort and share in the responsibility for promulgating performance standards. A systems engineer must be designated to coordinate the specifications of each project in the best interests of the occupants, including the individual patients. Architects, engineers, contractors, microbiologists, epidemiologists, physicians, and administrators can no longer distance themselves from the public health problem created by a fouled HVAC system that pumps morbidity and mortality along with "comfort."

## REFERENCES

ASHRAE Standard. 1981. Ventilation for acceptable indoor air quality. ASHRAE 62-1981. American Society of Heating, Refrigerating, and Air-Conditioning Engineers, Inc., 1791 Tullie Circle NE, Atlanta, GA 30329.

Baldwin, J. S., Jr. Baldwin Health Control. 413½ Avenue B, Melbourne Beach, FL 32951 (305/724-8055).

Banaszak, E. F., W. H. Thiede, and J. N. Fink. 1970. Hypersensitivity pneumonitis due to contamination of an air conditioner. *N. Engl. J. Med.* 283:271–76.

Bernstein, R. S., W. G. Sorenson, D. Garabrant et al. 1983. Exposures to respirable, airborne *penicillium* from a contaminated ventilation system: Clinical, environmental and epidemiological aspects. *Am. Ind. Hyg. Assoc. J.* 44(3):161–69.

Center for Disease Control, Dept. of Health, Education, and Welfare. 1975. *Isolation techniques for use in hospitals.* 2d ed. Publication no. (CDC) 76-8314. Washington, DC: U.S. Government Printing Office.

———. 1983a. Guideline for infection control in hospital personnel. *Infection Control* 4(4):326–49.

———. Hospital Infections Program, Center for Infectious Diseases. 1983b. Guideline for isolation precautions in hospitals. *Infection Control* 4(4):245–325.

DeRoos, R. L., R. S. Banks, D. Rainer et al. 1978. *Hospital ventilation stan-*

*dards and energy conservation: A summary of the literature with conclusions and recommendations, final report.* Springfield, VA: Dept. of Commerce, National Technical Information Service.

Division of Facilities Utilization, Health Resources Administration, Dept. of Health, Education, and Welfare. 1978. *Minimum requirements of construction and equipment for hospital and medical facilities.* (H)79-145000. Rockville, MD: Government Printing Office.

Edwards, J. H. 1980. Microbial and immunological investigations and remedial action after an outbreak of humidifier fever. *Brit. J. Ind. Med.* 37:55–62.

Feeley, J. C. 1984. Impact of indoor air pathogens on human health. In *Indoor Air and Human Health.* Chelsea, MI: Lewis Publications, pp. 183–87.

Fink, J. N., E. F. Banaszak, J. J. Barboriak et al. 1976. Interstitial lung disease due to contamination of forced-air systems. *Ann. Int. Med.* 84:406–13.

Fink, J. N., E. F. Banaszak, W. H. Thiede, and J. J. Barboriak. 1971. Interstitial pneumonitis due to hypersensitivity to an organism contaminating a heating system. *Ann. Int. Med.* 74:80–83.

Finnegan, M. J., C.A.C. Pickering, and P. S. Burge. 1984. The sick building syndrome: Prevalence studies. *Brit. Med. J.* 289:1573–75.

Foster, Larry. Air duct de-contamination. P.O. Box 409, Union City, GA 30291 (404/438-9355; 404/346-7300).

Hales, C. A., R. E. Greene, and R. H. Rubin. 1979. Hypersensitivity pneumonitis due to thermophilic actinomycetes. *N. Engl. J. Med.* 301:1168–74.

Ingels, Margaret. 1952. Willis Haviland Carrier: Father of air conditioning. Garden City, NY: Country Life Press, Doubleday.

Kumar, P., R. Marier, and S. H. Leech. 1981. Hypersensitivity pneumonitis due to contamination of a car air conditioner. *N. Engl. J. Med.* 305:1531–32.

Smith, P. W., and R. M. Massanari. 1977. Room humidifiers as the source of *Acinetobacter* infections. *J. Am. Med. Assoc.* 237(8):795–97.

Solley, G. O., and R. E. Hyatt. 1980. Hypersensitivity pneumonitis induced by *Penicillium* species. *J. Allergy Clin. Immunol.* 65:65–70.

Spengler, J. D., and K. Sexton. 1983. Indoor air pollution: A public health perspective. *Science* 221:9–17.

Thacker, S. B., et al. 1978. An outbreak in 1965 of severe respiratory illness caused by Legionnaires' disease bacterium. *J. Infect. Dis.* 138:512–19.

Walter, C. W. 1966. Cross-infection in hospitals. *ASHRAE J.* 8:41–45 (Oct.).

———. 1978. The surgeon's responsibility for asepsis. *Med. Instrum.* 12:149–57.

———. 1980. Prevention and control of airborne infection in hospitals. *Ann. New York Acad. Sciences* 353:312–30.

Walter, C. W., R. B. Kundsin, L. Page, and A. L. Harding. 1967. The infector on the surgical team. *Clin. Neurosurg.* 14:361–379.

Wells, W. F. 1933. Apparatus for study of the bacterial behavior of air. *Am. J. Public Health* 23:58–59.

Woods, J. E., and P. H. Morey. Honeywell Indoor Air Quality Diagnostics. Honeywell, Inc. 1985 Douglas Drive North, Golden Valley, MN 55422 (612/542-7043).

# 2

# The Architect's Concern about Indoor Pollution

PETER S. HOCKADAY

## INTRODUCTION: THE ISSUE EMERGES

Indoor pollution has clearly arrived as a unique issue in the fields of architecture and interior design. In the 1960s, the notion that our indoor air may be unhealthy was virtually unknown; but a proliferation of events in the 1970s and 1980s awakened the profession of architecture and brought awareness of indoor pollution to every architect in the country.

Examples are many.

In the 1970s, asbestos, an inert reliable product specified liberally by architects for insulation, piping, and many other uses, was shown decisively to be a carcinogenic killer and was banned by the Environmental Protection Agency (EPA) in 1978 for many of its uses.

In 1977 a mysterious disease struck and killed twenty-nine American Legion conventioneers attending a function at one hotel in Philadelphia. Subsequent investigation proved the disease agent to be bacteriologic. The new bacteria was ultimately named *Legionella* and the source of the bacteria was found to be within the hotel building itself, where deadly cultures had formed in the air-cooling system.

In the late 1970s and early 1980s, the phenomenon of "sick building syndrome" or "tight building syndrome" was noticed and named to describe the illnesses that were frequently reported (nausea, rashes, watery eyes, hoarseness, coughing, dizziness, lethargy, skin problems, stiff shoulders, and lung problems) by occupants of new, tightly sealed office buildings.

Several new highly publicized award-winning buildings were named among the sick structures in one incident or another—and it was discovered that these problem buildings had been deliberately designed with very low ventilation rates for energy conservation purposes.

As these examples indicate, indoor pollution is a health and safety issue. By the time the tragic history of asbestos has run its course, 2 million deaths will be attributed to this single pollutant alone. Indoor pollutants can range from products of combustion such as carbon monoxide, to organic chemicals such as formaldehyde, to radionuclides such as radon gas. Indoor microbes are responsible for fatal illnesses such as Legionnaire's disease and for flu-like outbreaks of hypersensitivity pneumonitis and humidifier lung reaction.

Indoor pollution is also a productivity issue. In the workplace, a small, nearly undetectable decrease in office worker productivity as might be caused by tight building syndrome could result in significant costs to the employer. For example, a 5 percent productivity loss is equal to a loss of $2,000 to $3,000 per employee per year. Yet it can be shown that a doubling of the ventilation rate in a typical office building would cost about five cents per square foot per year, or only about $12.50 per employee per year.

## THE ISSUE DEFINED

Public awareness of indoor pollution has never been greater. After several articles appeared in professional architecture and engineering journals, a variety of topical articles have appeared in the general media, such as *Newsweek's* "Beware Sick-Building Syndrome," of 17 January 1985.

Local television and newspaper reporting of indoor pollution incidents has mushroomed. During a one-month period in early 1986 in the San Francisco Bay Area, four separate air pollution incidents were extensively reported locally (with headlines such as "Mystery Vapors Sicken Scores in Concord," *San Francisco Chronicle,* January 17, 1986.) Follow-up articles included a detailed piece titled

"Indoor Pollution Tearful Problem for New Builders" in the Sunday Real Estate Section, *San Francisco Examiner and Chronicle*, 9 February 1986.

From the architect's perspective, real concern over indoor pollution began to arise in 1981–82. The earlier problems of the 1970s surrounding asbestos, for example, seemed to have been simple enough to solve by stopping its use (although it has turned out that the safe removal of asbestos from the environment is expensive, disruptive, time-consuming, and anything but simple). But the well-publicized failures of some of the profession's most celebrated energy-efficient buildings created a different sort of problem. Were energy-efficiency and indoor pollution somehow linked?

A fine example was the Gregory Bateson State Office Building in Sacramento—a beautiful, thoughtful design for thoroughly contemporary, energy-efficient offices. Designed by the state architect's office as part of a unique, forward-looking state program of energy-efficiency under the Jerry Brown administration, the Bateson Building opened with fanfare in 1981, but was nearly closed shortly thereafter when many of its occupants declared it unhealthy.

Although the Bateson health complaints were ultimately solved by improvements of the ventilation systems and by cleansing the rock thermal storage bed, the damage had been done. Lawsuits were filed, the California State Employees Association described occupancy as a "nightmare of health hazards," and several articles appeared in the architectural press. The general architectural reaction was one of confusion. The Bateson Building design was outstanding architecture and represented a well-meaning effort to solve an important problem for society—energy-efficiency. Yet if ventilation rates and outside air had to be increased to solve problems developing from formaldehydes, how much would this compromise the building's energy-efficiency?

Meanwhile numerous buildings in other locations were experiencing comparable (but not exactly similar) problems. The health symptoms reported from these buildings often seemed similar, but their causes would vary. A new Department of Transportation Building in Maine, extremely well scaled and energy-efficient, had problems with the fraying of fiberglass ducts. A new headquarters for the San Francisco Social Services Department developed excessive levels of industrial organic chemicals and solvents in office spaces. The source was normal cleaning and office operations, but the problem arose from faulty design of components of the ventilation system. Another new energy-efficient State of California Office Building in Long Beach developed near toxic levels of penta-chlorophenol indoors from unsealed wood preservative used on its indoor glulam structure.

The lessons that developed from these and other examples were varied, yet they can be characterized as follows. In the first place, architects and engineers have a lot to learn about indoor pollution—which can come from a wide variety of sources—and a process of education about this topic should begin immediately.

Second, indoor pollution and energy-efficiency are only indirectly linked. The minimal outside air ventilation rates, which in the late 1970s were embraced by the mechanical engineering profession in the name of energy-efficiency, proved to be inadequate to disperse indoor pollutants. Through subsequent action in 1983 of the mechanical engineers' professional organization, the American Society of Heating, Refrigeration, and Air Conditioning Engineers (ASHRAE), ventilation standards have been increased.

Third, architects and engineers must no longer use plans that specify toxic materials. Simple in concept, this is easier said than done. Levels of toxicity and levels of human response to materials very immensely. Architects and engineers are not physicians or health researchers, nor do they manufacture the products that may be toxic. Governmental response to indoor pollution has begun to develop since the late 1970s and systematic research and governmental action is being undertaken to learn more about the pollutants, their sources, and safe levels in the indoor environment.

In general, we may state that indoor pollution is caused by the use of toxic materials (or materials that temporarily release toxins) often combined with inadequate ventilation. This generalization does not, however, address microbial indoor pollution. It is possible to have a toxic condition of microbial pollution even though the building materials are totally nontoxic and the building ventilation rates are entirely adequate. Indoor microbial pollution—its special causes, controls, and concerns—will be addressed later in this chapter.

## THE ARCHITECT'S ROLE

The making of a building is the product of a large-scale team. The architect, or engineer in some cases, is the leader of the design team; the building design (but not its construction) is his or her responsibility.

The architect is a generalist. A team of specialists reports to the architect, who is not an expert in indoor pollution any more than he or she is a specialist in acoustics or air-conditioning or lighting. The architect's specialty, broadly, is the *built environment;* this definition is often used by attorneys. Colleges of Architecture are now frequently incorporated into Colleges of Environmental Design. The indoor environment is the architect's territory and the architect is in charge of creating it. This role affords both an opportunity and a potential liability.

The legal responsibilities that frame the work of the architect or engineer have evolved over the past decades. No specific ethical code is sworn to in licensing the professional; instead the standards of practice and responsibility to obey legal codes of design and construction are the architect's guidelines.

When a building is believed to be faulty and the designer is believed to be at fault, several legal concepts offer themselves. *Negligence* on the part of the designer may be provable. Another approach is to examine the faulty building as if it were a consumer product, with an implied warranty as to its safety, habitability, and so on. In avoiding charges of negligence, the standard is that the architect or engineer has a legal duty "to exercise the care, knowledge, and expertise in rendering the plans that an ordinary person with such schooling and experience would exercise." Negligence is not easy to prove; it usually requires the plaintiff to introduce expert opinion as evidence. From the architect's point of view the question will rest on "the foreseeability of injury arising from the act" of specifying certain products, such as asbestos, or of designing a building with extremely limited ventilation, or other concepts related to microbial pollution, which may in the future become part of the basic body of knowledge that is part of the architect's training.

The idea that an implied warranty attaches to a building as a consumer product is not universally endorsed. Building components may fit this definition, but their aggregate collective use in a building may not. Certain legal decisions suggest that a building is warranted to be habitable, and where proven to have been uninhabitable the provider would be at fault, depending on the conditions of sale. In a litigious world the architect's last defense is usually his or her professional liability insurance—an evermore expensive commodity as lit-

**Table 2.1** Indoor Pollutants

| Categories | Examples | Sources |
|---|---|---|
| Gases and vapors | Carbon monoxide | Combustion |
| | Nitrogen dioxide | Combustion |
| | Formaldehyde | Insulation, particle board |
| | Benzene | Cleaners, paint remover |
| | Penta-chlorophenol | Wood preservatives |
| Inert particulates | Asbestos | Insulation, pipe |
| Biologic | Legionnaire's bacteria | Cooling towers, evaporative condensers |
| Radiologic | Radon gas | Earth, concrete |

igation and awards escalate. Virtually all architectural or engineering professional liability insurance policies exclude coverage of indoor pollution claims and asbestos claims. The insurance companies explain that future pollution or asbestos claims are unpredictable—and therefore uninsurable—and suggest that such companies insure only predictable situations.

## THE POLLUTANTS

Table 2.1 is a sample of some of the substances that can contribute to indoor pollution. A complete reference source that tabulates the pollutants and describes guideline standards is the *Indoor Air Quality Handbook* prepared by Sandia National Laboratories for the Department of Energy, 1982. Table 12, on pp. 63–68 of the handbook tabulates the health effects of these pollutants.

Microbial pollution in buildings is a matter of separate investigation. Research findings as to the microbial pollutants themselves, their concentrations, sources, and controls are discussed in other chapters of this book. What follows is a perspective on these findings of indoor biologic pollution from an architectural design point of view.

## INDOOR MICROBIAL POLLUTION

If a common thread exists in the many case histories of biologically "sick" buildings, it is related to the lack of control of breeding places for fungi, bacteria, and other microorganisms. The illnesses described, Legionnaire's disease, Pontiac fever, hypersensitivity pneumonitis, and others, have as their source bacteria that are cultured in moisture. These cultures need a moist place to breed and in the faulty buildings investigated a great variety of incubation sources have been discovered. Case histories point to the following sources and breeding grounds for microbes:

- Stagnant water and slimes in drain pans of fan coil units and other elements of the heating, ventilation, and air-conditioning (HVAC) system.
- Water sprays as components of HVAC systems.
- Excessive relative humidities, above 70 percent in rooms or air supply systems, resulting in wet, moldy walls, ceiling tiles, and so on.
- Flooding or excessive leakage from internal sources, such as drainage systems, cafeterias, bathrooms, and drain and condensate pans.
- Flooded carpets or other materials difficult to dry out.
- Acoustic duct liners and other permeable materials hidden in the air supply system.
- External polluted microbial sources drawn into the air supply system by improper, faulty locations for air intakes.
- Roof leaks and other external water leak sources.

Some of these problems are easy to prevent or cure and others are avoidable with a little common sense, but several are worthy of special note because they are common components of standard, everyday architectural practice. For example, acoustic duct liners are a common solution of noise transmission difficulties through ductwork between rooms. The very properties that allow good acoustic absorption also allow concealed crevices for pollutants to collect; no equally good solution exists.

Control of rain leakage into any building is more complicated than it might seem. Buildings must be built in panels or pieces, because of factors such as thermal expansion, wind or seismic movement, and air pressure alleviation and deliverability. Joints between panels create paths for moisture entry. In addition, seemingly solid materials such as plaster, brick, and concrete are in fact quite porous. What architects must discover is how to deal with the moisture that will eventually enter and how to lead it back out, rather than allowing moisture to collect.

Beyond dealing with moisture entry or internal leakage, the problem of improper locations for fresh air intakes continues to crop up frequently. All sorts of incredible examples of foolish intake locations exist in case histories, such as:

- Adjacent to toxic fume hood exhaust stacks
- Adjacent to parking garage vents
- Adjacent to research-animal room exhausts
- Near cooling tower or moisture pan drifts

Problems often arise when pollutant sources are placed near air intakes of already existing buildings. And wind flow changes from buildings in the airstream can alter the path of intake air, causing it to pick up pollutants if a source exists nearby.

## THE ARCHITECT'S RESPONSE

Long-term efforts aimed at achieving healthy buildings are under way in many areas. The first step in the architectural and engineering professions has been to educate the professionals through publications, special conferences on indoor pollution with published findings, and a variety of other sources. Beyond a continuation of education and research on indoor pollution—which needs improved support—the building industry is taking specific actions to produce consistently healthy buildings.

### Improved Ventilation Standards and Better Mechanical Engineering

Mechanical engineering is becoming much more sophisticated about indoor pollution, as it benefits from recent research. Now that ventilation standards have been fine-tuned, we can look to future use of increased levels of fresh outside air as heat exchange equipment becomes more economical and cost-effective. Heat exchange technology allows us to pass outside air directly to rooms (without mixing in the tired internal exhaust air) and to heat (or cool) it from the heat in the building.

Another developing technology relates to pollution sensors. The concept is comparable to smoke detectors; the goal is to develop sensing equipment that will detect tract amounts of pollutants and warn occupants of a problem before health damage can occur.

## Bake-Out

A current topic of discussion but not yet a code requirement is the idea of "bake-out." Here, the HVAC systems of a building are run at full blast for several weeks after construction is complete but before occupation. This is supposed to "bake-out" the initial, most critical off-gassing, and in tests the technique has proved beneficial. In Scandinavia, certain codes require a six-month preoccupancy testing period, a concept that few American real estate developers are likely to support.

## Specification of Safe Products

The organizations that have the most influence on the architects' specification documents are the Construction Specifications Institute and the American Institute of Architects. Each organization writes its own fully computerized guide specifications. Most architects subscribe to one or the other. Architects then modify the specification as they see fit. Legally, the responsibility is with the architect, not the specification institutions.

Improved specifications will require more data from product manufacturers, such as test results of off-gassing. Ultimately, better standards for off-gassing will allow the architect to specify the time period to bake-out directly.

## Manufacture of Safe Products

Manufacturers carry a strong product safety liability, as witnessed by the legal actions that have arisen over claims against asbestos manufacturers. This situation is monitored and controlled by the EPA and other federal regulatory agencies.

# 3

# Experience on the Contribution of Structure to Environmental Pollution

PHILIP R. MOREY

Indoor air quality problems and complaints are being reported with increasing frequency (ACGIH, 1984; ORNL, 1985) and those in large office buildings are often referred to by the term "sick building syndrome" (Bardana and Montanaro, 1986; Finnegan, Pickering, and Burge, 1984). A sick building is one in which a substantial number of occupants experience discomfort as evidenced by symptoms such as eye and upper respiratory irritation, headache, fatigue, and sinus congestion. Occupants experience relief almost immediately after they exit the building. Symptoms recur upon reentry. Sick building syndrome has been ascribed to exposure to volatile organic compounds, unpleasant odors, smoke, and other contaminants that are characteristically found in the air of naturally and mechanically ventilated buildings. Increasing the rate or the effectiveness of outdoor air ventilation is generally successful in alleviating most occurrences of sick building syndrome.

Portions of this paper are reprinted with the permission of the American Conference of Governmental Industrial Hygienists (ACGIH). Some of the information presented in this paper first appeared in the symposium "Evaluating Office Environmental Problems," *Ann. Am. Conference of Governmental Industrial Hygienists* (1984) 10:21–35 and 10:121–27.

Although some sick buildings may also be microbially contaminated, it is important to recognize that microbial contamination can occur independently of the conditions (inadequate and ineffective ventilation) generally associated with sick building syndrome (Finnegan, Pickering, and Burge, 1984). The primary requirement for the growth and amplification of microorganisms in the indoor environment is the presence of moisture, and this can occur in a building regardless of the amount of outdoor air being supplied to the space. The percent of the United States building stock with indoor air pollution problems has not been scientifically determined. Likewise, the fraction of problem buildings with microbial contamination is unknown. However, in the more than 350 indoor air quality investigations that have been carried out since 1979 by the National Institute for Occupational Safety and Health (NIOSH), microbial contamination was considered to be an important air contaminant in about 5 percent of the buildings evaluated (Wallingford, 1986).

Microbial contaminants in the indoor environment may cause illness of two general types, namely, those that are infective and those that are allergic in nature. *Legionella pneumophila* may be infective in that it causes legionellosis among susceptible persons. In this illness the microorganism invades or colonizes an organ such as the lung. Allergic respiratory diseases, on the other hand, are caused by a hypersensitivity response to inhaled particles containing viable microorganisms, nonviable spores, or nonliving components of these organisms. In Europe and North America there have been numerous reports of building-associated outbreaks of influenza-like illness (often called humidifier fever or humidifier disease in Europe; sometimes called hypersensitivity pneumonitis in North America) in which affected individuals manifest acute symptoms such as malaise, fever, shortness of breath, cough, and muscle aches (Ager and Tickner, 1983; Kreiss and Hodgson, 1984; Morey et al., 1984). These illnesses usually occur as a response to microbial antigens aerosolized from heating, ventilation, and air-conditioning (HVAC) system components such as humidifiers (e.g., *Acanthamoeba* sp., or endotoxins from a humidifier reservoir; see Edwards, 1980; Rylander et al., 1978) or air washers (e.g., thermophilic actinomycetes; see Banaszak et al., 1970; Scully et al., 1979; Weiss and Soleymani, 1971) which may be contaminated or from other building components that may have been damaged by recurrent floods or moisture. Affected

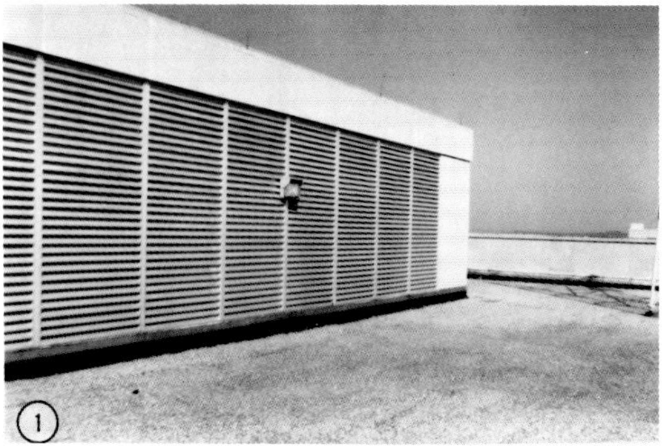

**Figure 3.1.** The outdoor air intake for the HVAC system of this building is located on the roof. Outdoor air moves through the louvers and into the mixing plenum of the air handling units (AHUs) located directly behind the intake wall.

individuals usually experience relief when they leave the building for several days.

Microorganisms that may cause allergic illnesses are ubiquitous in both outdoor and indoor environments. The presence of microorganisms or microbial materials in the indoor environment in sufficient amounts or kinds to cause hypersensitivity reactions in susceptible individuals depends on a number of factors, including the type of mechanical components that constitute the HVAC system as well as the program in place for the maintenance of mechanical systems. However, the most important of all factors affecting microbial contamination in the indoor environment is the presence of water. Water is required for the amplification of the microbial population that may be present. In large buildings, a HVAC system may serve to transport microorganisms from the locus of contamination (e.g., a humidifier or air washer) to the vicinity of sensitive occupants. HVAC systems are complex and offer many environments where microbial populations flourish. Water spray systems, humidifiers containing stagnant water, moist filters containing organic dusts, and interiors characterized by excessive humidity, all may offer suitable environments for microbial proliferation (Morey et al., 1984).

The objectives of this chapter are to (1) describe the basic (generic) components of the HVAC system that is likely to be found in large North American office buildings, (2) give examples of office buildings where microbial contamination has occurred, and (3) describe difficulties and procedures associated with the quantification of airborne microorganisms in office environments. Finally, corrective actions thought to be effective in alleviating microbial contamination will be reviewed.

## DESCRIPTION OF A GENERIC HVAC SYSTEM

The quality of air present in a modern office building is highly dependent upon the operation of its HVAC system. HVAC systems are designed to mix a given amount of outdoor air with a larger amount of recirculated air, condition this air mixture, and distribute it to the occupied space.

The outdoor air intake for the HVAC system of a large office building is generally located on the roof (Figure 3.1) although some may be located on the side or at ground level. Outdoor air entering the building may be contaminated by nearby sources of bioaerosols such as those from cooling towers, evaporative condensers, and sanitary vents (Figure 3.2).

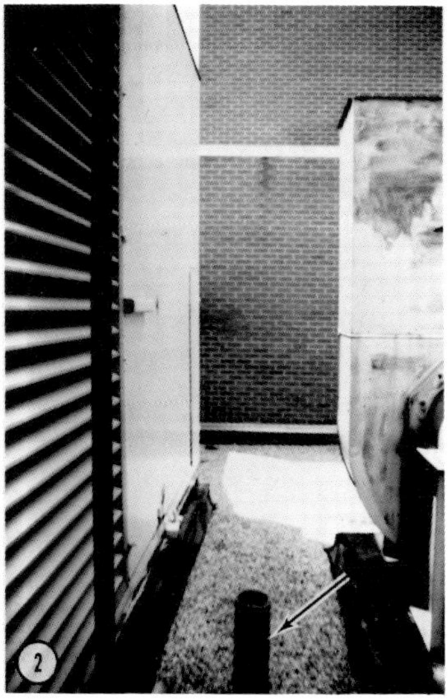

**Figure 3.2.** Outdoor air intake louvers on the roof of another building. A sanitary vent (arrow) is located less than a meter from the lower portion of the intake.

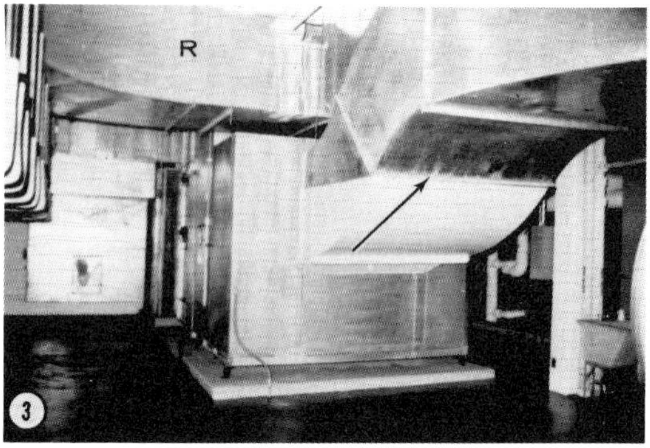


**Figure 3.3.** A primary AHU in a large office building. Outdoor air enters through a louvered intake in the wall behind this AHU. Return (R) air enters from the duct located above. After conditioning, air exits the AHU through the large (high-pressure) duct in the foreground (arrow).

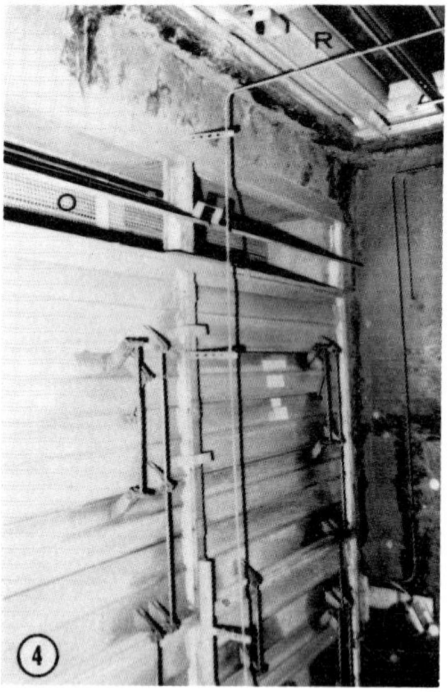


**Figure 3.4.** Mixing plenum of AHU shown in Figure 3.3. Outdoor (O) and return (R) air enter this plenum through separate inlets.

The air entering into a building's HVAC system passes through a series of louvers (Figure 3.1) and into one or more air handling units (AHUs) (Figure 3.3). Outdoor air enters the mixing plenum of the AHU in Figure 3.3 through one or more louvered intakes (Figure 3.4). Here outdoor air is blended with return air which, in the example illustrated, enters from the inlets in the ceiling of the mixing plenum.

The air exiting the mixing plenum of the AHU passes through one and sometimes two sets of filters (Figures 3.5 and 3.6). Filters are rated in terms of weight arrestance and dust spot efficiency (ASHRAE, 1983). Arrestance refers to the ability of the filter to capture a coarse synthetic dust, whereas efficiency (dust spot efficiency test) is used to classify filters according to their ability to remove finer airborne dusts that have the capacity to visually soil interior surfaces in the occupied space. The AHU filter illustrated in Figure 3.5 has as its main function the protection of the downstream heat exchange equipment and has an arrestance of about 80 percent and no (<20 percent) rated dust spot efficiency. This filter would therefore be a poor collector of small spores (e.g., *Penicillium* sp.) that might be entering the AHU from an outdoor source such as dead vegetation.

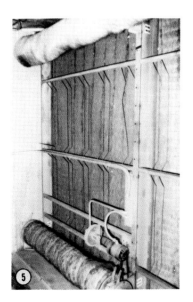


**Figure 3.5.** Roughing filter in downstream wall of AHU mixing plenum. Air exiting the plenum passes through this filter which is rated at <20 percent efficiency (atmospheric dust spot test) and about 80 percent arrestance.

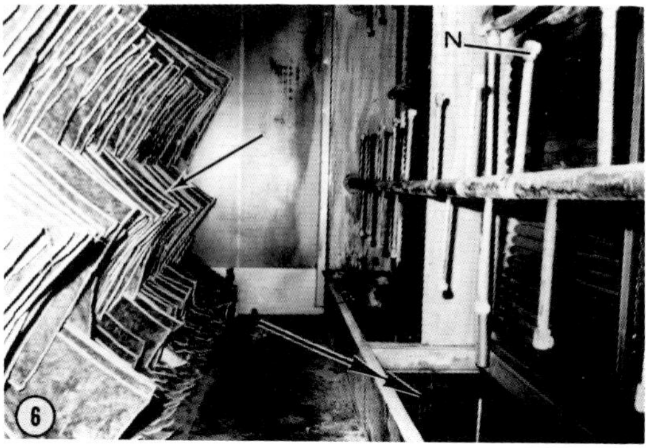


**Figure 3.6.** Bag filters (single arrow) in this AHU have an efficiency of about 80 percent, and are located in a plenum downstream of roughing filters. The upstream surface of the AHU's heat exchanger is visible on the right. A humidifier containing stagnant water in a sump is visible near the heat exchanger. Double arrow = stagnant water. N = spray nozzle of humidifier.

In a few buildings, higher-quality filters capable of removing respirable particulate are installed, usually because of the need to protect computer facilities or other special building contents. Figure 3.6 shows a view of an AHU plenum housing bag filters that are located downstream of "roughing" filters of the type shown in Figure 3.5. The bag filters have an efficiency of about 80 percent and can be expected to remove a significant portion of airborne spores and other bioaerosol particulate that may enter the AHU from either the outdoor or return air streams.

The filtered mixture of outdoor and return air now passes through the heat exchange coil section (upstream and downstream view of two heat exchangers, Figures 3.6 and 3.7, respectively) where it is heated or cooled as required to meet the comfort requirements in the occupied space. During the summer air-conditioning season, moisture condenses from the airstream as it passes over the cooling coils. Cooling coils contain a separate closed, water system which is maintained at a temperature of about 5–13 °C (42–55 °F) (depending on sensible and latent loads in the building) by a refrigeration or chiller system. Moisture from the airstream passing around cooling coils condenses on the outside coil surface when the coil surface temperature is below the dew point of the airstream. Condensed water collects in drain pan (Figure 3.7, arrow) and exits the AHU through drain lines with deep sealed traps. Drain pans should be constructed so that water does not collect and stagnate and become a potential reservoir and amplification site for microorganisms (Figure 3.8). Fans in AHUs may be located either upstream (blow through) or downstream (draw through; Figure 3.8) of heat exchangers. Care must be exercised so that the velocity of air over coil surfaces does not cause droplets of condensed water to be blown off and sent on to downstream sites within the AHU or in the air supply ductwork.

Humidifiers that may be components of office building HVAC systems are located downstream of filter banks and near heat exchange equipment. The humidifier illustrated in Figure 3.6 operates by aerosolizing water (from nozzles, Figure 3.6 N) into the airstream passing from the filter bank through the heat exchange coils. In the example illustrated, water that is not taken up by the air stream falls into a sump (Figure 3.6) and is circulated to nozzles for reaerosolization. This type of humidification system is subject to extensive microbial contamination. Humidification systems that emit steam into the air-

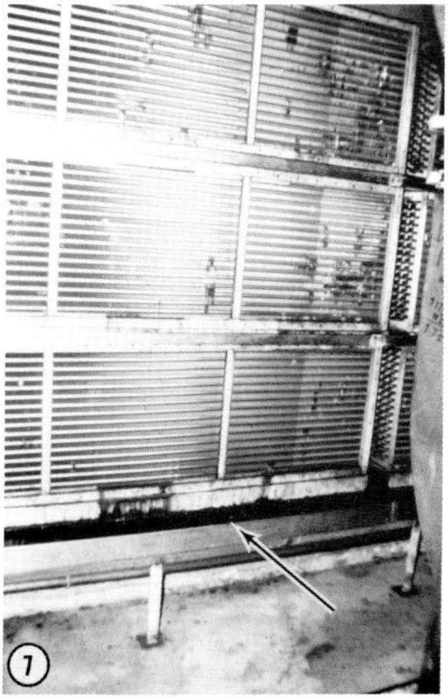


**Figure 3.7.** The downstream surface of a different AHU heat exchanger seen from inside the plenum housing the fan. Drain pans (arrow) located beneath cooling coils (summer mode of operation) collect water that condenses on coil surfaces.

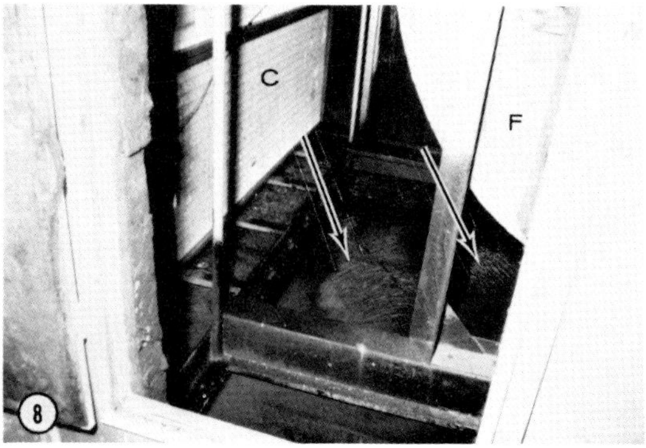


**Figure 3.8.** Cooling coil (C) section and fan (F) of an AHU. Stagnant water (arrows) has collected under the cooling coils and fan.

stream are found in some office building HVAC systems. While steam humidification systems offer no or little opportunity for microbial contamination, some steam systems contain boiler chemicals (e.g., volatile amines) which may be irritating and which may cause adverse health effects if aerosolized with the steam (National Research Council, 1983).

Conditioned air leaving the AHU-fan plenum is transported to the space by a system of high-pressure (Figure 3.3) and low-pressure (Figures 3.9 and 3.11) ducts. Air enters the space through grilles or diffusers (Figures 3.10 and 3.12) and, if the latter are designed properly, mixes with room air. Air exits or escapes from the space either through a system of return ducts (grilles located in ceilings or walls), or, more commonly in office buildings, by entrance into and passage through a common return plenum (Figures 3.9 and 3.11; the open space above the suspended ceiling). Figure 3.13 shows the location in the ceiling (above a fluorescent lamp) in one office building zone

**Figures 3.9–3.12.** Conditioned air is transported from the AHU to the occupied space through a system of ducts. The terminal low-pressure ducts transporting conditioned air are indicated in Figures 3.9 and 3.11 by single arrows. Air from the duct in Figure 3.9 enters the occupied space through a square ceiling diffuser (Figure 3.10, arrow). The air in the supply duct shown in Figure 3.11 enters the occupied space through a long rectangular plenum (Figure 3.11, double arrow) and slot diffusers (Figure 12, arrows) along one side of a suspended ceiling tile.

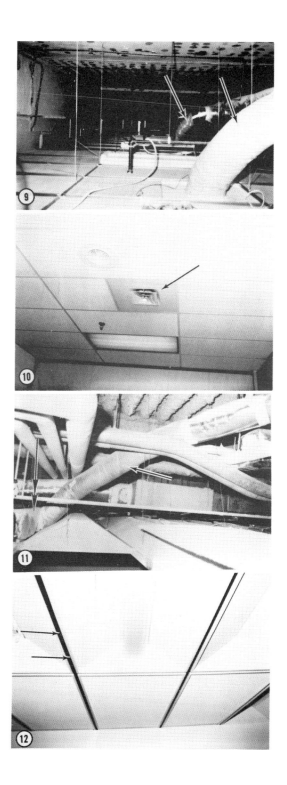

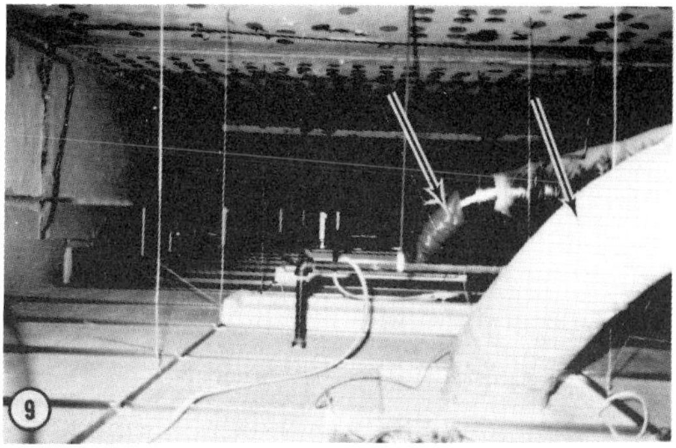
9

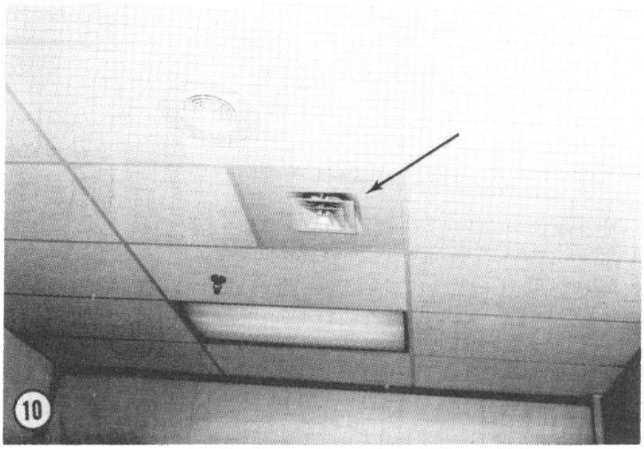
10

11

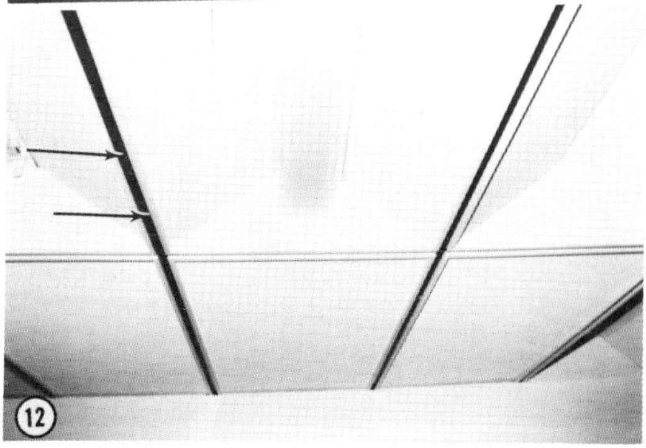
12

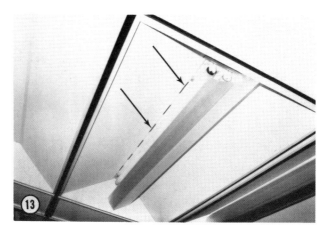


**Figure 3.13.** Location (arrows), above fluorescent light fixture, where air from the occupied space enters the common return plenum (space above ceiling tiles in Figures 3.9 and 3.11).

where air from the occupied space enters the common return plenum. Porous man-made insulation (in pre-1974 buildings sometimes asbestos) is applied as a fire-proofing material to structural components above the suspended ceiling (Figure 3.11). In large office buildings, air from the common return plenum enters chases or risers (Figure 3.14) and then may be moved by a return fan (Figure 3.15) back to AHU as illustrated in Figure 3.3. Because of difficulty with regard to maintenance access, microbial contamination that may occur in the common return plenum as well as in building chases and risers (e.g., as a result of flooding) is removed only with great difficulty.

A significant portion of the heating and cooling load in a large building may be handled by peripheral fan coil units (FCUs) (Figure 3.16). These units usually contain a filter, fan, and heating and cooling coils. The drain pan of the FCU shown in Figure 3.17 contains stagnant water and a microbial slime. Porous man-made insulation applied as a sound attenuator to the inside metal housing of FCUs (Figure 3.16) is another potential niche for microbial contamination. Dirt and debris accumulate within the porous insulation and microorganisms may flourish on this substrate when it becomes moist during the FCU's air-conditioning mode of operation.

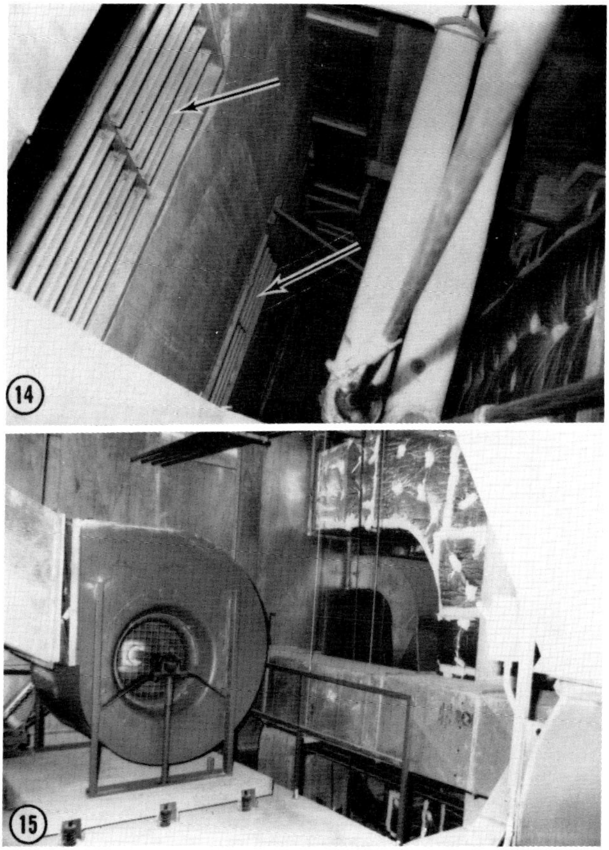


**Figures 3.14 and 3.15.** In this building return air from common return plenums on lower floors enters a riser at locations indicated by arrows (Figure 3.14) and then is transported up the shaft to a return fan (Figure 3.15) which moves the air to the primary AHU (Figure 3.3, R).

## CONTRIBUTION OF STRUCTURE TO MICROBIAL CONTAMINATION IN BUILDINGS

Table 3.1 summarizes the sites in the HVAC system or occupied space of six office buildings where microbial contamination was found. Outbreaks of humidifier fever or acute hypersensitivity pneu-

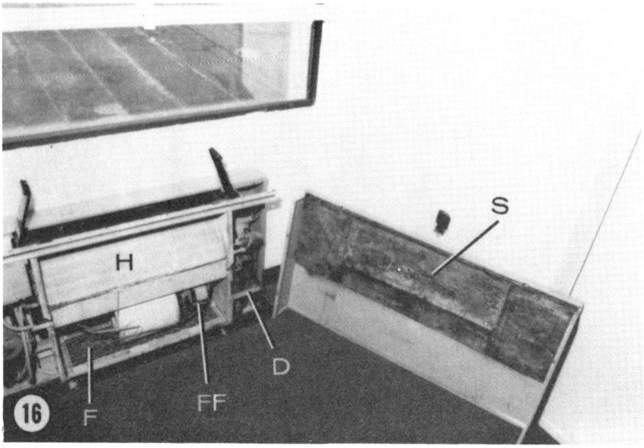


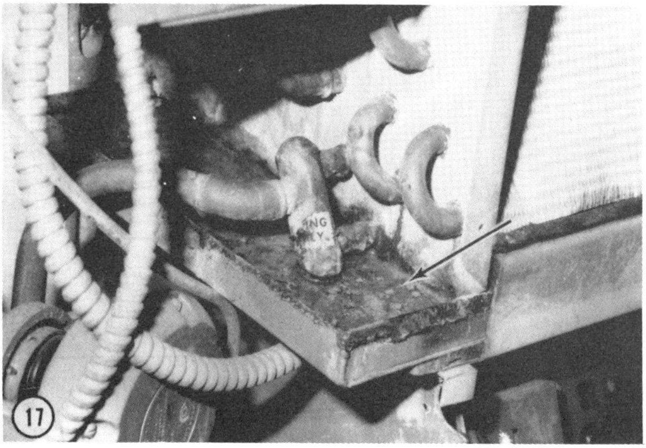


**Figures 3.16 and 3.17.** The following are integral parts of a fan coil unit located along a peripheral wall in an office building: filter (F), fan (FF), heat exchanger (H), sound insulation (S), and drain pan (D). The drain pan (Figure 3.17, arrow) of another FCU in the same building contains stagnant water.

monitis were documented in two buildings (A and C; see Hodgson et al., 1987; Hodgson et al., 1985, respectively). In the other four buildings, workplace-related outbreaks of allergic illness were alleged or suspected, but confirmatory epidemiologic (medical) studies were not undertaken.

**Table 3.1** Structural and Environmental Parameters Associated with Microbial Contamination in Six Office Buildings

| | |
|---|---|
| *Building A* | 1. Water spray system in AHUs; water in spray system recirculated.<br>2. Slime on floor, walls, and ceiling of plenum in which AHUs are located; slime on demisters.<br>3. Water/microbial aerosol enters air supply ductwork.<br>4. High relative humidity in HVAC system and in occupied space (reported to exceed 90% in occupied space). |
| *Building B* | 1. Bacterial aerosol emitted from air washers/water spray system.<br>2. Dew point temperature may exceed 62° F (17° C) in occupied space and return air stream.<br>3. Humidity in air supply stream exceeds 80%. |
| *Building C* | 1. Repeated floods in occupied space from cafeteria drain system.<br>2. Microorganisms or microbial products in furnishings in occupied space.<br>3. Slime in AHU drain pans. |
| *Building D* | 1. Massive flood on three lower floors from rupture of pipes serving heat pumps located above suspended ceiling.<br>2. Drain pan overflows from heat pumps.<br>3. Flooded carpet acts as reservoir for mesophilic fungi.<br>4. Sanitary vent located within 18 inches of building outdoor air intake. |
| *Building E* | 1. Slime in drain pans and on cooling coils of all primary AHUs.<br>2. Sound lining on inside surfaces of AHUs and on inside surfaces of downstream ductwork deteriorated; microorganisms in sound lining.<br>3. Drift from cooling tower enters AHU through outdoor air intake.<br>4. Heat exchange coils of primary AHUs freeze in winter; repeated floods in HVAC system and in occupied spaces.<br>5. Slime in FCU drain pans. |
| *Building F* | 1. Relative humidity in occupied space exceeds 70% in summer.<br>2. Drain pans of AHUs and FCUs contain stagnant water and slime; drain pans of small AHUs totally enclosed in interior walls making maintenance impossible.<br>3. Water permeates masonry ceiling slabs; drain pan of small AHUs and FCUs overflow; wet, moldy suspended ceiling tiles.<br>4. AHUs and FCUs are sources of microorganisms; filters not replaced with adequate frequency-filters act as microbial reservoirs and amplifiers; porous sound lining on inside surfaces of AHUs and FCUs permeated by microorganisms. |

## Contaminated Air Washers (Water Spray Systems)

### *Building A*

At least one-third of the 350 employees in a building located in a southern city experienced recurring outbreaks of humidifier fever that led to a permanent evacuation of the facility. This building's HVAC system was installed in 1941 and contained two systems for spraying water over finless direct expansion evaporator coils for summer cooling. A mixture of return and outdoor air that was essentially unfiltered passed through the water spray system. The spray water was collected in two 3,000-gallon tanks, chilled, and then reaerosolized. Conditioned air from each spray water-direct expansion system passed through demister plates, into fans, and then was transported via ducts to occupied space throughout the building.

The HVAC system was turned off on 18 September 1981, as cool weather was expected shortly. Because the temperature in the building had reached 30 °C (85 °F) three days later, the HVAC system was turned back on. During that day and evening illness occurred in approximately 40 percent of the employees. It consisted of headaches, muscle aches, fever, chills, nausea, wheezing, and chest tightness. In most individuals the symptoms resolved by the next morning. Since there was a temporal relation between illness and turning the HVAC system on, the latter was shut down and water spray systems were cleaned with steam and a quaternary ammonium compound. The HVAC system was then operated without effect upon building occupants until 10 October when it was shut down for repairs.

The HVAC system, including water sprays, was turned on again on 12 October (Columbus Day, a holiday); on 13 October a second outbreak of febrile illness occurred. The HVAC system was then turned off and remained off until 15 October. On that day the HVAC fan system was turned on, a third outbreak of illness occurred, and building occupants were moved into other office facilities.

Inspection of HVAC system air washers showed that their baffle plates were coated with a microbial growth. Similarly, microbial growths (slimes) were found on the surfaces of water spray sumps, on both pipe insulation and masonry wall surfaces located between water spray systems and fans, and on the floor in the vicinity of the fans. A number of microorganisms were identified in the slimes present in Building A's HVAC system. These included *Flavobacterium* sp., *Bacillus* sp. (including thermophiles), thermophilic actinomycetes, amoebae (e.g., *Acanthamoeba* sp.), many fungal genera, ciliates, and nematodes (see Morey et al., 1984, for details).

The microbial contamination found in the HVAC system of Building A was considered to be responsible for the three outbreaks of humidifier fever. If the source of the agent responsible for this disease outbreak was the aerosolization of microorganisms in or near the water sprays, the high relative humidity associated with the operation of Building A's HVAC system (water in the sump was apparently not being chilled; occupants reported humidities exceeding 90 percent) would be conducive to the survival of viable particles at locations throughout the ductwork and in occupied space of this building. Consequently, it was recommended that all nondisposable building contents, including books, desks, carpets, drapes, HVAC system ductwork, and water spray-direct expansion system surfaces be cleaned with a vacuum incorporating a high-efficiency particulate air (HEPA) filter. It was further recommended that building contents that could not be adequately cleaned be discarded.

### *Building B*

Environmental studies described for Building A did not involve a meaningful aerobiologic component because the HVAC system had already been somewhat cleaned and decommissioned, and the occupants had been moved to other offices prior to the initiation of studies. During the course of an environmental study in another office building (Building B), it was observed that several air washers (Figure 3.18) were functioning as HVAC system components. Studies in this building did not involve an extensive medical or epidermologic component. However, it was observed that air washers utilized a spray of chilled water [10–13 °C] (50–55 °F) both to remove sensible heat and airborne particulate from ventilation air being moved through the units. Water from spray droplets was collected in a large (>1,000 gallons) sump, pumped to a chiller for cooling, and returned to the air washer unit from reaerosolization. Maintenance of water spray systems in Building B was excellent; microbial slimes were not readily evident on mechanical components of the air washers.

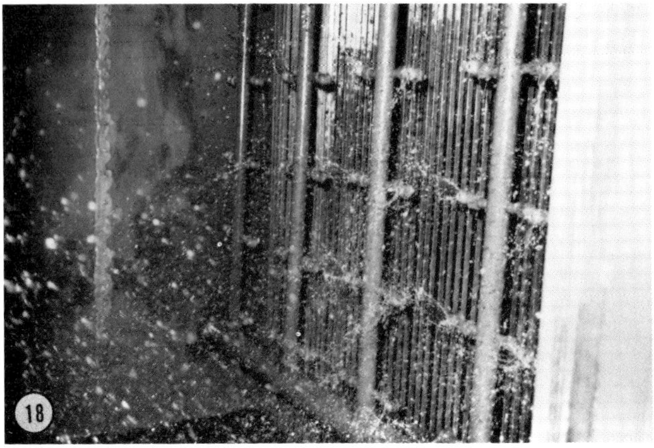

**Figure 3.18.** View of the inside of an air washer (water spray) in a primary AHU. Filtered air (roughing filters only) passes from right to left through a water spray prior to movement to the fan and transport to occupied spaces.

Nevertheless, it was of interest to determine whether the water spray units were sources of bioaerosols.

A modified single-stage Andersen viable sampler (Jones et al., 1985) was utilized to measure levels of microorganisms in air entering (almost 100 percent recirculated air) the air washer, conditioned air exiting the air washer, air entering an office, and outdoor air (Table 3.2). Levels of bacteria and fungi in return air entering the air washer were low, about ten colony-forming units (CFU)/m$^3$. After

**Table 3.2** Airborne Bacterial and Fungal Levels in Building B and in Outdoor Air

| | CFU/m$^3$, Mean (SE) | |
|---|---|---|
| Location | Bacteria | Fungi |
| Outdoor air, roof | 115 (10) | 1,350 (130) |
| Plenum where return air enters air washer | 12 (0) | 9 (0) |
| Plenem where conditioned air exits air washer | 5,475 (750) | 40 (35) |
| Office being supplied with conditioned air | 105 (30) | 135 (10) |

conditioning in the air washer, levels of bacteria increased by more than two orders of magnitude; there was only a slight elevation in airborne fungal counts. Levels of bacteria in office air were similar to outdoor counts. This study was interpreted as showing that the HVAC system air washer was a source of bacterial aerosol. Whether the lower bacterial count (Table 3.2) in the office as compared to the level in the HVAC system just downstream from the air washer was due to dilution of conditioned air by the volume of air in the office or due to the death of bacteria by desiccation in the airstream was not determined.

## Chronic Floods

### *Building C*

In an eight-story building, twelve of forty-one office workers in a central zone on one floor experienced hypersensitivity pneumonitis (HP) symptoms consisting primarily of fever, chills, muscle aches, and chest tightness. The affected zone had been the site of a series of floods, one of which occurred in January 1982. Over the following months, several persons in this office experienced a subacute febrile illness. Ill persons were more likely than healthy persons to occupy desks near water leaks (Hodgson et al., 1985). The cafeteria kitchen on the floor directly above and its water-drainage system runs through the common return air plenum above the suspended ceiling over offices occupied by personnel experiencing illnesses. The plumbing for the cafeteria dishwasher had no grease traps. Consequently, grease periodically clogged drain pipes, causing water to back up and eventually flood the underlying office zone.

Eighteen primary AHUs and over 900 FCUs condition the supply air in Building C. Primary AHUs condition a mixture of outdoor and return air whereas FCUs condition only recirculated air. Conditioned air from each primary AHU is transported to offices through ducts that terminate in slots around the periphery of ceiling light fixtures (Figures 3.11 and 3.12) and in long slot-type supply outlets at some building perimeter locations. Each AHU in Building C provides supply air to vertically superimposed zones on several floors. Return air from occupied space passes into slots above ceiling lighting fixtures (Figure 3.13) and enters the common return air plenum. Return air from zones and on each floor moves through this common plenum and then through shafts and is transported (by return fans) to main AHUs or is expelled from the building during economizer operation. Air interchange between AHUs occurs because of mixing both in common return plenums and in building return air shafts. Thus, once an air contaminant enters a common return plenum it could be distributed into other AHUs and then throughout the building.

Microorganisms were isolated from damaged ceiling tiles and carpets obtained from the zone where illness had occurred. In addition, similar analyses were carried out from debris obtained from the outside surface of pipes (Figure 3.19, arrows) in the common return air plenum above this zone and from a sample of water collected during a flood. All samples examined for protozoa contained *Acanthamoeba polyphaga* (Hodgson et al., 1985). Other predominant microorganisms isolated included *Rhodotorula* sp. and *Aureobasidium* sp. Sampling for airborne fungi was carried out in this office but, unfortunately, four to six weeks after major floods. On all occasions levels of airborne fungi were found to be low, being less than 100 CFU/m$^3$. Dust samples collected from primary AHUs and FCUs throughout the building contained *Thermoactinomyces* sp. as predominant iso-

**Figure 3.19.** Drain pipes (arrows) in common return plenum above an office zone where an outbreak of acute HP occurred. Dirt and debris from pipe surfaces contained *Acanthamoeba* sp. and numerous other microorganisms.

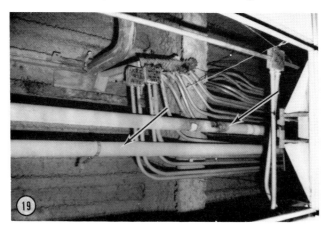

lates. Attempts to use serologic techniques to determine whether *Acanthamoeba, Aureobasidium, Thermoactinomyces,* and other microorganisms isolated in Building C were disease agents proved inconclusive (Hodgson et al., 1985). Additional studies revealed that up to $1 \times 10^8$ bacteria/mL were present in flood waters reaching the office zone where illness occurred. Stagnant water containing microbial slimes was present in the drain pans of some primary AHUs.

Because disease was related to working near water leaks and because the affected office was contaminated with a variety of microorganisms, some of which are known to cause HP-lung disease (Hodgson et al., 1985; MRC, 1977) it was thought that the affected persons experienced respiratory exposure to an unidentified microbial agent associated with flooding from the overhead cafeteria.

Only minimal levels of airborne fungi were recovered by air sampling. However, in both instances, aerobiologic sampling was carried out at least one month after the office zone had been flooded, at a time when airborne levels of viable spores may have been dissipated by such variables as desiccation, clean-up activities in occupied spaces, and filtration by the HVAC system. In another office building where HP was shown to be caused by spores emanating from contaminated FCUs (Bernstein et al., 1983), the time at which air sampling was carried out was shown to be critical in attempts to relate disease prevalence to airborne levels of microorganisms. In that study, sampling conducted on the day that FCUs were first operated in their heating mode showed that airborne fungal spore density was 50- to 80-fold above background levels; on the previous day when FCUs were quiescent, spores in occupied space were present only at background levels. By analogy, air sampling in Building C might have been a more useful indicator of disease prevalence had it been carried out during or within a few days after the major floods.

Clean-up measures recommended for the affected office zone in Building C included the following: (1) Make structural changes in cafeteria plumbing so that flooding in offices is prevented. (2) Discard damaged carpeting (Figure 3.20) and ceiling tiles; clean (with dilute bleach) the outside surfaces of pipes from which floods originated; clean all upholstered furniture, wall partitions, and office materials that need to be reused with vacuums incorporating HEPA filters. (3) Disinfect the floor with dilute bleach and then refurnish and reoccupy the office.

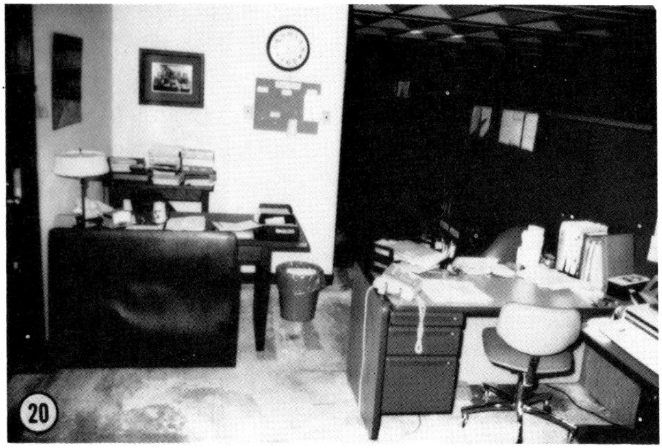

**Figure 3.20.** Office zone where an outbreak of acute HP occurred. The office zone had been vacated and carpet discarded. All other office furnishings were removed before disinfection of masonry with dilute bleach.

During the clean-up of the affected office in May 1982, large amounts of dust were liberated when office partitions were handled. Illness recurred in previously ill individuals. Even though the studies cited earlier were unsuccessful in identifying the etiologic agent, it was probably still present in office partitions in May. There are many reasons for the difficulty in identifying the specific disease agent, and these include the following. First, the agent may be an organism other than the predominant ones that were isolated. Second, the agent may not be viable and therefore was not cultured from bulk samples and was absent from the antigens used in serologic studies. Illness may also have been caused by microbial toxins such as endotoxin. Third, the exact etiology of this disease may be demonstrable only by provocative challenge of affected individuals and this was not attempted in this study.

### *Building D*

The eighteen-story office building was constructed in 1972 and houses about 1,900 occupants. In November 1982, plumbing lines serving a heat pump located in the common return plenum above a second-floor office in Building D ruptured and caused a massive flood on the second, first, and mezzanine floors. Carpet in flooded zones was subsequently vacuumed and treated with a germicidal chemical. Complaints offered by occupants throughout the building included headaches, eye and throat irritation, and a perception that indoor air was stuffy or poorly ventilated. Employees located in zones that had been flooded in November 1982 reported chills and flu-like symptoms.

Air within Building D is conditioned by more than 360 heat pumps (about 20 per floor) located in the plenum above the suspended ceiling. Conditioned air from heat pumps is ducted to zones and enters occupied space through diffusers located in the suspended ceiling. Air from occupied space returns to the ceiling plenum through slots around light fixtures, and then is reconditioned by heat pumps. Some air from the ceiling plenum on each floor is removed from the building through a single riser that terminates in plenums housing rooftop exhaust fans. Additional air is removed from the building by restroom and cafeteria exhausts (fans on roof). Make-up air is ducted into several locations within the ceiling plenum on each floor from risers that connect with rooftop plenums housing make-up air fans.

Heat exchange between the outside environment and building heat pumps is accomplished by evaporative condensers located outdoors on the seventeenth floor. Heat pumps operate in a closed-loop system with pipes (water containing a corrosion inhibitor [sodium nitrite] in pipes) in each unit continuous with pipes that pass through evaporative condensers. Water in evaporative condenser reservoirs never mixes with water in the closed loop-heat pump system. The flood on the lower floors of Building D in November 1982 was caused by a rupture in the closed-loop system serving heat pumps.

Two sanitary vents and one restroom and one cafeteria exhaust stack were located on the roof within 3 meters of intake louvers where outdoor air enters the plenums housing make-up air fans. One of the sanitary vents was less than 1 meter from a louvered outdoor air intake (Figure 3.2). Contamination of make-up air with exhausts from vents and stacks occurred whenever fans supplying make-up air to the building were operated.

Sampling for airborne mesophilic and thermophilic fungi and for airborne bacteria was carried out in Building D in December 1983 (Table 3.3; Morey, 1984). The average number of mesophilic fungi

**Table 3.3** Concentration of Airborne Fungi in Flooded and Nonflooded Offices and in Outdoor Air*

| | Mesophilic Fungi, CFU/m³ Mean (SE)** | Thermophilic Fungi, CFU/m³ Mean (SE)† | Bacteria, CFU/m³ Mean (SE)† |
|---|---|---|---|
| Flooded | 10,200 (2,945) | 3,090 (2,615) | 4,440 (1,880) |
| Nonflooded | 3,020 (865) | 650 (155) | 1,920 (446) |
| Outdoor air | 1,290 (600) | 200 (115) | 267 (80) |

*Mesophilic fungi incubation at 28–30 °C (82–86 °F); thermophilic fungi incubation at 42–45 °C (108–113 °F); bacteria incubation at 35–37 °C (95–98 °F). Group means are an average of ten to fifteen samples. For collection methods, see Morey, 1984; Morey et al., 1984.

**Mesophilic fungi: means of three groups are significantly different at the 1% level by one way analysis of variance; flooded versus nonflooded and flooded versus outdoor air group means are significantly different at the 5% level.

†Thermophilic fungi and bacteria: no significant differences between group means.

in air samples from locations that had been flooded was 10,200 CFU/$m^3$. Levels of fungi in air from nonflooded floors were about 3,000 CFU/$m^3$, whereas average outdoor concentrations were 1,290 CFU/$m^3$. The variable number of fungi recovered within each of the three locations was likely the result of collecting samples over a three-day period from different building locations. In spite of the variability noted, statistical analysis showed that levels of airborne mesophilic fungi in flooded locations were significantly greater than those found either in nonflooded locations or in the outdoor air.

Levels of airborne thermophilic fungi and bacteria found in flooded locations were also higher than those present in nonflooded zones (Table 3.3). However, significance of difference between group means could not be demonstrated.

Microbial sampling conducted in Building D showed that numbers of airborne mesophilic fungi were higher in flooded compared with nonflooded offices. The concentration of fungi present in indoor air both in flooded or in nonflooded locations was higher than that found outdoors (Table 3.3). Mechanical ventilation is usually associated with a lowering of the indoor concentration of airborne fungi compared with levels encountered outdoors or in naturally ventilated (open windows) structures (Hirsh et al., 1978; Rose and Hirsch, 1979; Solomon et al., 1980). Since the levels of microorganisms recovered in Building D were higher than those outdoors, it may be concluded that an internal source(s) of fungi exists especially in offices that were flooded. That carpet might be a source of indoor fungi was suggested by data (Morey, 1984) which show that carpet from zones that had been flooded contains significantly more entrained fungi than carpet from nonflooded locations.

The remedial action suggested for Building D was to replace the carpet or remove fungi from the carpet. If, as a result of flooding, fungi proliferated in the carpet, vacuuming with instruments incorporating HEPA filters should remove spores and other microbial products that may become airborne. A common feature of office buildings with HP-like illnesses may be moisture incursion into occupied space or into the HVAC system. For this reason, regardless of whether the carpet in Building D is replaced or cleaned, it is essential that additional flooding in occupied space be prevented.

## Stagnant Water in Air Handling Units

### *Building E*

Complaints of respiratory illnesses were studied among office workers in a nine-story building located in a southern city. One employee who worked on the seventh floor of Building E had symptoms suggestive of HP. An industrial hygiene survey was carried out in this building to determine if there was an environmental basis for the complaints.

Conditioned air is supplied to office areas by a HVAC system that contains five primary AHUs. Each primary AHU supplies air to an adjacent pair of floors. The unit supplying the seventh floor also provides air to the floor below. Supplemental heating and cooling in occupied spaces was provided by FCUs located next to the outside walls on all floors. Air from occupied space enters the common return plenum on each floor through slots in light fixtures, moves through a large riser along with return air from three or more floors, and is subsequently transported to primary AHUs by return fans. Therefore, it is possible that a contaminant from one primary AHU might enter additional AHUs because of the mixing of return air streams.

The cooling deck of the primary AHU serving the seventh floor lacked an adequate drain pan necessary for the collection and removal of condensed water. As a result, condensed water pooled to a considerable depth and stagnated on the deck of the plenum housing the cooling coils and the air supply fan (Figure 3.8). Microbial slime covered the wetted surfaces of this AHU. The drain pan in FCUs found in the office occupied by the complainant were also coated with a layer of slime.

Water and slime samples from the primary AHU serving the seventh floor and from an FCU located on this floor were analyzed for content of viable fungi and bacteria. For comparison purposes, similar analyses were carried out on water collected from a cooling tower on the roof of Building E. Condensate water from the AHU and water from the reservoir of the cooling tower contained equivalent numbers of microorganisms (Table 3, Morey et al., 1984). However, slime collected from wetted surfaces of the AHU drain pan contained concentrations of bacteria and fungi several orders of magnitude greater than cooling tower water. Slime from the drain pan of the FCU was also more heavily contaminated with microorganisms. Cooling towers are well-known microbial incubators (Miller, 1979). Since contamination within AHUs and FCUs is equal to or greater than that found within cooling towers, and because air flow within the HVAC system has a direct impact upon microbially contaminated surfaces, it is likely that at least some microbial particulate is aerosolized directly into the conditioned air supplied to occupied space. Although no experiments were done to test this hypothesis, it is important to recognize that cooling coil drain pans in primary AHUs in office buildings are located downstream of filter banks that might be effective in removing some airborne microbial particulate.

Two remedial recommendations were made for Building E. (1) Provide adequate drainage for condensed water in drain pans. For drains originating in the vicinity of cooling coils, install deep sealed water-filled traps (AIHA, 1975). Trap depth should exceed the maximum suction pressure head created by the fan, which in a draw-through type of AHU should prevent intake of drain line gasses into the HVAC system air stream. (2) Clean and disinfect cooling coil surfaces and drain pans of AHUs and FCUs.

## Excessive Humidity, Contaminated Insulation and Filters

### *Building F*

An environmental study was carried out in a fifteen-story office complex housing more than 2,000 employees. Some occupants on lower floors of the building reported symptoms including eye, nose, and throat irritation, persistent cough, shortness of breath, and fatigue. The building has had a long history of environmental problems including floods, a relative humidity that often exceeds 70 percent during the summer, and a general absence of preventive maintenance for the HVAC system.

The HVAC system of Building F contains a number of primary AHUs that supply 100 percent outdoor air to occupied space. Conditioned air moves through pressurized supply plenums formed by the suspended ceiling and the slab of the floor above. Supply air enters occupied space through diffusers located in the suspended ceiling. Air within Building F is further conditioned by more than 350 small AHUs and more than 1,000 peripheral FCUs. Each small AHU is located in an interior zone and it provides conditioned air (cooling only) to occupants in several adjacent rooms. Peripheral FCUs are located in rooms along outside walls. These units condition (heat or cool) air within peripheral offices.

Inspection of lower floors of Building F revealed evidence of moisture incursion into occupied space such as wet ceiling tiles and wet masonry. Ceiling tiles in some offices were partially covered by colonies of sporulating fungi. During the air-conditioning season it was additionally observed that stagnant water and microbial slimes were present in drain pans in some primary AHUs (Figure 3.21) and in some FCUs (Figure 3.17). Bacteria were present at a concentration of $1 \times 10^7$/mL in stagnant water in a drain pan in one primary AHU. The extent to which microbial contamination occurred in drain pans of small AHUs could not be ascertained because the cooling coil section of each unit was totally inaccessible (sealed in room walls) for maintenance purposes.

Filters within AHUs and FCUs were seldom replaced. In one small AHU, dust removed from a filter contained in excess of $1 \times 10^7$ viable fungi/g (Morey et al., 1984). Thus, filters appeared to be a reservoir for microbial particulate and possibly an amplification site for microbial growth given the high relative humidity characteristic of the building. Sequential sampling for airborne fungi was carried out in an office where most of the conditioned air was provided by a small AHU whose filter was encrusted with dirt and debris. Air samples were collected in the center of the room during various operating conditions, including when the fan was turned on, when the ductwork was pounded, and when the filter was replaced (see Table 4 of

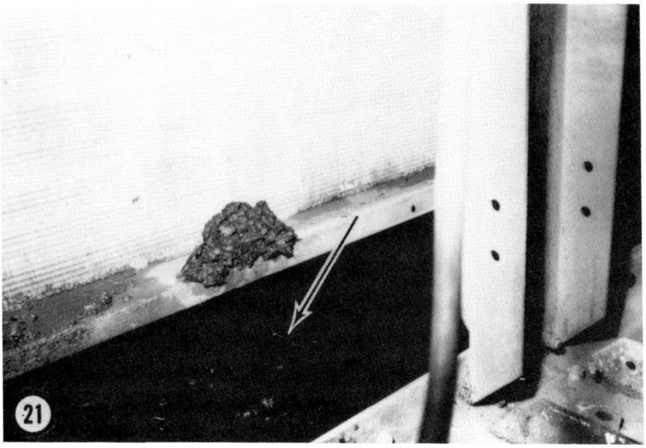


**Figure 3.21.** Drain pan under cooling coil in a primary AHU. A thick microbial slime is present in the pan (arrow). Some of the material has been placed on the horizontal metal surface in the center for purposes of better visualization.

Morey et al., 1984). A sevenfold increase in the level of airborne fungi was associated with turning on the unit's fan. Pounding the AHU's ductwork during fan operation additionally doubled the level of airborne fungi. Fungal levels in the conference room rose more than an order of magnitude when the unit's dirty filter (which up to this time had been kept out of the AHU; see Table 4, Morey et al., 1984) was replaced and subsequently agitated.

Fungal levels present in the air in office rooms served primarily by FCUs varied from $<100$ to about 100,000 CFU/$m^3$ (outdoor levels approximately 1,000 CFU/$m^3$). Thus, in one office with an FCU that had not been operated for some time, the concentration of airborne fungi was 165 CFU/$m^3$ (Table 5, Morey et al., 1984). In a nearby room with an inactive FCU, but with a very characteristic "barn-yard-like" odor, the level of fungi was 7,360 CFU/$m^3$. The drain pan of the FCU in the latter room contained stagnant water and microbial slime (Figure 3.17). In addition, the inside metal surface of the front housing of this FCU was lined with a porous, and obviously dirty, sound-dampening insulation (Figure 3.16). When the fan of the FCU was turned on and its outside surface was agitated, the level of airborne fungi approached 100,000 CFU/$m^3$. It was not determined whether the source of fungi in this FCU was the drain pan containing stagnant water and/or the porous dirty insulation lining the inner surface of the unit.

The generic composition of the airborne fungi collected in the room with the dirty FCU and in the outdoor air was determined (Table 6, Morey et al., 1984). *Penicillium* sp. comprised approximately 98 percent of the isolates when the FCU was operating (total airborne count for fungi approximately 70,000 CFU/$m^3$; 98 percent *Penicillium* sp.). Two percent of the isolates were *Cladosporium* sp. Outdoor air at the same time was characterized by the following rank-order of fungal isolates: *Cladosporium* sp., 49 percent; *Penicillium* sp., 12 percent; *Alternaria* sp., 12 percent; *Aspergillus* sp., 1 percent; other, 26 percent. Clearly, the FCU with its dirty drain pan and insulation served as a reservoir for the accumulation and amplification of *Penicillium* sp.

Peripheral FCUs and small AHUs in Building F were characterized by the presence of a dirty porous insulation found on the interior housing surfaces of the units especially in the vicinity of fans and heat exchange components (Figure 3.22). This insulation is placed on the inside metal housing of these units to reduce the transmission

**Figure 3.22.** Porous insulation (arrows) on the inside surfaces of the metal housing of a small AHU. This insulation is encrusted with dirt and debris. Insulation of this type can act as a source of airborne fungi and bacteria in the occupied space. C = cooling coils.

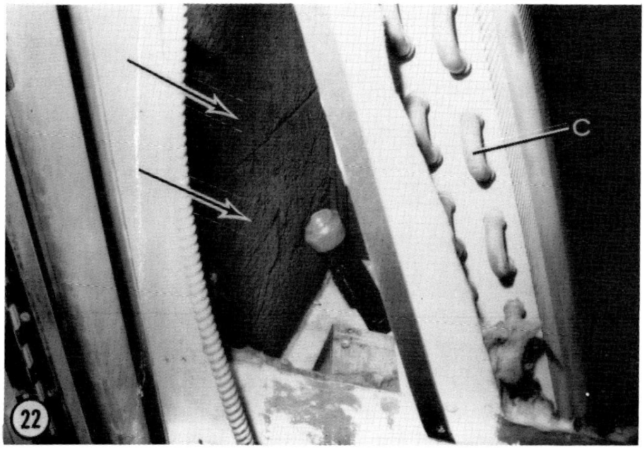

of fan noise to the occupied space. One small AHU was used in an experiment to determine whether dirty porous insulation can release airborne microbial particulate into the indoor environment. The access door to the cooling coil section of the unit was opened and the suction end of a portable microbial sampler was positioned about 2–6 inches (5–15 cm) away from insulation that lined the unit's housing. Counts of bacteria and fungi collected from air within the otherwise undisturbed unit were 39 and 27 CFU/$m^3$, respectively (see Table 3, Morey et al., 1986). The sampler was removed from the small AHU, sound lining was agitated by vigorous pounding along its inside surface and the sampler was reinserted into the vicinity (2–6 inches) of the insulation surface. Counts of airborne bacteria and fungi increased to 8,600 and 1,850 CFU/$m^3$, respectively. After this phase of sampling was completed, the AHU's access door was closed and bolted shut (elapsed time was five minutes), the unit's fan was turned on, and air samples were collected in the room at a location about 2–3 ft (0.6–0.9 m) from the unit's air supply register. Levels of bacteria and fungi found in room air were 600 and 5,400 CFU/$m^3$, respectively. At the time that the sampling was being carried out indoors, the levels of bacteria and fungi in the outside air were 380 and 160 CFU/$m^3$, respectively. This experiment shows that the porous insulation in AHUs does offer a niche for the accumulation and amplification of microbial populations in mechanical systems. Since air sampling was carried in February, it was likely that the bacteria and fungi from porous insulation were surviving populations (hardy spores) of microorganisms that had proliferated in the very humid environment to be expected near the cooling coil section (Figure 3.22) during the summer air-conditioning season. During a subsequent visit to this building in August 1985, interior insulation in the vicinity of the cooling coil section of this as well as several other small AHUs was examined and found to be wet. Porous insulation thus offers a physical niche for the growth and proliferation of microorganisms. Presumably, they grow on the nutrients present in and on the particulate trapped within the insulation.

## MICROBIAL EXPOSURES IN OFFICE ENVIRONMENTS

A common feature in the six office buildings described is moisture incursion into the occupied space or its HVAC system. Buildings C,

D, and F were characterized by a history of repeated floods. All HVAC systems examined contained AHUs with pools of stagnant water and microbial slimes. That moisture incursion into the indoor environment can lead to elevated microbial levels that are associated with respiratory disease is evident in a residential case study of an individual with rhinitis (Kozak et al., 1980). Airborne sampling conducted subsequent to a roof leak and the growth of microorganisms on room walls revealed levels of viable fungi exceeding 5,000 CFU/$m^3$. A level of only 260 CFU/$m^3$ was present before flooding. Since microorganisms are ubiquitous in the atmosphere, and since substrate that supports microbial growth, such as paper, plasterboard, ceiling tiles, carpet, and organic dusts are commonly found in office buildings, prevention of moisture incursion into occupied space and within HVAC systems is probably the best means of preventing microbially induced, allergic respiratory illness.

No scientifically based criteria exist to show whether a measured level of fungi or bacteria is a risk factor with regard to HP or other allergic diseases. Any quantitative criteria must take into account the qualitative nature of the diverse viable and nonviable etiologic agents thought to be responsible for these illnesses. Problems associated with quantitative microbial standards have been previously reviewed (Greene et al., 1962). For example, is air containing a total of 500 fungal spores/$m^3$ of which 20 percent are *Penicillium* inherently safer than that with 1,000 fungal spores/$m^3$ but with only 10 percent *Penicillium*? Establishment of a quantitative standard for viable particulate is further complicated because nonviable spores (Kozak et al., 1980) and microbial products (Flaherty et al., 1984; Rylander et al., 1978) may cause illness, variable numbers and types of microorganisms may be present in single airborne particles, human susceptibility to these agents varies greatly, and large doses of organic dust may be needed to produce sensitization whereas a subsequent response may be evoked by a small quantity of material (MRC, 1977).

Nevertheless, several suggestions have been made concerning normal or hygienically acceptable levels of airborne viable particulate found in office environments. In 1948 a level of approximately 1,775 bacteria-containing particles/$m^3$ was described as the threshold for clerical environments in need of investigation and improvement (Bourdillon et al., 1948). Levels of about 700 bacteria/$m^3$ were considered more normal. It has been stated (Wright et al., 1969) that levels of viable microorganisms in the indoor environment seldom exceed 1,700/m$^3$ and indeed, background levels in a number of the buildings described here never (Buildings A, B, C) or seldom (Buildings E and F) exceeded 1,000 CFU/m$^3$. Japanese studies indicate that levels of viable particulate in occupied space of office buildings with HVAC systems normally range from 100 to 300 CFU/m$^3$ (Ikeda, 1986; Yoshizawa and Sugawara, 1985). A level of viable particles in occupied spaces in office buildings in excess of about 1,000 CFU/m$^3$ has been suggested as indicative of an environment that may need further investigation or hygienic improvement (Bourdillon et al., 1948; Morey et al., 1984). However, the reader is cautioned that it is impossible, based on measurement of total bacterial or fungal particulate alone, to say that the air in an office is unsafe or hazardous. Illnesses such as HP can only be diagnosed or identified by medical or epidemiologic studies.

The difficulty of correlating microbial sampling data (alone) with an outbreak of allergic illnesses can be seen by considering several literature reports together with the illness reported here for Buildings A and C. During an outbreak of humidifier fever in a Swedish office 3 of 7 occupants became ill at a time when levels of *Flavobacterium* sp. rose to approximately 3,000/m$^3$; this bacterium was absent from the air when the humidifier serving the office was turned off (Rylander et al., 1978). During an outbreak of HP where 2 out of 14 occupants in a small office became ill, levels of airborne fungi from a contaminated FCU (mostly *Penicillium* sp.) rose to 5,000 to 10,000 CFU/m$^3$ (Bernstein et al., 1983). On the other hand, in Building A where approximately 40 percent of an office force of 325 workers developed symptoms of acute humidifier fever, subsequent microbial sampling (Hodgson et al., 1987; Morey et al., 1984) indicated that levels of fungi were less than 1,000 CFU/m$^3$. In the office zone in Building C, where approximately 25 percent of the 40 occupants developed symptoms of acute HP, sampling failed to detect levels of airborne fungi or bacteria exceeding 100 CFU/m$^3$ (Hodgson et al., 1985; Morey et al., 1984). In Buildings A and C, sampling was undertaken only a week to six weeks after the outbreak of illness, at a time when environmental conditions in the occupied space may have changed. The studies in Buildings A and C indicate the inappropriateness of using a given level or concentration of viable particulate as the sole indicator of an illness threshold. Just as it is impossible to say that a level of viable particulate exceeding 1,000/$m^3$ is unsafe or hazardous, so too the presence of lower counts as in Buildings A and C does not mean that an indoor environment is free of allergic illnesses. In these two buildings, microbial air sampling by itself would not have been indicative of the outbreak of humidifier fever or acute HP that had occurred.

Numerous unpredictable variables affect results of aerobiologic sampling carried out in office buildings. Among these are the following:

1. Sampling should occur simultaneously with the event that triggers illness.
2. Respiratory diseases such as HP are caused by a wide variety of microbial particulates that may require special sampling instrumentation (Kozak et al., 1980; Reed et al., 1983) and special collection media (Edwards, 1980).
3. Sampling is affected by the variable contamination and variable operational parameters of HVAC system components including AHUs, FCUs, humidifiers, and water sprays.
4. Viable sampling indoors is affected by the sedimentation of airborne particles (McNall, 1975), the effect of HVAC filtration units (McNall, 1975), and the infiltration of seasonally varying loads and types of microorganisms in the outdoor air (Solomon, 1975).

The ACGIH Bioaerosols Committee is developing a generic protocol (ACGIH, 1986) for collection and analysis of viable microorganisms in office environments. Listed here are some of the most salient points of their protocol, with some personal views of the author.

1. *Qualitative preassessment.* One should eliminate the possibility that the complaints of occupants are due to nonmicrobial causes such as thermal discomfort; acoustic, lighting, smoke, and odor problems; and inadequate or inefficient HVAC operation. Before sampling is carried out, obtain medical opinion that occupant problems are likely due to allergic bioaerosols. If there appears to be microbial contamination in the building,

see if remedial action (see the next section) can eliminate the problem before expensive microbial sampling is initiated.

2. *Sampler selection.* The Andersen impactor is generally accepted as the standard instrument for collecting viable particles in environments such as offices where bioaerosol concentrations are low. However, other impactors (e.g., Spiral Air System, Biotest, Microban, and slit samplers) as well as impingers and filter cassettes may be successfully utilized.
3. *Culture media.* Malt extract and trypticase soy agar provide good general support for the growth of microorganisms. A quality assurance program is needed to make sure that the media utilized will support the growth of common microorganisms such as *Cladosporium cladosporioides* and *Staphylococcus epidermidis* as well as certain microorganisms that may be suspect in a building (e.g., immunologic evidence may indicate that the affected occupant has a high titer to a *Thermoactinomyces* antigen).
4. *Sampling strategy.* The objective of sampling is to identify the source of microbial contamination so that effective corrective action may be undertaken.
5. *Interpretation.* Compare outdoor versus indoor levels of 25 °C (77 °F) fungi, 25 °C (77 °F) bacteria, and 55 °C (131 °F) thermoactinomycetes. Is there an amplification (of numbers) indoors? Carry out rank order identification of predominant fungi and bacteria. Is there evidence of amplification of a particular microorganism indoors? For example, in Building F *Penicillium* accounted for 98 percent of the almost 100,000 fungal CFU/$m^3$ found in an office versus only 12 percent *Penicillium* among the 165 fungal CFU/$m^3$ outdoors. *Penicillium* were being amplified (in the office FCU) indoors.
6. *Remedial action.* Carry out corrective actions (see next section) after the indoor source has been located. Additional air samples should be taken to document that remedial actions were effective.
7. *Additional tests.* Allergic responses of occupants may be caused by other agents such as nonviable fungal spores (Kozak et al., 1980; Solomon et al., 1980), protozoans (Edwards, 1980), endotoxins (Rylander et al., 1978), and submicron particulate antigens (Burge and Solomon, 1987; Reed et al.,

1983). Special sampling techniques will be required to measure these microbial agents.

## CORRECTIVE ACTIONS FOR OFFICE BUILDINGS

Very little scientifically based information is available on preventive and remedial measures that are effective in reducing building-associated microbial contamination. Listed here are some preventive measures that may be effective in reducing building-associated microbial contamination. It would be prudent for building engineers and managers to incorporate these measures into their preventive maintenance programs.

1. Repair all external and internal leaks promptly and permanently.
2. Stagnant water should not be allowed to accumulate under cooling coils in AHUs. Proper inclination and continuous drainage of drain pans is necessary. Cooling coils should be run at a low enough temperature so that adequate dehumidification can result to keep space relative humidities at proper levels (30–50 percent is best for comfort) and so that spores and substrate impacted on coils may be washed away in condensate water. The AHU components should be inspected for the presence of stagnant water and microbial contamination. The AHUs should be constructed or modified so that maintenance personnel have easy and direct access to the heat exchange components as well as to drain pans. If contamination with microbial slime is found, it should be removed. Mechanical or detergent cleaning may be required to remove slime before using microbiocidal chemicals. Steam lancing can be used to remove slime providing that the treatment does not damage the heat exchanger (Brundrett et al., 1981). Chlorine-generating slimicides and proprietary biocides may be used for disinfection provided that chemicals are removed before AHUs are reactivated (Brundrett et al., 1981). Aerosolization of microbiocidal chemicals into occupied space must be avoided.
3. Humidifiers in HVAC systems should preferentially use steam

as a moisture source. A dedicated "dry steam" system is preferable to systems that use raw steam from a central boiler system. The latter may contain corrosion inhibitors that are meant to carry over into condensate return lines. For steam humidifiers, avoid steam sources that contain volatile amines. Consult the recommendations of the National Research Council (1983) for minimizing exposure to volatile amines that may be present in steam from plant boilers. Humidifiers utilizing recirculated water are not recommended, as these can become rapidly contaminated with organic dusts and microorganisms (Ager and Tickner, 1983). Treatment of this type of humidifier with biocides has been ineffective in controlling microbial contamination (Cockcroft et al., 1981; Ganier et al., 1980). If cold-water-type humidifiers are used, water should originate from a potable source and water after passing through the humidifier should be run into a drain line (Edwards, 1980) instead of being recirculated. Cold water humidifiers should be subject to a fastidious preventive maintenance program (Ager and Tickner, 1983; Brundrett, 1979) involving regular inspection, cleaning, and disinfection as outlined earlier in number 2. The use of portable cold mist vaporizers is discouraged, since these devices are known to contaminate room air with microorganisms (Solomon, 1974).

4. The use of water sprays as components of office building HVAC systems should be eliminated as these units have been associated with several outbreaks of HP (Arnow et al., 1978; Banaszak et al., 1970). If water sprays are to be utilized, a very rigorous preventive maintenance program must be employed to control microbial contamination. It should be kept in mind that some water spray units (air washers) were designed to operate with sterile water or water treated with a disinfectant (Carswell et al., 1938). The use of disinfectants in these units, however, is questionable because of their possible toxicity on occupants after prolonged exposure and because of their corrosiveness to HVAC mechanical equipment (Yaglou and Wilson, 1942). Water spray systems that are utilized in AHUs to enhance heat exchange capacity of coils should be subject to a preventive maintenance program as described earlier in number 2. Migration of water/microbial aerosols from water spray

systems into ductwork and occupied space should be prevented.

5. Relative humidity in occupied spaces should not exceed 70 percent. As relative humidity rises above this level, the increased moisture content of organic substances encourages fungal spore germination and proliferation (Block, 1953; Brundrett and Onions, 1980). This recommendation is contrary to generally accepted energy management techniques wherein occupied space relative humidities can exceed 70 percent during the summer months. Relative humidity can be lowered either by reducing the moisture content or by raising the dry-bulb temperature of the air. Cooling coils of AHUs should be run at a low enough temperature to dehumidify conditioned air. In buildings using economizer systems, where relative humidity outdoors is sometimes excessive, air taken into the building's HVAC system may require dehumidification. Reheat coils may then have to be utilized to raise the temperature of dehumidified supply air, as the dry-bulb temperature of this air may be too low due to the necessary prior dehumidification process.
6. Filters used in AHUs should ideally have a moderate to high (ASHRAE, 1983) efficiency (80–90 percent) as measured by the ASHRAE atmospheric dust spot test. To prolong the life of these filters and to improve cost-effectiveness, prefilters (such as roll-type low efficiency; high arrestance) should be used to clean the air prior to passage over the higher efficiency filters. Filters with a 80–90 percent efficiency will remove most spores as well as the organic dusts that support microbial growth. Electronic air cleaners have also been reported to be effective in removing microorganisms from the airstream (Kozak et al., 1979; Margard and Lodgsdon, 1965) but high initial cost and subsequent maintenance may prohibit their use. Care also should be exercised to ensure that these air cleaners do not liberate ozone into the airstream. The location of these air cleaners in the HVAC system is important. In most AHUs, filters are located upstream of the cooling or heating coil decks so as to protect the heat exchange capacity of these surfaces. Building occupants will not be entirely protected by these conventionally located filters if microbial con-

tamination occurs downstream (e.g., slime in cooling coil drain pan or in humidifier in air supply ductwork). Therefore, it may be necessary to provide downstream filtration to achieve suitable protection. Because dirty filters in AHUs may be sources of microorganisms, a preventive maintenance program must exist by which filters are inspected and replaced at regular intervals.

7. Microbial aerosols from cooling tower drift, sanitary, and other exhaust vents may enter improperly located outdoor air intakes. Remedial action may include relocation of sanitary or exhaust vents or increasing their heights, relocation of outdoor air intakes, or upgrading AHU filter efficiency. A preventive maintenance program to inhibit microbial build-up in cooling towers is essential. Outdoor microbial aerosols may also enter buildings through idle exhaust ducts and miscellaneous stacks and vents. For this reason, the building should be operated so that inside pressure is slightly positive with respect to that of the atmosphere.
8. In buildings or zones of buildings where carpet, upholstery, ceiling tiles, and other porous furnishings are obviously contaminated with microbial material, it is better to discard these items rather than to attempt disinfection (Building C). However, if the extent of microbial contamination is uncertain, disinfection may be attempted using vacuum cleaners with HEPA filters. Since it is almost impossible to clean contaminated suspended ceiling-return air plenums with porous spray-on fire insulation, these may have to be bypassed by installation of return air ductwork. A special maintenance program is needed to clean FCUs. This should include the removal of debris from beneath and within units and replacement of dirty porous insulation along inside surfaces. During building clean-up, microbially laden materials (e.g., carpets, porous insulation, filters) should be carefully removed so as to minimize aerosolization of inhalable particulate. Personnel assigned to clean-up operations should wear respirators with high-efficiency particulate filter media. Structural and other building surfaces should be vacuumed with instruments incorporating HEPA filters and then disinfected with dilute bleach or proprietary biocide.

## REFERENCES


Ager, B. P., and Tickner, J. A. 1983. The control of microbiological hazards associated with air-conditioning and ventilation systems. *Ann. Occup. Hyg.* 27:341–58.

American Conference of Governmental Industrial Hygienists (ACGIH). 1984. Evaluating office environmental problems. *Ann. Am. Conf. Gov. Ind. Hyg.* 10:1–136.

———. 1986. Bioaerosols committee report on airborne viable microorganisms in office environments: Sampling protocol and analytical procedures. *Appl. Industr. Hyg.* 1:R19–R23.

American Industrial Hygiene Association (AIHA). 1975. *Heating and cooling for man in industry.* 2d ed. Akron, Ohio, pp. 61–64.

American Society of Heating Refrigerating and Air Conditioning Engineers (ASHRAE). 1983. *Equipment Volume* 10.2–10.5.

Arnow, P.; Fink, J.; Schlueter, D.; Barboriak, J.; Mallison, G.; Said, S.; Martin, S; Unger, G.; Scanlon, G.; and Kurup, V. 1978. Early detection of hypersensitivity pneumonitis in office workers. *Am. J. Med.* 64:236–42.

Banaszak, E. F.; Thiede, W. H.; and Fink, J. N. 1970. Hypersensitivity pneumonitis due to contamination of an air conditioner. *N. Engl. J. Med.* 283:271–76.

Bardana, E. J., and Montanaro, A. 1986. Tight building syndrome. *Immunology and Allergy Practice* 8:74–88.

Bernstein, R. S.; Sorenson, W. G.; Garabrant, D.; Reaux, C.; and Treitman, R. 1983. Exposures to respirable, airborne *Penicillium* from a contaminated ventilation system: Clinical, environmental and epidemiological aspects. *Am. Ind. Hyg. Assoc. J.* 44:161–69.

Block, S. S. 1953. Humidity requirements for mold growth. *Appl. Microbiol.* 1:287–93.

Bourdillon, R. B.; Lidwell, O. M.; Lovelock, J. E.; and Raymond, W. F. 1948. Airborne bacteria found in factories and other places: Suggested limits of bacterial contamination. *Studies in Air Hygiene,* Medical Res. Coun. Spec. Rep. Series No. 262. London: HM Stationery Office, pp. 257–63.

Brudrett, G. W. *Maintenance of spray humidifiers.* 1979. Capenhurst, Chester, U.K.: Electricity Coun. Res. Ctr.

Brundrett, G. W., and Onions, A.H.S. 1980. Molds in the home. *J. Consumer Stud. Home Econ.* 4:311–21.

Brundrett, G. W.; Collins, J. B.; DaCosta, G. S.; Edwards, J. H.; Jones, W. P.; Newson, D. J.; and Stone, R. J. 1981. Humidifer fever. *J. Chart. Inst. Build. Serv.* 3:35–36.

Burge, H. A., and Solomon, W. R. 1987. Sampling and analysis of biological aerosols. *Atmo. Env.* 21:451–56.

Carswell, T. S.; Nason, H. K.; and Fleming, J. D. 1938. Studies on bacterial control in air conditioning. *Heating, Piping and Air Conditioning* 10:279–82.

Cockcroft, A.; Edwards, J.; Bevan, C.; Campbell, I.; Collins, G.; Houston, K.; Jenkins, D.; Latham, S.; Saunders, M.; and Trotman, D. 1981. An investigation of operating theatre staff exposed to humidifier fever antigens. *Brit. J. Ind. Med.* 38:144–52.

Edwards, J. H. 1980. Microbial and immunological investigations and remedial action after an outbreak of humidifier fever. *Brit. J. Ind. Med.* 37:55–62.

Finnegan, M. J.; Pickering, C.A.C; and Burge, P. S. 1984. The sick building syndrome: Prevalence studies. *Brit. Med. J.* 289:1573–75.

Flaherty, D. K.; Deck, F. H.; Cooper, J.; Bishop, K.; Winzenburger, P.A.; Smith, L. R.; Bynum, L.; and Witmer, W. B. 1984. Bacterial endotoxin isolated from a water spray air humidification system as a putative agent of occupation-related lung disease. *Infection and Immunity* 43:206–12.

Ganier, M.; Lieberman, P.; Fink, J.; and Lockwood, D.G. 1980. Humidifier lung: An outbreak in office workers. *Chest* 77:183–87.

Greene, V. W.; Vesley, D.; Bond, R. G.; and Michaelsen, G. S. 1962. Microbiological contamination of hospital air. II. Qualitative studies. *Appl. Microbiol.* 10:567–71.

Hirsch, D. J.; Hirsch, S. R.; and Kalbleisch, J. H. 1978. Effect of central air conditioning and meteorologic factors on indoor spore counts. *J. Allergy Clin. Immunol.* 62:22–26.

Hodgson, M. J.; Morey, P. R.; Attfield, M.; Sorenson, W. G.; Fink, J. N.; Rhodes, W. W.; and Visvesvara, G. V. 1985. Pulmonary disease associated with cafeteria flooding. *Arch. Env. Health* 40:96–101.

Hodgson, M. J.; Morey, P. R.; Simon, J.; Waters, T. D.; and Fink, J. N. 1987. An outbreak of recurrent acute and chronic hypersensitivity pneumonitis in office workers. *Am. J. Epidemiology.* 125:631–38.

Ikeda, K. 1986. Institute of Public Health, Tokyo. Personal communication.

Jones, W.; Morring, K.; Morey, P.; and Sorenson, W. 1985. Evaluation of a single stage viable sampler. *Am. Ind. Hyg. Assoc. J.* 46:294–98.

Kozak, P. P. Jr.; Gallup, J.; Cummins, L. H.; and Gillman, S. A. 1979. Factors of importance in determining the prevalence of indoor molds. *Ann. Allergy* 43:88–94.

———. 1980. Currently available methods for home mold surveys. II. Examples of problem homes surveyed. *Ann. Allergy* 45:167–76.

Kreiss, K., and Hodgson, M. J. 1984. Building-associated epidemics. In

*Indoor Air Quality*, P. J. Walsh, C. S. Dudney, and E. D. Copenhaver, eds. Boca Raton, Fla.: CRC Press, pp. 87–106.

McNall, P. E. 1975. Practical methods of reducing airborne contaminants in interior spaces. *Arch. Env. Health* 30:552–56.

Margard, W. L., and Lodgsdon, R. F. 1965. An evaluation of the bacterial filtering efficiency of air filters in the removal and destruction of airborne bacteria. *ASHRAE J.* 10:49–54.

Medical Research Council (MRC) Symposium. 1977. Humidifier fever. *Thorax* 32:653–63.

Miller, R. P. 1979. Cooling towers and evaporative condensers. *Ann. Int. Med.* 90:667–70.

Morey, P. R. 1984. Case presentations: Problems caused by moisture in occupied spaces of office buildings. *Ann. Am. Conf. Gov. Ind. Hyg.* 10:121–27.

Morey, P. R.; Hodgson, M. J.; Sorenson, W. G.; Kullman, G. J.; Rhodes, W. W.; and Visvesvara, G. S. 1984. Environmental studies in moldy office buildings: Biological agents, sources and preventive measures. *Ann. Am. Conf. Gov. Ind. Hyg.* 10:21–35.

Morey, P. R.; Jones, W. G.; Clere, J. L.; and Sorenson, W. G. 1986. Studies on sources of airborne microorganisms and on indoor air quality in a large office building. *IAQ '86 Managing Indoor Air for Health and Energy Conservation.* ASHRAE, Atlanta 92:Part 1, 399–419.

National Research Council. 1983. *An assessment of the health risks of morpholine and diethylaminoethanol.* Washington, D.C.: National Academy Press.

Oak Ridge National Laboratory (ORNL) 7th Life Sciences Symposium. 1985. *Indoor air and human health,* R. B. Gammage and S. V. Kaye, eds. Chelsea, Mich.:Lewis Publishers.

Reed, C. E.; Swanson, M. C.; Lopez, M.; Ford, A. M.; Major, J.; Witmer, W. B.; and Valdesz, T. B. 1983. Measurement of IgG antibody and airborne antigen to control an industrial outbreak of hypersensitivity pneumonitis. *J. Occup. Med.* 25:207–10.

Rose, H. D., and Hirsch, S. R. 1979. Filtering hospital air decreases aspergillus spore counts. *Am. Rev. Resp. Dis.* 119:511–13.

Rylander, R.; Haglind, P.; Lundholm, M.; Mattsby, I.; and Stengvist, K. 1978. Humidifier fever and endotoxin exposure. *Clin. Allergy* 8:511–16.

Scully, R. E.; Galdabini, J. J.; and McNeely, B. U. 1979. Case records of the Massachusetts General Hospital, Case 47-1979. *N. Engl. J. Med.* 301:1168–74.

Solomon, W. R. 1974. Fungus aerosols arising from cold-mist vaporizers. *J. Allergy Clin. Immunol.* 54:222–28.

Solomon, W. R. 1975. Assessing fungus prevalence in domestic interiors. *J. Allergy Clin. Immunol.* 56:235–42.

Solomon, W. R.; Burge, H. A.; and Boise, J. R. 1980. Exclusion of particulate allergens by window air conditioners. *J. Allergy Clin. Immunol.* 65:305–8.

Solomon, W. R.; Burge, H. A.; Boise, J. R.; and Becker, M. 1980. Comparative particle recoveries by the retracting Rotorod, Rotoslide, and Burkard spore trap sampling in a compact array. *Intern J. Biometeor.* 24:107–16.

Wallingford, K. 1986. NIOSH field experience overview: Investigating sources of IAQ problems in office buildings. *IAQ '86 Managing Indoor Air for Health and Energy Conservation.* ASHRAE, Atlanta: 448–53.

Weiss, N. S., and Soleymani, Y. 1971. Hypersensitivity lung disease caused by contamination of an air-conditioning system. *Ann. Allergy* 19:154–56.

Wright, T. J.; Greene, V. W.; and Paulus, H. J. 1969. Viable microorganisms in an urban atmosphere. *J. Air Poll. Cont. Assn.* 19:337–41.

Yaglou, C. P., and Wilson, U. 1942. Disinfection of air by air-conditioning processes. Am. Assoc. Adv. Sciences Publ. No. 17, pp. 129–32.

Yoshizawa, S., and Sugawara, F. 1985. Standards for airborne bacteria. In *Database of state-of-the-art technology for food bacteria control,* M. Haruta, S. Udagawa, and R. Yokayama, eds. Tokyo: Science Forum Co.

# 4

# Water in Health Care Facilities

ANITA K. HIGHSMITH

Health care facilities are communities unto themselves. The complex community that makes up a health care facility today may include, besides the hospital and clinics, research and clinical laboratories; departments of birthing and infertility, dialysis, radiation, oncology, burn, donor and transplant, and surgery; and rehabilitation, wellness, home and extended care, and hospice programs. New building construction and renovation have steadily increased to provide for expanded services. Critical to building design and basic services are engineering systems such as water, heating, and air-conditioning. In this chapter, special emphasis is placed on water systems in health care facilities.

Water systems in health care facilities operate continuously, every day, twenty-four hours a day, providing various grades or types of water. Incorporation of state-of-the-art water systems in health care building design followed by a program for operation and maintenance is one method for ensuring water quality after treatment and distribution.

Water quality is critical to scientific research and health care. Although the design and operation of a water system contributes greatly to the water quality, chemically pure water is nonexistent. However, it is possible and cost-beneficial to produce a grade of water for general and specific use. Potable water can be treated by a variety of water purification systems to meet specific water quality parameters for use in research and diagnostic laboratories and for special purpose water in health care facilities where impurities in the water can interfere with or alter laboratory tests or be life-threatening to patients.

Recognition of the occurrence and persistence of contaminants in potable water is important in establishing criteria for assessing water quality and controlling potential health effects. Environmental and nosocomial waterborne illness have been reported after ingestion, inhalation, and skin contact with contaminated water. Water sources containing a variety of microorganisms that are able to multiply have been shown to be potentially hazardous, sometimes causing epidemics of infection or endotoxemia.

## WATER SYSTEM DESIGN

State, local, and federal agencies provide regulations for the construction, design, and operation of health care facilities, and national committees have published guidelines for water quality. However, providing water quality through systems design is an interdisciplinary responsibility: the architect, engineer, planner, scientist, and occupant are accountable for comprehensive service in systems design. Youngberg (1986a and b) published a list of criteria for selecting potential vendors for high-purity water systems, thereby providing buyers with an unbiased approach to obtaining the system most suited for their facility.

Generally water contains four types of contaminants: dissolved inorganics, dissolved organics, suspended particles, and microorganisms. A combination of water treatment systems can be used to achieve the desired level of water quality in research and diagnostic laboratories and for special purposes in health care. Some important features of water systems may include (1) a central distribution system with a minimum of dead-end points, (2) a central system produced by a point-of-use on-demand system that can recirculate, (3) water inlets of an absolute minimum length, (4) stored water that can be covered and decontaminated periodically, (5) mechanism(s) that provide for monitoring or measuring water quality periodically, (6) projected water needs over the next ten or more years, and (7) a system that can ensure biosafety for service/maintenance personnel. These features are discussed in the following sections.

## Central Water Systems

Most health care facilities are supplied with chlorinated potable water from municipal water systems that is distributed throughout the facility, stored until use, or treated with deionization or distillation before distribution. Incoming water is used primarily for drinking and food preparation, patient care, laundry, and building maintenance. Central water systems are a major investment and require professional design and maintenance. To minimize health hazards to personnel, patients, and visitors, plumbing should be designed and operated to provide an adequate and safe supply of water for all required operations, including safe removal of wastewater.

Factors that affect the overall quality in a central water supply are taste, odor, appearance, turbidity, and the presence of chemicals, as well as inadequate disinfection, biofouling, construction of distribution system, cross-connections, storage facilities, blow-offs and vacuum or air relief valves, and biologic degradation.

Central water systems have numerous problems with extended distribution lines, inadequate drains, and dead-ends. Oftentimes, recirculating systems are recommended. Acceptable piping materials include components of certain metals (stainless steel, tin-lined, or titanium); and nonmetals (Teflon, polypropylene, polyethylene). Glass is a nonacceptable piping material and polyvinyl chloride (PVC) is not recommended for distribution by the National Committee for Clinical Laboratory Standards (NCCLS). NCCLS Type 1 water is considered the highest purity produced with currently available water treatment technology and is used at the time of production. Biofilms are formed when microorganisms or certain chemicals attach to pipe interiors. The interior surface of a pipe with microbial colonization is shown in Figure 4.1.

Disinfection may prove inadequate in water distribution systems extending over large areas. Dead-end sites and cross-connections in distribution systems can contribute to bacterial contamination in potable water supply systems. Since plumbing blueprints are rarely amended after years of reconstruction an effort should be made to keep them current and to eliminate dead-end sites and cross-connections.

Storage tanks for potable water should be covered or sealed with

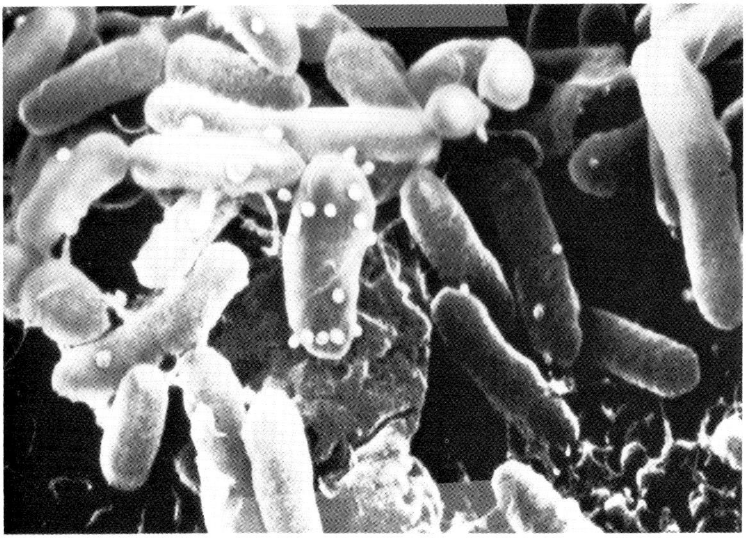

**Figure 4.1.** Interior surface of a pipe with microbial colonization (6000 ×).

an air vent, cleaned, and decontaminated periodically. This will help to prevent the accumulation of slime and other impurities on the interior surface or lining of a tank, which can be difficult to remove and can contaminate the water.

Proper operation and maintenance of water systems and disposal of wastewater are important. Water systems with a negative pressure indicator can pose potential problems. Adequately maintained pumps help to prevent backflow of foreign materials or liquids from such items as bedpan washers, toilets, laboratory sterilizers, and siphon apparatus into a system. Requirements for water used for boiler operations and hot water supply are promulgated in the *Accreditation Manual for Hospitals* (JCAH, 1985). Aerators attached to water faucets become reservoirs for bacterial colonization unless removed and cleaned periodically. Excess moisture build-up in carpets, around sinks, and equipment can become contaminated with microorganisms over time. Special procedures should be implemented for handling contaminated water, including transport systems, storage areas, and treatment facilities containing hazardous wastes.

## Point-of-Use Water Systems

High-purity water is critical in research and diagnostic laboratories and in some areas of the hospital and health care facility. Potable water treated by one or more processes removes critical contaminants and provides different grades of high-purity water. In general, components used in the typical water purification system are shown in Figure 4.2.

Distillation, one of the oldest means of purifying water, removes most contaminants and produces water continuously. Generally, point-of-use water is purified at the time of use or "on-demand" and should be recirculated continuously to retard microbial contamination. The grade or type of water quality depends on the treatment process. Each process functions independently, but in sequence each renders a high-purity water free of certain contaminants. Water quality is compromised on storage.

Purification processes used to treat potable water include membrane filtration for removal of bacteria or colloidal particles of a given pore size, generally 0.45 $\mu$, 0.22 $\mu$, or 0.1 $\mu$; reverse osmosis to remove dissolved organic, dissolved ionic, and suspended impurities

**Figure 4.2.** Components used in typical water purification system for producing high-purity water.

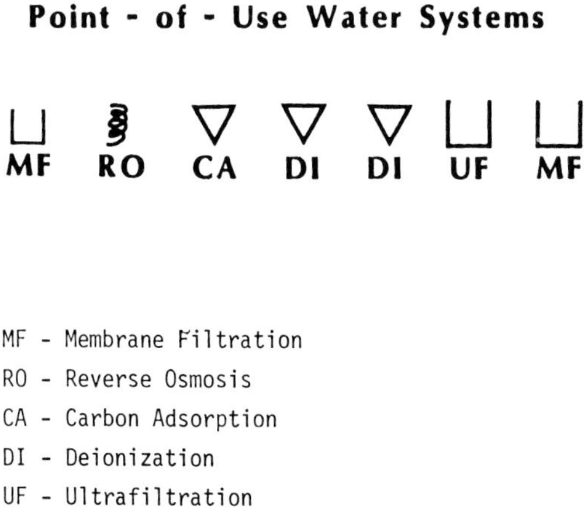

**Table 4.1** Water Purification Processes

| | Major Classes of Contaminants* | | | | | |
|---|---|---|---|---|---|---|
| Process** | Dissolved Ionized Solids | Dissolved Ionized Gasses | Dissolved Organics | Particulates | Bacteria | Pyrogens |
| Distillation | $G–E_{(1)}$ | P | G | E | E | E |
| Deionization | E | E | P | P | P | P |
| Reverse osmosis | $G_{(2)}$ | P | G | E | E | G–E |
| Carbon adsorption | P | $P_{(3)}$ | $G–E_{(4)}$ | P | P | P |
| Filtration | P | P | P | E | E | P |
| Ultrafiltration | P | P | $G_{(5)}$ | E | E | E |
| Ultraviolet oxidation | P | P | $G\text{-}E_{(6)}$ | P | $G_{(7)}$ | P |

*From* NCCLS, 1988.

*E = *Excellent* (capable of complete of near total removal). G = *Good* (capable of removing large percentages). P = *Poor* (little or no removal).

**1. Resistivity of water purified by distillation is an order of magnitude less than water produced by deionization (DI), due mainly to the presence of $CO_2$, $H_2S$, and $NH_3$.
2. The resistivity concentration of dissolved ionized solids is dependent on the original concentration in feedwater.
3. Activated carbon will remove chlorine by adsorption.
4. When used in combination with other purification processes, special grades of activated carbon and other synthetic adsorbants exhibit excellent capabilities for removing organic contaminants. Their use, however, is targeted toward specific compounds and applications. We recommend consultation with the manufacturer before use.
5. Ultrafilters, being molecular sieves, have demonstrated usefulness in reducing specific feedwater organic contaminants based on the rated molecular weight cut-off of the membrane.
6. 1985 nm ultraviolet (UV) oxidation (batch process systems) has been shown to be effective in removing trace organic contaminants when used as post-treatment. Feedwater makeup plays a critical role in the performance of these batch processors. They should not be confused with in-line UV sterilizers which utilize 254 nm UV light to inactivate bacteria.
7. 254 nm UV sterilizers, while not physically removing bacteria, may have bactericidal or bacteriostatic capabilities limited by intensity, contact time, and flow rate.

such as particles, bacterial, colloidal, and pyrogens; carbon adsorption for attaching molecules, atoms, ions such as chlorine, and chloramines to the surfaces of solids and liquids; deionization (working and polishing units) that selectively exchange $H^+$ or $OH^-$ ions for the ionized impurities in the water; and ultrafiltration for removal of dissolved organic and suspended impurities based on molecular weight and size. Ultraviolet (photochemical) oxidation is a process by which an ultraviolet light source is used to convert carbon to carbon dioxide.

The major classes of contaminants and the efficiency of the process used for removal are given in Table 4.1. Dissolved ionized solids and gasses in high-purity water consists of heavy metals, calcium, magnesium, zinc, iron, and other inorganic salts and gasses. On-line total oxidizable carbon (TOC) analyzers now measure laboratory-grade water at higher sensitivity levels in the parts per million or parts per billion range.

## WATER QUALITY AND NATIONAL WATER STANDARDS

Regulations, standards, and guidelines have been established for potable water, processed water, and pharmaceutical water used in the health care environment. Regulations for water are the standards by which a water supply is judged; standards for water quality are designed to ensure that a measured comparison is possible for qualitative and quantitative values, whereas guidelines are recognized statements of policy or procedure. In the hospital and health care facility setting local, state, and federal agencies, and the Joint Commission on Accreditation of Hospitals issue specifications for water systems. The following organizations issue specifications for water quality: American Society for Artificial Internal Organs, Association for Advancement of Medical Instrumentation, United States Pharmacopoeia, National Committee for Clinical Laboratory Standards, College of American Pathologists, American Society for Testing and Materials, and the Centers for Disease Control. Methods and procedures used to measure water quality parameters are included in each organization's publication.

Different grades or types of water are used in health care facilities. Potable water from a main water supply is used for food preparation, drinking, bathing, laundry, other housekeeping needs, and recreational use. Water is used in the clinical laboratory to prepare media, standards, reagents, and sample dilutions. High-purity water is used in critical care areas, special care units, and dialysis, fertility, or donor departments where impurities in water can be life-threatening; and in some research laboratories.

## National Interim Primary Drinking Water Regulations

Current potable or drinking water regulations for maximum contaminant levels were described by the Environmental Protection Agency (EPA) in 1977 in accordance with the Safe Drinking Water Act (Public Law 93-523). The microbiologic and chemical standards are based on the National Interim Primary Drinking Water Regulations which estimate that the average adult in the United States consumes 2 liters of water each day. The standards for safe drinking water described in *The Interim Drinking Water Report* of 1977 provides limits on chemical and physical parameters.

### *Drinking Water*

Historically, the coliform test has been the microbiologic index for safe drinking water, whereas the chemical quality of water has been based on substances representing adverse health effects at the lowest practical level for lifetime limits. Potable water is not routinely monitored by building occupants but can be examined by local, state, or federal agencies when deemed necessary.

Waterborne diseases caused by bacteria, viruses, and protozoan cysts are controlled by treating potable water with disinfectants. In a 1986 EPA project summary, Hoff reviews the inactivation of microbial agents by chemical disinfectants (free chlorine, chloramine, chlorine dioxide, and ozone) in terms of individual characteristics, effects of laboratory tests, and performance in the field.

### *Housekeeping*

One of the primary objectives in good housekeeping practice is to provide and maintain a healthy environment for staff, patients, and visitors. Potable water is generally mixed with cleaning agents to process certain items in central supply, to clean equipment, or to wet-mop, wet-vacuum, or spray-clean hallways and patients' rooms. Aerators should not be used in patient care areas, however. If aerators are used in a health care facility, a scheduled cleaning and sterilization (preferably steam autoclaving) should be implemented. If there are any doubts, the type or quality of water used for cleaning medical devices, instruments, and patient care equipment or articles should be reviewed by members of the health care facility infection control committee to ensure compliance.

### *Laundry*

The *Accreditation Manual for Hospitals* (JCAH, 1985) and the Centers for Disease Control (CDC) *Guidelines for Handwashing and Hospital Environmental Control* (1985) describe recommendations for handling clean and soiled laundry. Dirty laundry facilities are usually separated from other areas of a health care facility to minimize microbial dissemination into the environment. In addition, soiled laundry from isolation areas and septic surgical cases is separated from other laundry before processing. Washing laundry in potable water heated to 71 °C (160 °F) for twenty-five minutes appears to be more effective in reducing microbial contamination than chemical sanitization. Lower water temperature [71.6–122 °F] (11–50 °C) requires chlorine bleach to obtain the same results (Buford et al., 1977).

### *Physiotherapy*

Most health care facilities provide staff and patients with a variety of recreational and therapeutic bathing facilities. These tubs or tanks are supplied primarily with potable water and may be cleaned periodically or after each use. Guidelines are available on swimming pools, whirlpools and spas (CDC, 1983 and 1985).

Microbiologic, chemical, and physical parameters for physiotherapy are outlined in a collection of papers dealing with pool operation, clinical and epidemiologic aspects of disease associated with whirlpool use, host factors, characteristics of microorganisms isolated from whirlpools and bathers, and public health implications of whirlpool use (Castle, 1985; Davis, 1985; Geldreich et al., 1985a; Highsmith et al., 1985b; Jacobson, 1985; Schiemann, 1985; Solomon, 1985).

### *Recreational*

Swimming pools, whirlpools, and hydrotherapy tanks are used by patients and employees for exercise, relaxation, and physical therapy. They are constructed in a variety of shapes and materials. Inadequate chlorine levels or malfunction of the disinfecting equipment can result in increased levels of microbial contaminants in the water (Castle, 1985; Davis, 1985). Microorganisms become attached to surfaces and form biofilms or excellular materials, such as glycocalyx, which can shield the bacteria from germicidal action (Costerton et al., 1985).

Although national standards have not been determined for levels of microbial contaminants in recreational water, some states use the following criteria: "The presence of organisms of the coliform group, or standard plate count of more than 200 bacteria per milliliter, or both, in 2 consecutive samples or in more than 10 percent of the samples in a series shall be deemed as unacceptable water quality" (CDC, 1985b). Table 4.2 lists water quality parameters for whirlpools.

### *Therapeutic*

Hydrotherapy pools, Hubbard tanks, and immersion tanks are used by patients for therapeutic purposes. Although microbiologic parameters have not been set for therapeutic water, patient exposure or contact with contaminated water should be minimized. It is recommended that water for hydrotherapy be heated to approximately 37 °C (98.6 °F), filtered a minimum of three times a day, and maintained at a pH of 7.2 to 7.6 with a chlorine residual of 0.5 mg/L. Hubbard and immersion tanks are generally drained and cleaned after each patient use.

### *Special Purpose*

In order to meet the requirements for high-purity water in the pharmacy, research laboratory, or for critical patient care, additional water treatment is sometimes necessary to remove trace contaminants. As in the research laboratory, a variety of grades or types of water are used in the pharmacy, from laboratory-grade water for cleaning and rinsing to water for additives or for injection. Although the operation and maintenance of medical devices can depend on

**Table 4.2** Water Quality for Whirlpools

| | Recommended Optimum Standards | | |
|---|---|---|---|
| | Minimum | Range | Maximum |
| Disinfectant levels | | | |
| Free chlorine mg/L (ppm) | 2 | 3–5 | 5 |
| Combined chlorine mg/L (ppm) | none | none | 0.2 |
| Bromine (ppm) | 2 | 3–5 | 5 |
| Iodine (ppm) | | levels not confirmed | |
| Chemical values | | | |
| pH | 7.2 | 7.4–7.6 | 7.8 |
| Total alkalinity (buffering) ppm as $CaCO_3$ | 60 | 80–100* | 180 |
| | none | 100–120** | none |
| Dissolved solids (ppm) | 300 | none | 2,000 |
| Hardness ($CaCo_3$) (ppm) | 150 | 200–400 | +500 |
| Cyanuric acid (optional) | 10 | 30–50 | 100 |
| Heavy metals | none | none | none |
| Biologic values | | | |
| Algae | none | none | none |
| Bacteria | none | none | none† |
| Parasites | none | none | none |
| Viruses | none | none | none |
| Physical values | | | |
| Temperature | none | none | 104 °F (40 °C) |
| Turbidity (nephelometric turbidity units) | 0 | ≤0.5 | 1.0 |

*From* CDC, 1985.

*Range for calcium hypochlorite, lithium hypochlorite, and sodium dichlor.

**Range for sodium hydrochlorite, trichlor, chlorine gas, and bromione gas.

†National specifications not determined. Some states use as criteria: "The presence of organisms of the coliform group, or standard plate count of more than 200 bacteria per milliliter, or both, in 2 consecutive samples or in more than 10 percent of the samples in a series shall be deemed as unacceptable water quality."

high-purity water, not all medical devices or critical care areas require the same water quality. For example, water used for inhalation therapy should be sterile (Favero et al., 1978) whereas water for dialysis should not exceed 200 colony-forming units (CFU)/mL (Petersen and Favero, 1981). Guidelines should be reviewed periodically for latest specifications (NCCLS, 1988; USP, 1980).

### *Laboratory- or Reagent-Grade Water*

Guidelines for water quality used in the laboratory are described by the National Committee for Clinical Laboratory Standards (NCCLS, 1985), the College of American Pathologists (CAP, 1978), and the American Society for Testing and Materials (ASTM, 1985). The presence of trace organics and other impurities in laboratory tests can cause baselines to shift unpredictably. In other procedures, minute quantities of contaminants in the water, such as minerals, microorganisms, and endotoxins, can interfere with or alter laboratory test results or can contaminate medical equipment used for patient care. Each of these committees has prepared analytical tests methods to referee water quality. Definitions are based on general classes of water use, for example for reagent, analytic, and general purposes. Table 4.3 lists the specifications for NCCLS reagent-grade water for use in the clinical laboratory.

### *Tests for Potable Water*

Detection of pathogenic microorganisms in water requires specialized methods and techniques. Although numerous microorganisms have on occasion been isolated from potable water supplies, the water in a health care facility is not routinely tested for microbial content, viruses, or protozoa. Microbial parameters may be deter-

**Table 4.3** Specifications for Reagent Grade Water

| | Type I | Type II | Type III |
|---|---|---|---|
| Bacterial content, CFU/mL, maximum | 10 | $10^3$ | NA |
| pH | NA | NA | 5.0–8.0 |
| Resistivity, megohm-cm, 25 °C | 10 (in-line) | 1.0 | 0.1 |
| Silicate, mg/L $SiO_2$, maximum | 0.05 | 0.1 | 1.0 |
| Particulate matter* | 0.22 μm (filter) | NA | NA |
| Organics* | Activated carbon | NA | NA |

*From* NCCLS, 1988.

*These are process specifications not measured by the end user.

mined in critical care areas (such as the dialysis center or the clinical laboratory) or in the cases of a suspected problem or illness-outbreak investigation. Methods for collecting water samples and isolating and recovering microorganisms are described by several national committees (APHA, 1985; NCCLS, 1985).

Water is sometimes tested for pyrogens or endotoxins. With the acceptance of the *Limulus* amebocyte assay as the official test, more hospitals and laboratories are using this assay to rapidly detect contamination of fluids, equipment, and supplies (Highsmith et al., 1982), in hemodialysis (Carson et al., 1983; Favero et al., 1971; 1975), in cardiac and hepatic catheterization (Kundsin and Walter, 1980; Lee et al., 1973; Trapana, Y., 1981), and respiratory therapy (Favero et al., 1975; Reinhardt et al., 1981).

The occurrence in and isolation of viruses from drinking water is rare and may be limited to infectious hepatitis, poliomyelitis, and Norwalk agent (Metcalf, 1983). Viruses may fail to survive in water due to the presence of an oxidizing or disinfecting agent; the water's pH, temperature, physical dilution; or the relatively short survival time of viruses.

Potable water is rarely examined by health care facilities for chemical contamination. Generally the local, state, or federal health department is consulted for assistance where problems are suspected.

### Tests for High-Purity Water

The 1988 NCCLS *Guidelines for Preparation and Testing of Reagent Water in the Clinical Laboratory* describes specific water quality levels and uses, methods for processing types of water, and techniques for monitoring water quality (bacterial content, resistivity, pH, silica, organic content, and particulate matter).

High-purity water should be defined according to water quality parameters and should be tested accordingly. Most high-purity reagent water should not contain bacterial (organic) contaminants. Another example of a process that requires specific water quality requirements is high-performance liquid chromatography, which requires water void of organic impurities that could concentrate in columns. In addition, the presence of soluble silica in the water supply adversely affects most enzyme determinations, trace metal analyses, electrolyte assays, and spectrophotometric measurements.

The municipal water supply to most laboratory facilities contains a wide spectrum of simple and complex organic compounds, particularly the low-boiling-point and low-molecular-weight organics. Industrial waste products, including alcohols and halogenated hydrocarbons, are detected more frequently in municipal water supplies when specific compounds are identified in treated water. Since the operating procedures in some areas of the health care facility are more critical than originally anticipated, water purification equipment designs can provide extremely low levels of total oxidizable carbon (TOC).

## EFFECTS OF CONTAMINATED WATER IN HEALTH CARE FACILITIES

Contaminated water in health care facilities has been shown to cause endemic and epidemic cases of disease. Numerous microbial species have been isolated from contaminated faucets, aerators, and sinks; physiotherapy tanks and medical equipment have also been implicated in disease epidemics (Alyffe et al., 1974; Baird et al., 1976; Baker et al., 1979; Branson and Consodine, 1973; Saepan et al., 1975).

### Endemic Disease

In 1967, Winstead reported on the effects of contaminated water on certain laboratory results. First, Winstead observed problems with laboratory tests directly traceable to water quality, and then, the effects on tests when water was specifically contaminated. The results of her studies are classic examples of how contaminated water, system design, and maintenance influence laboratory data. Significant effects on laboratory results were shown to occur in the following tests: bilirubin, chloride, colloidal gold, Coulter counting, fibrinogen, glucose, oxyhemoglobin, protein-bound iodine, prothrombin, sodium and potassium, total protein, urea, uric acid, and the enzymes amylase, lipase, lactic dehydrogenase, phosphatase, and transaminase.

Water has been the source of endogenous contamination and has served as a secondary route of disease transmission. Microorganisms such as *Pseudomonas* and *Staphylococcus* have been isolated in water and uncooked foods, and other investigations have implicated the water in flower vases in hospitals as potential reservoirs of pathogenic bacteria (Kominos et al., 1972; Schroth et al., 1973; Taplin and Mertz, 1973).

Contaminated water or moisture has also been related to less-defined illnesses such as the "sick building syndrome" (Finnegan et al., 1984). A "sick" building is a building in which complaints of ill health are more common than might reasonably be expected. In some buildings, up to 90 percent of the air may be recirculated to conserve energy. Infrequent filter replacement has resulted in the isolation and recovery of high numbers of polymicrobial flora. The affected buildings are usually offices with aerosols in the air-conditioning system. Postulated causes for discomfort include moisture formation, formaldehyde from cavity wall insulation, furniture or carpet adhesives, cigarette smoke, excess airborne particles and carbon dioxide, bacteria in the air from contamination of the humidifiers, poor air circulation, mixes used for janitorial services, and the lack of negative ions. Symptoms of sick building syndrome include blocked, itchy, or runny noses; itchy, irritated, or watering eyes; drying of mucous membranes (dry throat, stuffy nose); asthma (chest tightness, difficulty in breathing, shortness of breath, wheezing); humidifier fever (fever, joint, and muscle pains, fatigue, headache); lethargy; nosebleeds; dry skin; rashes; itchy skin; and headache.

Recognition of the occurrence and persistence of bacteria in potable water is important in establishing criteria for assessing the quality of water and for controlling potential health effects. It is unclear whether hospital potable water systems are reservoirs of bacterial pathogens causing endemic nosocomial infections. The CDC and the EPA conducted a collaborative study to identify and quantitate specific bacteria found in hospitals' potable water supply, and to determine whether similar bacteria were associated with nosocomial infections in patients in the intensive care unit of ten hospitals (Highsmith et al., 1985; 1987). In twenty-three (5 percent) instances, temporal association was demonstrated between a patient with a nosocomial infection and a bacterial isolate of the same species from water (Table 4.4).

## Epidemic Disease

Compared with healthy persons, hospitalized patients with decreased resistance to infections may be one of the populations at

**Table 4.4** Microorganisms Isolated from Water Before, After, or Index Week of Onset of Nosocomial Infection

| | No. Bacterial Species Identified | | | | |
|---|---|---|---|---|---|
| | | Water Sample | | | |
| Microorganism | Nosocomial Infection(s)* (N)** | Hot | Hot (1 min after flush) | Cold | Main |
| *Pseudomonas* | | | | | |
| *aeruginosa* | 127(10) | | 2 | | 2 |
| *cepacia* | 4 | | | | |
| *maltophilia* | 3 | | | | |
| species | 7 | | | | |
| *Enterobacter* | | | | | |
| *aerogenes* | 38 | | | | |
| *agglomerans* | 4 | | | 1 | |
| *cloacae* | 53(2) | | 1 | | 1 |
| species | 13(1) | 1 | 2 | 1 | 1 |
| *Klebsiella* | | | | | |
| *pneumoniae* | 75(4) | 1 | 2 | 2 | |
| *oxytoca* | 2 | | | | |
| species | 1 | | | | |
| *Acinetobacter* | | | | | |
| *anitratus* | 7 | | | | |
| *lwoffi* | 2(1) | 1 | | | |
| species | 6 | | | | |
| *Serratia* | | | | | |
| *marcescens* | 37(1) | | | | |
| species | 4 | | | | |
| *Enterococcus* | 80(4) | 2 | | 3 | |
| Unidentified | 4 | — | — | — | — |
| Total | 467(23) | 5 | 7 | 7 | 4 |

*From* Highsmith et al., 1985, 1988.

*Number of nosocomial infections with selected bacteria.

**Number of nosocomial infections with water isolate of same species identified during pre-, post-, or index week of onset of nosocomial infection.

highest risk of secondary health effects. During their hospital stay patients may receive numerous exposures to possible pathogens and undergo multiple procedures and types of care. Outbreaks have occurred as a result of contaminated distilled water, storage and cooling tanks, and equipment including physiotherapy pools, pharmacy-purified water, and medical devices. Table 4.5 lists some nosocomial infections caused by contaminated water. Over the years, illnesses have been associated with contaminated water in hospitals. For instance, an outbreak of disease occurred in a hospital when pharmacy-purified water, contaminated with *P. aeruginosa* and *P. thomasii,* was used to cool fluids (Baird et al., 1976). Water collected from nebulizer reservoirs on six pediatric wards was contaminated with gram-negative bacteria that multiplied rapidly in distilled water reaching levels of $3 \times 10^8$ CFU/mL (Favero et al., 1971). In 1979, Baker and colleagues published a report on illness related to waterborne contamination of intrauterine pressure transducers. Pyrogenic reactions occurred in patients during cardiac catheterization with catheters cleaned with contaminated hospital-prepared water before sterilization (Reyes et al., 1980). The epidemiology and microbiology of whirlpools has been discussed in a series of publications already mentioned.

Central water systems have also been implicated in outbreak investigations; two examples were *Pseudomonas* and *Legionella* epi-

**Table 4.5** Nosocomial Infections Due to Ingestion, Inhalation, and Body Contact with Contaminated Water

| Etiologic Agent | Water Source | Illness | Reference |
|---|---|---|---|
| *Pseudomonas multivorans* | tap + disinfectant | wound infection | Bassett, 1970 |
| *P. aeruginosa* | tap + disinfectant | peritonitis | Parrott, 1982; Berkelman, 1984 |
| *P. aeruginosa* | hydrotherapy tank | cellulitis | McGuckin, 1981 |
| *P. aeruginosa* | tap | meningitis | Ho, 1981 |
| *Acinetobacter calcoaceticus* | water bath | peritonitis | Abrutyn, 1978 |
| *Staphylococcus epidermidis* | basin splash | wound infection | Baird, 1976 |
| *Legionella pneumophila* | potable water | Legionnaire's disease | Cordes, 1981 |

demics. In 1981, Ho and colleagues demonstrated that *P. aeruginosa* in a hospital water system was the cause of meningitis in patients receiving ventricular shunt tubing. *Legionella* species have been implicated in hospital water distribution systems as the etiologic agent in ongoing epidemics of Legionnaire's disease (Shands et al., 1985). Although air-conditioning cooling towers are not uniformly constructed, they act as heat exchangers for large facilities and have been the source of nosocomial outbreaks, particularly of *Legionella* (Cordes et al., 1981; Dondero et al., 1980; Orrison et al., 1980).

## SUMMARY

Factors that contribute to overall water pollution include (1) increased population demands on water for domestic use, health care, industrial, agricultural, and recreational purposes, (2) land congestion and less ground for natural water run-off retention or absorption into the underground supply and, (3) improper treatment and distribution of water.

Providing and maintaining an adequate water supply is important in the health care facility. Water systems with improper design, operation, and maintenance procedures have impacts on the water quality at all levels. In particular they are a potential source of infection to those with a high risk for illness. Outbreaks of infection associated with contaminated water are a significant public health concern in health care institutions. Although committees have provided specifications for water in many of the areas now a part of the health care facility, the prime responsibility for designing and maintaining good water quality standards belongs to everyone.

## ACKNOWLEDGMENT

Permission to reprint Tables 4.1 and 4.3 from C3-P2, "Preparation and Testing of Reagent Water in the Clinical Laboratory—Second Edition; Proposed Guideline," has been granted by the National Committee for Clinical Laboratory Standards. The NCCLS is not responsible for errors or inaccuracies. Copies of the complete guideline are available from NCCLS, 771 E. Lancaster Avenue, Villanova, PA, 1988.

## REFERENCES

Abrutyn, E., G. L. Goodhart, K. Ross et al. 1978. *Acinetobacter calcoaceticus* outbreak with peritoneal dialysis. *Am. J. Epidemiology* 107:328–35.

American Public Health Association (APHA). 1985. *Standard methods for the examination of water and wastewater.* 16th ed. New York: APHA.

American Standard Testing Methods (ASTM). 1985. *Part 31, Water: Atmospheric analysis.* Philadelphia: Am. Soc. for Testing and Materials.

American Water Works Association, Inc. 1985. *Water quality and treatment.* New York: McGraw-Hill.

Ayliffe, G. A., B. J. Collins, J. R. Babb, E. J. Lowbury, and S. W. Newsom. 1974. *Pseudomonas aeruginosa* in hospital sinks. *Lancet* 1:578–80.

Baird, R. M., K. M. Elhag, and E. J. Shaw. 1976. *Pseudomonas thomasii* in a hospital distilled water supply. *J. Med. Microbiology* 9:493–95.

Baker, D. A., P. B. Mead, J. M. Gallant et al. 1979. Waterborne contamination of intrauterine pressure transducers. *Am. J. Obstet. Gynecol.* 133:923–24.

Bassett, D.C.J., K. J. Stokes, and W.R.G. Thomas. 1970. Wound infections with *Pseudomonas multivarans:* Waterborne contaminant of disinfectant solutions. *Lancet* 1:1188–91.

Berkelman, R. L., R. L. Anderson, B. J. Davis, A. K. Highsmith, N. J. Petersen, W. W. Bond, E. H. Cook, D. C. Mackel, M. S. Favero, and W. J. Martone. 1984. Intrinsic bacterial contamination of a commercial iodophor solution: Investigation of the implicated manufacturing plant. *Appl. Environ. Microbiol.* 47:752–56.

Branson, D., and T. J. Consodine. 1973. Unexpected results of changing a hospital water treatment system. *Laboratory Medicine* 4:27–29.

Buford, Linda, M. S. Pickett, and P. A. Hartman. 1977. Sanitation in self-service automatic washers. *Appl. Environ. Microbiol.* 33:74–78.

Carson, L., G. Bolan, N. J. Peterson et al. 1983. Antimicrobial and formaldehyde resistance patterns of non-tuberculous *Mycobacteria* associated with reprocessed hemodialysers. *Proc. of the Ann. Mtg: Interscience Conf. on Antimicrobial Agents and Chemotherapy.* Am. Soc. Microbiol., Washington, D.C.

Carter, H. C., and G. E. Martin. 1975. An engineer's guide to medical plumbing systems. *Actual Specifying Engineer* May: 57–60.

Castle, S. P. 1985. Public health implications regarding the epidemiology and microbiology of public whirlpools. *Infect. Control* 6:418–20.

Centers for Disease Control (CDC). Reprinted 1983. *Safety and disease control for swimming pools through proper design and operation.* Atlanta: CDC, June 1976.

———. 1985a. *Guideline for handwashing and hospital environmental control.* Washington, D.C.: Public Health Service, U.S. Government Printing Office, pp. 5–20.

———. Revised 1985b. *Suggested health and safety guidelines for public spas and hot tubs.* Atlanta: CDC, April 1981.

College of American Pathologists (CAP). 1978. *Reagent water specifications.* Chicago: Commission of Laboratory Inspection and Accreditation.

Cordes, L. G., A. M. Wiesenthal, G. W. Gorman, J. P. Phair, H. M. Sommers, A. Brown, V. L. Yu, M. H. Magnussen, R. D. Meyer, J. S. Wolf, K. N. Shands, and D. W. Fraser. 1981. Isolation of *Legionella pneumophila* from hospital showerheads. *Ann. Int. Med.* 94 (2):195–97.

Costerton, T. W., J. C. Nichel, and T. J. Marrie. 1985. The role of the bacterial glycocalyx and of the biofilm mode of growth in bacterial pathogenesis. Roche Seminars on Bacteria No. 2.

Davis, B. J. 1985. Whirlpool operation and the prevention of infection. *Infec. Control* 6:394–97.

Dondero, T. J., R. C. Rendtorff, G. F. Mallison, R. M. Weeks, J. S. Levy, E. W. Wong, and W. Schaffner. 1980. An outbreak of Legionnaires' disease associated with a contaminated air-conditioning cooling tower. *N. Engl. J. Med.* 302:365–70.

Favero, M. S., F. X. Brey, D. G. Brown, and N. E. Dewar. 1978. Proposed microbiologic guidelines for respiratory therapy equipment and materials. *Health Lab. Sci.* 15:117–79.

Favero, M. S., L. A. Carson, W. W. Bond, and N. J. Petersen. 1971. *Pseudomonas aeruginosa:* Growth in distilled water from hospitals. *Science* 173:836–38.

Favero, M. S., N. J. Peterson, L. A. Carson, W. W. Bond, S. H. Hindman. 1975. Gram-negative water bacteria in hemodialysis systems. *Health Lab. Sci.* 12:321.

Finnegan, J., C. A. Pickering, and P. S. Burge. 1984. The sick building syndrome: Prevalence studies. *Brit. Med. J.* 289:1573–75.

Geldreich, E. E., A. K. Highsmith, and W. J. Martone. 1985a. Public whirlpools: The epidemiology and microbiology of disease. *Infec. Control* 6:394–97.

Geldreich, E. E., R. H. Taylor, J. C. Blannon, and D. J. Reasoner. 1985b. Bacterial colonization of point-of-use water treatment devices. *AWWA:* 72–80.

Highsmith, A. K., R. L. Anderson, and J. R. Allen. 1982. Application of the *Limulus* amebocyte assay in outbreaks of pyrogenic reactions associated with parenteral fluids and medical devices. In *Endotoxins and their detection with the Limulus amebocyte lysate test,* S. W. Watson, J. Levin, and T. J. Novitsky, eds. New York: Alan R. Liss, pp. 465–71.

Highsmith, A. K., T. G. Emori, S. M. Aguero, M. S. Favero, and J. M. Hughes. 1987. Heterotrophic bacteria isolated from hospital water systems. In *Proceedings of the international Meeting on Water-Related Health Issues, Atlanta,* C. L. Tate, ed. American Water Resources Assoc., Bethesda, Md.: pp. 181–88.

Highsmith, A. K., T. G. Emori, S. M. Aguero, J. M. Hughes, and M. S. Favero, 1985. The relationship of bacteria in hospital water systems to nosocomial infections. *Proc. Ann. Mtg. Am. Soc. Microbiol.* L-39, p. 419.

Highsmith, A. K., P. N. Le, R. F. Khabbaz, and V. P. Munn. 1985b. Characteristics of *Pseudomonas aeruginosa* isolated from whirlpools and bathers. *Infect. Control* 6:407–12.

Ho, J. L., A. K. Highsmith, E. S. Wong et al. 1981. Common source *Pseudomonas aeruginosa* infection in neurosurgery. *Proc. Ann. Mtg. Am. Soc. Microbiol.* L-10, p. 80.

Hoff, J. C. 1986. *Inactivation of microbial agents by chemical disinfectants.* EPA/600/52-86/067. Washington, D.C.: U.S. Environmental Protection Agency.

Jacobson, J. A. 1985. Pool-associated *Pseudomonas aeruginosa* dermatitis and other bathing associated infections. *Infect. Control* 6:398–401.

Joint Commission on Accreditation of Hospitals (JCAH). 1985. *Accreditation Manual for Hospitals.* Chicago, Ill.

Kominos, S. D., L. E. Copeland, B. Grosiak, and B. Postic. 1972. Introduction of *Pseudomonas aeruginosa* into a hospital via vegetables. *Appl. Micro.* 24:567–70.

Kundsin, R. B., and C. W. Walter. 1980. Detection of endotoxin on sterile catheters used for cardiac catheterization. *J. Clin. Microbiol.* 11:209.

Lee, R. V., M. Drabinsky, S. Wolfson, L. S. Cohen. 1973. Pyrogen reactions from cardiac catheterization. *Chest* 63:757.

Mangione, E. J., R. S. Remis, K. A. Tait, H. B. McGee, G. W. Gormani, B. B. Wentworth, P. A. Baron, A. W. Hightower, J. M. Barbaree, and C. V. Broome. 1982. An outbreak of pontiac fever related to whirlpool use. *J. Am. Med. Assoc.* 253:535–39.

Metcalf, T. G. 1978. Indicators for viruses in natural water. In *Water pollution microbiology,* R. Mitchell, ed. New York: John Wiley and Sons, pp. 301–24.

McGucklin, M. B., R. J. Thorpe, and E. Abrutyn. 1981. Hydrotherapy: An outbreak of *Pseudomonas aeruginosa* wound infections related to Hubbard tank treatments. *Arch. Phys. Med. Rehabil.* 62:283–85.

National Committee for Clinical Laboratory Standards (NCCLS). 1988. *Guidelines for preparation and testing of reagent water in the clinical laboratory.* 2d ed. Villanova, Penn.

Parrott, P. L., P. M. Terry, E. N. Whiteworth, L. W. Frawley, R. S. Coble, I.

K. Wachsmuth, and J. E. McGowan. 1982. *Pseudomonas aeruginosa* peritonitis associated with intrinsic contamination of a poloxamer-iodine solution. *Lancet* 2:683–85.

Petersen, N. J., and M. S. Favero. 1981. Biologic and chemical quality of water used in reprocessing hemodialyzers. *AAMI* 4:11–14.

Orrison, L. H., W. B. Cherry, and D. Milan. 1980. Isolation of *Legionella pneumophila* from cooling tower water by filtration. *Appl. Environ. Microbiol.* 41:1202–05.

Reinhardt, D. J., W. Nabors, C. Kennedy, and B. Malecka-Griggs. 1981. *Limulus* amebocyte lysate and direct sampling methods for surveillance of operating nebulizers. *Appl. Environ. Microbiol.* 42:850–55.

Reyes, M. P., S. Ganguly, M. Fowler et al. 1980. Pyrogenic reactions after inadvertent infusion of endotoxin during cardiac catheterizations. *Ann. Intern. Med.* 93:32–35.

Saepan, M. S., H. O. Bodman, R. B. Kundsin et al. 1975. Microorganisms in heated nebulizers. *Health Lab. Sci.* 12:316–20.

Schiemann, D. A. 1985. Experiences with bacteriological monitoring of pool water. *Infection Control* 6:413–17.

Schlech, W. F., N. Simonsen, R. Sumarah, and R. S. Martin. 1986. Nosocomial outbreak of *Pseudomonas* folliculitis associated with a physiotherapy pool. *Can. Med. Assoc. J.* 134:909–13.

Schroth, M. N., J. J. Cho, and S. D. Kominos. 1973. No evidence that *Pseudomonas* chrysanthemums harms patients. *Lancet* 2:906–7.

Solomon, S. L. 1985. Host factors in whirlpool-associated *Pseudomonas aeruginosa* skin disease. *Infect. Control* 6:402–6.

Taplin, D., and P. M. Mertz. 1973. Flower vases in hospitals as reservoirs of pathogens. *Lancet* 2:1279–81.

Trapana, Y. 1981. Personal Communication.

U.S. Environmental Protection Agency (EPA). 1977. *National interim primary drinking water regulations.* EPA-570/9-76-003. Washington, D.C.:EPA.

United States Pharmacopeia (USP) XX. 1980. Rockville, Md.: U.S. Pharmacopeial Convention.

Winstead, M. 1967. *In reagent grade water: How, when and why?* Ann Arbor: American Society of Medical Technologists, pp. 1–139.

Youngberg, D. A. 1986a. Determination of potential vendors for an Ultra-Pure water system. BDX-613-3359. Bendix Aerospace, Kansas City Division, Kansas City, Mo.

———.1986b. Equipment evaluation prior to shipment. BDX-613-3397. Bendix Aerospace, Kansas City Division, Kansas City, Mo.

# 5

# The Microbiologist's Role in Evaluating the Hygienic Environment

RUTH B. KUNDSIN

The microbiology of the hospital has been studied extensively. Because the hospital is essentially a microcosm of the community at large, the information can be extrapolated to any environment where people congregate. While the hospital's microbiology is geared to resolving problems of nosocomial infections, cross-infections occur in the community as well, and an understanding of the transmission and interception of infections in a hospital can also serve to explain disease transmission in a community. Airborne microorganisms exist in all occupied spaces. Fallout is present in all areas, whether occupied or not. Basically, therefore, microorganisms have the same aerodynamics wherever they are, in the office, in the home, in the airplane, or in the hospital.

Environmental contamination falls into two major categories. Contamination may be inherent in the building's design and construction. Thus filters in air-conditioning units, accumulations of water or condensate around cooling coils, air intake plenums, and linings of air ducts can all disseminate microorganisms into the building's occupied space. The types of organisms originating from these sources are typically gram-negative rods such as *Legionella* or spore-formers such as *Aspergillus*.

The second type of contamination arises from the building's occupants. This may take the form of gross contamination such as body secretions or excretions; a more subtle type of contamination occurs when droplet nuclei are exhaled by infected or colonized humans. Bacteria and viruses are also potential pathogens for other occupants of the building.

Recognition of the source of the environmental problem is essential in order to focus on the resolution. Microbiologic sampling of the environment is the only way to ascertain whether contaminants originate from the building's innate construction or its occupants.

The hygienic impact of the environment is shown in Table 5.1. This table, taken from Wells (1955) describes where the microorganisms can be found, their mode of production and suspension, their diameter, and their settling velocity.

Microorganisms in the environment are associated with particles of differing sizes. The three categories are droplets, dust, and droplet nuclei. Droplets are the large particles (>100 μm) expelled on speaking, coughing, or sneezing which are too large to evaporate before settling to the floor. Some equipment can also produce large droplets, as occurs with splashing from faucets, fountains, and sprinklers.

Dust (10–100 μm) is produced by accretion of particles from textiles, feathers, wood, paper, and so on. In a hospital the dust consists predominantly of cellulose arising from the manipulation of textiles.

**Table 5.1** Comparison of Dust, Droplets, and Droplet Nuclei

| | Dust | Droplets | Droplet Nuclei |
|---|---|---|---|
| Sources | Solid matter, fabrics, etc. | Fluids from nose and throat | Solid residues of evaporated droplets |
| Production | Attrition | Atomization of fluids | Evaporation of droplets |
| Mode of suspension | Air wafted | Projected into air by sneezing, coughing, etc. | Caught in air by evaporation |
| Particle diameter | 10–100 μm | >100 μm | 2–10 μm |
| Settling velocity | 1 ft/min to 1 ft/sec | >1 ft/sec | <1 ft/min |

*From* Wells, 1955.

Droplet nuclei (2–10 $\mu$m in diameter) are the residues of expired droplets, droplets that evaporate before reaching the ground. These droplet nuclei, because of their small size, drift in air currents, like cigarette smoke, until they are inhaled or vented. The microorganisms they carry may die in time, depending on such factors as relative humidity, temperature, and protective protein.

The differences between the various particles as to size and aerodynamics is a basic concept that must be appreciated before any evaluation of indoor air can be made. The state of suspension of the microorganisms associated with these particles is critical in determining the role the microorganisms play in the transmission of disease. Their state of suspension also defines the best method for controlling survival and intercepting dissemination.

Particle size also determines the methods necessary for detection of the microorganisms associated with the particle. Volumetric air samplers are needed for recovery of droplet nuclei. These machines are essentially artificial lungs that recover the air-wafted bacteria which remain suspended and cannot be detected on a settling plate because their settling velocity is too low. For the recovery of these particles, devices employing centrifugal force to multiply the force of gravity are essential. The centrifugal force flings the droplet nuclei onto an agar medium. After incubation, the resultant colonies are counted as colony-forming units (CFUs) per unit of air, that is, cubic foot or cubic meter depending on the sampling device.

Dispersed dust and droplets can be recovered on settling plates because of their larger size and rapid settling velocity. Petri dishes equal approximately one-fifteenth of a square foot; a fifteen-minute sample can be considered to show fallout per square foot per minute, that is, CFUs recovered per square foot per minute.

To evaluate the total accumulations of organisms on a surface, another type of culture needs to be done. This culture can demonstrate how well an area has been cleaned and how many microorganisms have accumulated since the last cleaning. The best and the simplest method involves the use of the Rodac plate. This is a shallow plastic dish filled to the brim with nutrient agar. The 3.8-sq in agar surface can be directly pressed against the area to be sampled. All samples are incubated at 36 °C (96.8 °F) and counted at forty-eight and ninety-six hours and reported as CFUs.

Each of the three methods of culture yields different information. The small droplet nuclei contain microorganisms that can be distributed by air currents to other occupants of the area. The larger dust particles and droplets fall onto horizontal surfaces where they remain until they are destroyed by germicides or resuspended by air currents and activity. The quantity and types of microorganisms recovered are also useful in solving problems and in predicting new ones.

With such data, we can compare environments and make intelligent observations about the air hygiene of an area. The source of the contaminating microorganisms can also be surmised and documented.

The settling velocity of particles associated with bacteria can be ascertained by dividing the CFUs falling out per square foot per minute (on the fallout plate), by the CFUs in one cubic foot of air sampled by a volumetric air sampler in the same environment.

$$V_g = \frac{\text{area CFU per sq ft}}{\text{volumetric CFU per cu ft}}$$

The $V_g$ (settling velocity) is the distance in feet through which the bacteria-laden particles actually fall in one minute.

Riley and O'Grady (1961) have compiled a series of settling velocities related to different environments which indicate that a particle-settling velocity of approximately 0.1 ft/min describes an environment in which droplet nuclei predominate as opposed to an environment with a particle-settling velocity of 1 ft/min or greater where dust particles predominate.

A simple, useful method for visualizing fungal spores and house dust mites is with the use of clear cellophane tape. The sticky surface of the tape is pressed against the area to be examined. The tape is then placed sticky side down on a glass microscope slide. The imprint can be examined for fungal spores, insects, fiberglass, and other debris (Figure 5.1).

House dust mites are the most important group of allergen-producing arthropods contained in house dust. They live on fungi and skin scales. Rugs that have become wet and contaminated with fungi provide an environment for the proliferation of these dust mites. They are also found in areas where skin squames accumulate, that is, on mattresses, mattress pads, bedding, and on the floor in bedrooms. Large numbers have also been found in filters in air conditioners, demonstrating a potential for airborne dissemination.

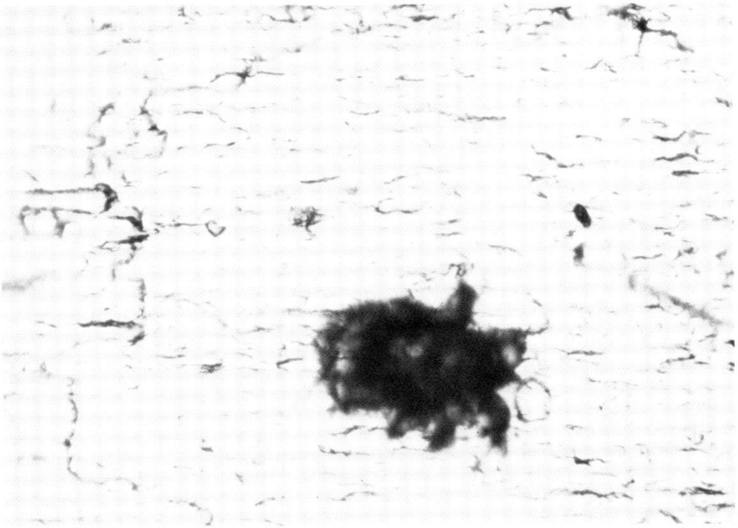

**Figure 5.1.** Cellophane tape impression of house dust mite (Dermatophagoides-like mite, 0.5 mm long) recovered from top of a bookcase in an allergic patient's home.

Sampling air currents with chemicals does not approximate how live organisms would react. Live organisms are influenced by relative humidity, temperature, protective protein from secretions, and ultraviolet irradiation. Live organisms also become embedded in moist environments where they can proliferate with an average generation time of twenty minutes. Thus linings of ducts, filters, any surfaces moistened with condensate, rugs wetted by flooding or spatter from faucets are all ideal reservoirs for microbial proliferation. And, again, infestation by dust mites follows fungal proliferation.

New building design and construction frequently can have an innate source of microbial pollutants. Air-conditioning ducts are often lined with materials such as fiberglass to serve as acoustical barriers. On one construction site, many such ducts piled up on the exterior of the building were exposed to the weather prior to installation (Figure 5.2). The fiberglass lining was found to contain $1 \times 10^3$ microorganisms/g of fiberglass. The predominant organisms were *Bacillus* sp., fungi, and gram-negative rods. After a rainstorm,

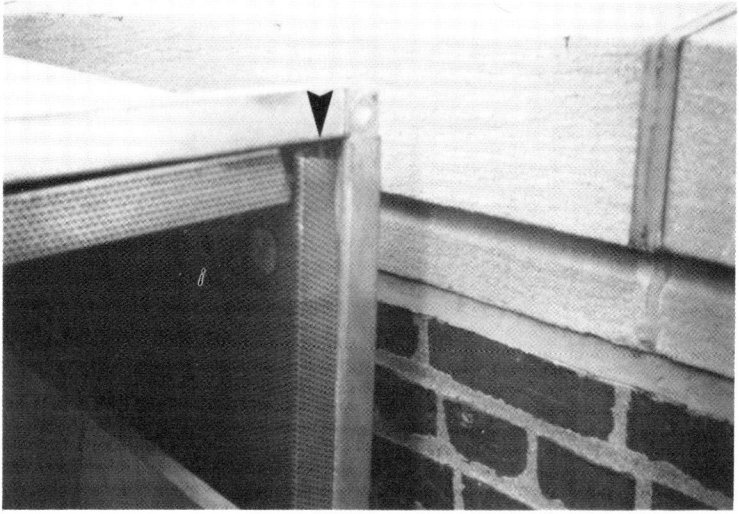

**Figure 5.2.** Arrowheads indicate fiberglass lining the interior of air-conditioning ducts, with $1 \times 10^3$ microorganisms per gram of fiberglass; this became $1 \times 10^5$ per gram after a rainstorm.

the same fiberglass contained $1 \times 10^5$ microorganisms/g. The predominant organisms were *Morganella morganii,* micrococci, *Bacillus* sp., and fungi. This demonstrates that microorganisms are inherent in the fiberglass that lines the ducts of new installations and they multiply in the presence of moisture.

This finding has serious implications, in that installations with such lined ducts will be constantly disseminating microorganisms into the circulating air of the building. Because many ducts are situated after the filters, the microorganisms will not be filtered out but will be redistributed. There is also the likelihood of house dust mites proliferating in ducts contaminated by fungi.

The American Hospital Association and the Centers for Disease Control suggest surveillance as the means by which to deal with nosocomial infections. This essentially consists of counting patients with infections or, in other words, using patients as sampling devices. It would be more logical as well as more humane to use sampling devices instead.

Respiratory tract infections, wound infections, and urinary tract infections are the three most common hospital-acquired infections. Instead of volumetric air sampling devices, we are using the respiratory tracts of patients and hospital personnel to inform us that a problem exists. Instead of settling plates, patients' wounds collect the bacteria and fungi. Urinary tract infections have been shown to be associated with indwelling urinary tract catheters. When the connection of the indwelling catheter is disturbed, infection is more apt to occur. This again implicates microbial contamination from the environment.

## DETERMINATIONS USING ENVIRONMENTAL CULTURES

### Ventilation: Air Changes per Hour

Architects construct buildings with definite calculated air changes per hour in each area. These air changes per hour can actually be verified using bacterial aerosols and collecting them with a volumetric air sampler. The bacterial die-away, essentially a regression line, can be calculated using viable aerosols under varying environmental conditions. Ultraviolet installations in an operating room can be easily tested in a similar fashion. In an intensive care unit with ultraviolet irradiation as a curtain over the doorway and as barrier lights at lower levels, biologically equivalent air exchanges were doubled even though no direct irradiation existed in the room itself. That is, the rate of removal of bacteria, an *Escherichia coli* aerosol, by normal room ventilation was doubled with the use of such irradiation.

### Detection of Carriers Implicated in Infections

Specific shedding carriers can be detected by microbial sampling of the environment. One such report (Walter et al., 1963) demonstrated that a shedding carrier in the operating room could be detected by any one of the environmental samples. *Staphylococcus aureus* of the carrier's phage type was found in volumetric air samples in 11 percent of operations, on fallout plates on the aseptic field in 33 percent of the operations, on fallout plates on the floor in 25 percent. The carrier's *S. aureus* was recovered from one or more environmental samples in 49 percent of the operations he attended. His *S. aureus*

**Table 5.2** Environmental Isolations of Staphylococcus Aureus from a Carrier during 169 Operations

| Source of Specimen* | No. Pos./Total Done (%) |
|---|---|
| Settling plates on aseptic field | 56/169 (33%) |
| Settling plates on the floor | 42/169 (25%) |
| Volumetric air samples | 19/169 (11%) |
| Operations during which *S. aureus* recovered | 82/169 (49%) |
| Two wound infections | 2/169 (1%) |

**S. aureus* phage type 52/52A/79/7/70/73/80.81/82/47C.

was also isolated from two postoperative wound infections. These results are shown in Table 5.2.

In an outbreak of postoperative Group A streptococcal infections, an operating room nurse recovered a Group A streptococcus on a fallout plate on a Mayo stand in the operating room. The source was an anesthesiologist who was an anal carrier of the streptococcus of the same type as that which had infected 13 (7 percent) of 183 patients and caused 1 death (Gryska and O'Dea, 1970).

Actual testing for bacterial dissemination is the only scientific way to ascertain the need for patient isolation. Currently, decisions about the isolation of patients are made empirically in all hospitals. This is neither rational nor scientific. If a patient has a *Staphylococcus aureus* infection, for example, isolation should only be maintained as long as the patient continues to shed staphylococci. Effective antibiotic therapy should be validated by actual testing of the environment for staphylococci. When shedding has ceased, isolation is no longer required.

## Documentation of the Source of Symptoms

Employees in an administration office in a hospital complained of headaches and malaise which they felt were related to their environment. Cultures of the environment were done. The number of CFUs in the volumetric air samples and on fallout plates were well within the normal range until the room air conditioner was turned on. Thereupon, overwhelmingly high counts were found on all samples, and a spectacular burst of many species of fungi and *Pseudomonas* were recovered both in volumetric air samples and on fallout plates. The results are shown in Figure 5.3. Upon opening the unit, layers of dirt and dust were found coating the sides and refrigerating coils. The filter had been dutifully changed routinely, but no one had cleaned the unit since its installation. The microorganisms in the dust and dirt corresponded to the ones recovered from the air in the room when the unit was turned on. The condensate on the cooling coils had permitted proliferation of microorganisms. The coils dried when the unit was turned off. Subsequently, when the unit was turned on again the dried dust was disseminated into the room. Cleaning of the interior of an air-conditioning unit with germicides should be as routine as changing the filters.

Pediatricians recommend volumetric air sampling in homes where children have allergic rhinitis and asthma. A typical example cited by Kozak and colleagues (1980) describes a two-and-a-half-year-old patient with severe asthma requiring hospitalization. It was found that carpeting in the child's room was constantly being wetted by water seeping through a wall. Mold on the jute backing of the rug had caused extensive damage to the carpet and the pad underneath. Removal of the carpeting eliminated the child's asthma.

Rug or carpet shampooing has been associated with outbreaks of Kawasaki syndrome in the United States. This is an acute illness that occurs predominantly in children under five. It is characterized by high fever, rash, swollen hands and feet, reddened eyes, and inflamed mucous membranes. Most children recover in two to three weeks. Some 20 percent may go on to develop serious complications. The largest outbreak to date in the continental United States occurred between August 1984 and January 1985. Sixty-one confirmed cases of Kawasaki syndrome occurred in the area extending from Colorado Springs, Colorado, to Cheyenne, Wyoming. Eighty-five percent of these cases were in the Denver metropolitan area (Patriarca et al., 1982). Another cluster of cases was reported in Harris County, Texas, by Rauch et al. (1985). Kozak and co-workers (1980) suggest that shampooing of carpets created the problem, as carpets remain wet for several days after shampooing and the opportunity for fungal proliferation and dissemination of spores is created.

Building construction and renovation present fungal problems. Deaths have been attributed among immunosuppressed patients to *Aspergillus* spores released during such activities.

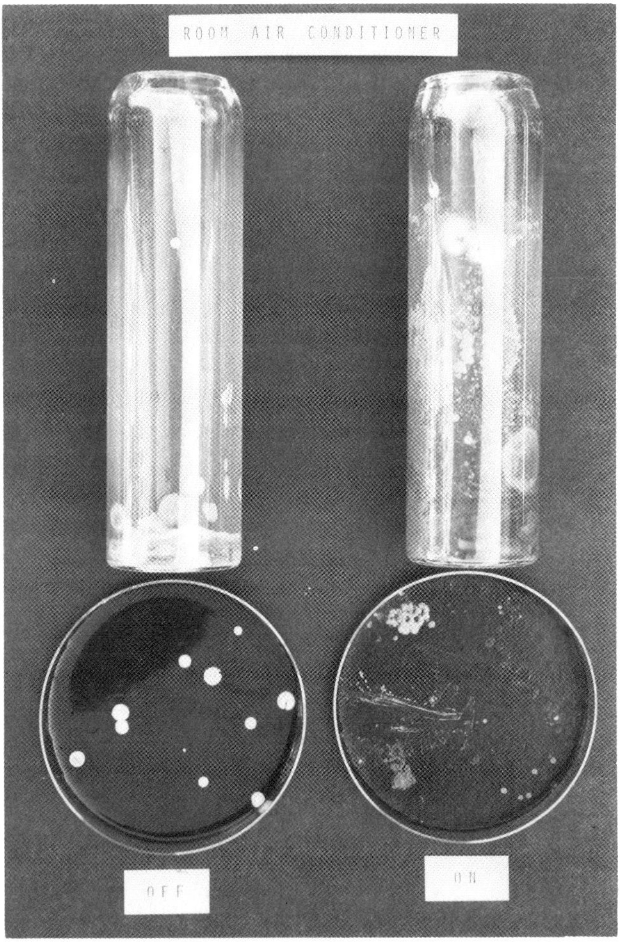


**Figure 5.3.** Volumetric air samples and fallout plates in an office with a room air conditioner. Samples on the left were taken before turning on the air conditioner. Samples on the right were taken immediately after turning on the room air conditioner. The rise in bacterial contamination upon turning on the air conditioner is obvious.

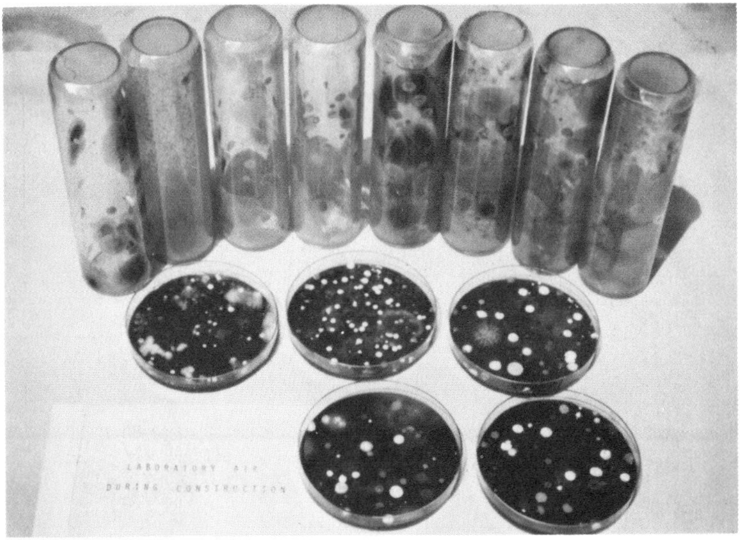


**Figure 5.4.** Volumetric air samples and fallout plates taken in a microbiology laboratory during major reconstruction on the floor below. The high level of fungi is readily discernible in both types of cultures.

During renovation in a building housing a microbiology laboratory, excessive contamination of cultures with fungi was encountered. Investigation revealed high fungal counts on fallout plates and in air samples. The results are shown in Figure 5.4.

## Tracing Microbial Dissemination

Debridement of a severely burned patient with known bacteriology in the operating room presented an opportunity to demonstrate how the patient's particular organisms were disseminated in the operating room. *Pseudomonas aeruginosa* of the same pyocine type as the patient's was distributed throughout the room (Figure 5.5). The bacteria were found on the floor, in the air, and on all horizontal surfaces. The recovery of these organisms on the open shelves on top of sterile supplies used for subsequent procedures demonstrated unequivocally the requirement for the elimination of all open shelving in such critical areas. We did not test for the dissemination of

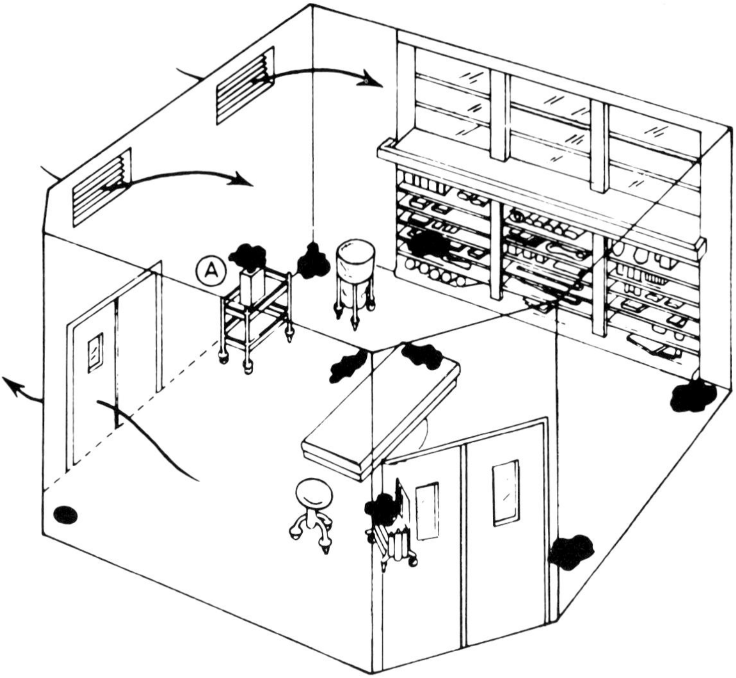


**Figure 5.5.** *Pseudomonas aeruginosa* of the same pyocine type as the patient's found in all the areas indicated by black splotches, demonstrating contamination of the operating room after a debriding procedure.

these organisms into other operating rooms via the recirculating air of the air-conditioning system. We did recover them in our volumetric air samples, indicating that such aerial dissemination is conceivable.

## Evaluation of the Total Environment

The evaluation of an environment can be done with comparisons of the amount of microbial contamination. In a study done at a West Coast hospital where an unusually high number of infections had been observed among patients undergoing cardiac surgery, it was possible to demonstrate through bacteriologic cultures that not only could the problem microorganisms be recovered from the environment but that one environment where cardiac catheterization was done had excessively high levels of bacteria. The cultures are shown in Figures 5.6 and 5.7.

## Standards for the Microbiology of the Operating Room

No official standards exist for microorganisms that are airborne, that fall out, or that have accumulated on horizontal surfaces in the operating room. However, many years' experience has enabled our laboratory at the Brigham and Women's Hospital to set up standards to describe a clean operating room. These are shown in Table 5.3. In addition to quantitation, the types of microorganisms recovered in the environmental samples is also important. A predominance of fungi, or pseudomonads would suggest a different source than the predominance of *S. aureus.*

Industry has resolved the problem by designating requirements for

**Figure 5.6.** Volumetric air samples, fallout plates, and surface cultures. Upper series taken in the cardiac catheterization room, compared with the lower series taken in an operating room in the same hospital.

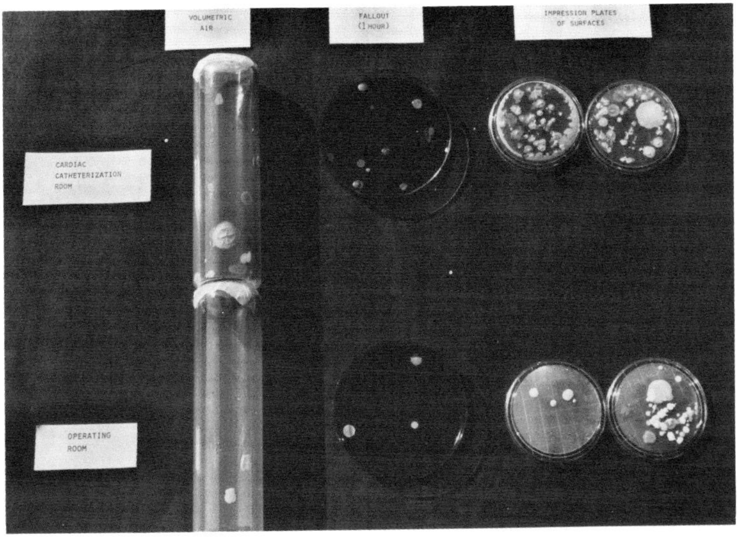

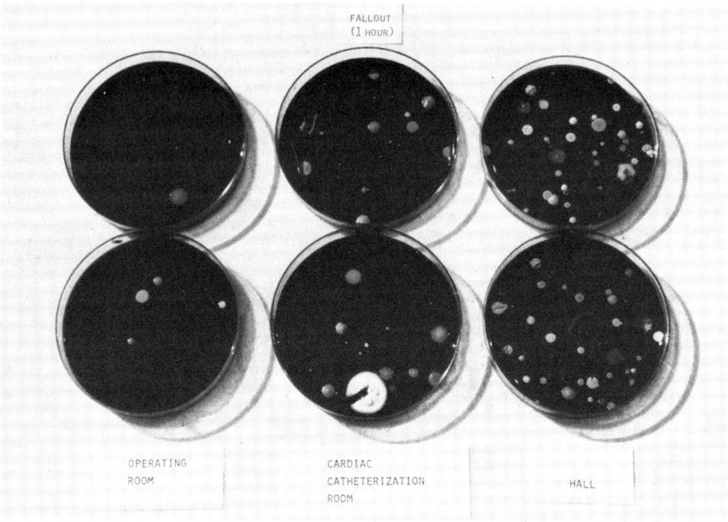


**Figure 5.7.** Comparison of fallout plates taken in the operating room, the cardiac catheterization room, and the public hallway, directly outside the operating suite.

categories of clean rooms. The manufacture of microchips demands a Class 10 clean room, because freedom from dust particles is critical for the assembling of microprocessors. Buildings are being designed so that access to ductwork from the exterior is available for repairs.

The Food and Drug Administration recommends monitoring of the microorganisms in the environment where aseptic filling of injectables or processing of pharmaceuticals is done.

No comparable recommendations exist for any part of the hospital environment.

**Table 5.3** Microbiologic Standards for Operating Room

| | |
|---|---|
| Volumetric air samples | 0–5 CFU/cu ft |
| Fallout | 0–5 CFU/sq ft/min |
| Accumulation | 0–5 CFU/Rodac plate |

## Evaluation of the Efficacy of Ultraviolet Irradiation

The installation of direct ultraviolet irradiation in the operating room of the orthopedic service at the Brigham and Women's Hospital was first tested using microbiologic sampling. The results of volumetric air samples are shown in Figure 5.8. A concomitant and dramatic decrease in postoperative wound infections was also noted. A survey in the Brigham and Women's Hospital reported that the percent of wound infections on the orthopedic service are currently less than half of those on the other services that do not use ultraviolet irradiation.

Direct irradiation is feasible for the operating room where irradiation of the wound and the displayed instruments is desirable and essential. It is not feasible for occupied spaces where people congregate. For such areas either upper air irradiation or installations in ducts is the solution.

Examples of spread of infection throughout whole buildings has been amply documented; rubella, influenza, measles, and tuberculosis are but four examples (Levine et al., 1973, Morbidity and Mortality Weekly Reports, 1986, 1984, and 1980). There is therefore no

**Figure 5.8.** Volumetric air samples taken at the site of the incision during a total hip replacement procedure done under direct ultraviolet irradiation.

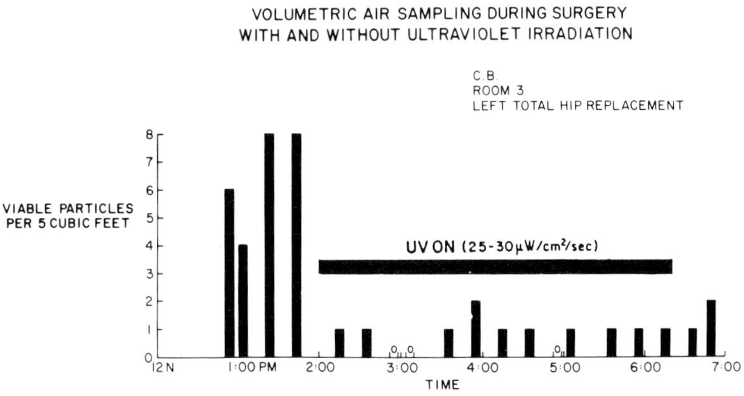

question that the agents of respiratory tract infections are distributed with efficient air-circulating systems. Ultraviolet irradiation in the ducts or upper air irradiation are the suggested solutions. These problems must be addressed by the professionals involved in building design.

## Correlation of Human Infections with Environmental Microbiology

Our laboratory is currently doing research on newborns. We have observed that babies are born with no bacteria in their nasopharynxes. During their first few days in the nursery they begin to be colonized with the bacteria in their environment. Although colonization is a natural phenomenon, it is debatable whether hospital flora are the ideal organisms with which to start one's life.

Several studies have demonstrated that the length of an operation determines the percent of postoperative wound infections. This clearly demonstrates that an exposed wound is essentially the equivalent of a settling plate. Cruse and Foord (1973), in a five-year prospective study of 23,649 procedures, found that each minute of surgery increased postoperative wound infections by .025 percent. Altemeier and colleagues (1976) showed the same phenomenon in a series of 15,613 operations. Each minute of surgery resulted in a .032 percent increase in the incidence of infections.

The incidence of infection was related to the duration of the operation. Thus, a six-hour operation in the first hospital would result in a 9.6 percent infection rate; in the second hospital the same procedure would result in a 15.2 percent infection rate. The difference is highly significant. What is being measured is the microbiology of the environment, that is, the fallout into the wound. Involved in the microbiology of the air in the operating room is the microbiology of the occupants. Whatever the source, it is clear from the statistical evidence that the microbial burden of the air is consistently 158 percent higher in the hospital of one study over the hospital in the other study. This cumulative evidence shows that the exposure of the wound to the environment determines infection. Only careful microbial evaluation can determine the source, which in many cases is a carrier in the operating room.

## Monitoring Isolated Environments

Patients may be isolated in a hospital for two reasons. One reason is to contain microorganisms, as in the case of a patient with tuberculosis, hepatitis, or acquired immune deficiency syndrome (AIDS). Second, patients who are immunosuppressed and susceptible to infection must be isolated to exclude microorganisms.

Bone marrow transplantation procedures are only one example of the use of these techniques. Bacterial monitoring of both the patient and the environment is done throughout the period of patient confinement, beginning eleven days before actual transplantation. Before the transplant, the patient receives doses of chemotherapeutic agents or total body irradiation to suppress existing abnormal bone marrow and to promote engraftment. This treatment causes the patient to become extremely susceptible to fungal, viral, bacterial, and parasitic infections. Lavish use of germicides for cleaning the room, extreme care on the part of personnel to minimize microbial exposure by donning masks, caps, surgical scrub suits, and booties, and the use of laminar air flow all serve to maintain low bacterial counts on all horizontal surfaces.

The care of a burned patient is another situation in which the exclusion of microorganisms from the patient's environment has a salutary effect on prognosis. The fewer the microorganisms in the environment, the fewer are available to colonize the burned surface of the patient.

Levine and colleagues (1973), working with leukemic patients in a protected environment, reported that the use of nonabsorbable antibiotics alone did not reduce the frequency of severe infections or the rate of deaths in which infection was the proximate cause. Their experience demonstrated, however, that patients treated within a protected environment and given an extensive prophylactic antimicrobial regimen had one-half as many severe infections and one-fourth as many life-threatening infections as patients treated with antibiotics alone and patients not isolated and not receiving prophylaxis.

At the Brigham and Women's Hospital (then called the Peter Bent Brigham Hospital), twenty-one patients were followed intensively with personal and environmental cultures at regular intervals.

Twenty received bone marrow transplants. Stringent criteria for housekeeping were set up with simultaneous environmental cultures to ensure low levels of accumulated microorganisms on all horizontal surfaces and as fallout (Kundsin et al., 1979).

It was discovered that patients with clinically apparent infections on admission who were undergoing bone marrow transplants did not fare well even in a protected environment. They remained infected and eventually succumbed to this infection. The only two deaths due to acquired infection occurred in the least-protected environment. Four infections were acquired in the more-protected environments, but no deaths occurred among them. The protected environment did have a salutary effect on the outcome of patients with no infection at the time of admission.

## CONCLUSIONS

Concern for environmental pollutants has focused primarily on chemical and particulate pollutants. Indoor exposures to tobacco smoke, asbestos particles, formaldehyde, and radon have been the prime targets of governmental intervention. Microbial pollution has been relegated to a minor role. The reason for this may be that microbial pollution represents an enigma because of the complications involved in understanding both the source and the control of such pollution.

People are the source of some of these microorganisms and people are also the occupants of inhabited space. Other microorganisms arise from pools of water; contaminated construction materials; the movement of soil as in excavation sites; reservoirs such as filters, duct linings, and all materials wetted either by flooding or by the spatter created by water use; and hospitals by patient secretions or patient care procedures.

An analysis of the major causes of death in the United States has indicated that pneumonia and influenza deaths are increasing. Aside from the ultimate result—mortality—the morbidity associated with respiratory disease and influenza accounts for more than half of all acute conditions, including all illnesses and injuries. The incidence of respiratory illness is almost one person per year and the activity of that person is restricted for 4.5 days. If we consider the response to allergens such as fungi and dust mites, we can appreciate the impact of these microorganisms in terms of time lost from work or school and the consequent medical costs involved.

Architects must come to terms with the indisputable findings of the microbiologist. Air-conditioning systems must be scientifically designed not primarily for comfort but for microbiologic safety validated by testing of actual use conditions. Installations of carpeting and other materials primarily designed for aesthetics should be eliminated if such installations introduce health hazards into critical environments or into homes as allergens. Similarly, the linings of ductwork for acoustic considerations can develop into a reservoir for bacterial and fungal allergens to such an extent as to make our aesthetically pleasing interiors uninhabitable.

The Hippocratic oath to do no harm has been the ethical guide of the medical profession since antiquity. I propose that architects, the creators of the human indoor environment in which we all spend our lives, should take the same oath.

## REFERENCES

Altemeier, W. A., J. F. Burke, B. A. Pruitt, and W. R. Sandusky. 1976. *Manual on control of infection in surgical patients.* New York: J. B. Lippincott, p. 135.

Cruse, P.J.E., and R. Foord. 1973. A five year prospective study of 23,649 surgical wounds. *Arch. Surg.* 107:206.

Gryska, P. F., and A. E. O'Dea. 1970. Postoperative streptococcal wound infection: The anatomy of an epidemic. *JAMA* 213:1189–91.

Kozak, P. P. Jr., J. Gallup, L. H. Cummins, and S. A. Gillman. 1980. Currently available methods for home mold surveys. II. Examples of problem homes surveyed. *Annals of Allergy* 45:167–76.

Kundsin, R. B., H. A. Bodman, J. M. Rappeport. 1979. Clean room and laminar flow room microbiology in the treatment of bone marrow transplant patients. *J. Env. Sci.* 22:27–29.

Levine, A. S., S. E. Siegel, A. D. Schreiber, J. Hauser, H. Preisler, I. M. Goldstein, F. Seidler, R. Simon, S. Perry, J. E. Bennett, and E. S. Henderson. 1973. Protected environments and prophylactic antibiotics. *N. Engl. J. Med.* 288:477–83.

Morbidity and Mortality Weekly Report. 1986. Update: Influenza activity—United States. 35:135–41.

Morbidity and Mortality Weekly Report. 1984. Outbreaks of respiratory illness among employees in large office buildings. *JAMA* 252:1843–44.

Morbidity and Mortality Weekly Report. 1980. Rubella outbreak in an office building—New Jersey. 29:517–18.

Patriarca, P. A., M. F. Rogers, D. M. Morens, L. B. Schonberger, R. M. Kaminski, J. C. Burns, and M. P. Glode. 1982. Kawasaki syndrome: Association with the application of rug shampoo. *Lancet* September 11:578–80.

Rauch, A. M., E. S. Hurwitz, L. B. Schonberger, M. Nihill, S. L. Kaplan, D. E. Seavy, and G. R. Reeve. 1985. Cluster of Kawasaki syndrome cases, Harris County, Texas. *Abstracts of the 1985 Interscience Conference on Antimicrobial Agents and Chemotherapy,* p. 162.

Riley, R. L., and F. O'Grady. 1961. *Airborne infection, transmission and control.* New York: Macmillan.

Walter, C. W., R. B. Kundsin, and M. M. Brubaker. 1963. The incidence of airborne wound infection during operation. *JAMA* 186:908–13.

Wells, W. F. 1955. *Airborne contagion and air hygiene.* Cambridge: Harvard University Press.

# 6

# Heating, Ventilation, Air-Conditioning Systems: The Engineering Approach to Methods of Control

JAMES E. WOODS and DEAN R. RASK

The conflict between energy conservation and indoor air quality is as old as our human desire to protect and shelter ourselves. The earliest enclosures served primarily as shelter from the weather and protection from enemies. However, since the time when windows were first glazed by the Romans about 150 B.C., the sizes and functions of buildings began to vary from simple dwellings to large places of worship (Douglas and Frank, 1972; Foster, 1986). Thus, the use of windows in buildings for lighting and for natural ventilation has a history almost as old as buildings themselves.

During the Middle Ages, the indoor air quality was often noted to be unacceptable. To alleviate this problem, regulations were developed which specified the sizes of windows to be installed in buildings. In the 1600s, King Charles I of England promulgated what may have been the first ventilation code (Nevins, 1976; Winslow and Herrington, 1949). To improve ventilation for removal of smoke, odors, and heat, he specified that no house could be built with a ceiling height of less than 10 feet and that the heights of windows had to be greater than their widths.

Major scientific advances were made during the next two centuries, including the discovery of $O_2$ and $CO_2$, Dalton's Law of partial pressures, description of the composition of air, description of the respiratory function, and so on. Many of these discoveries subsequently led to new theories for ventilation requirements (Klauss et al., 1970; Winslow and Herrington, 1949). Obviously, this was a time when much controversy existed about these new theories. For example, Benjamin Franklin stated in response to concerns generally expressed about the difference between indoor and outdoor air quality: "I considered [fresh air] an enemy, and closed with extreme care every crevice in the room I inhabited. Experience has convinced me of my error. I am persuaded that no common air from without is so unwholesome as the air within a closed room that has been often breathed and not changed." He further stated: "You physicians have of late happily discovered, after a contrary opinion had prevailed some ages, that fresh and cool air does good to persons in the smallpox and other fevers. It is hoped, that in another century or two we may find out that it is not bad even for people in health" (Leeds, 1868).

A general definition of indoor air quality may be stated as "the nature of air that affects one's health and well-being." This definition incorporates the concept of "health" as defined in the Constitution of the World Health Organization: "Health is a state of complete physical, mental and social well-being, and not merely the absence of disease or infirmity" (1946). As a technical definition of indoor air quality, that used in a study for the Iowa Energy Policy Council (Woods and Maldonado, 1982) serves well: "The *quality* of the air in an enclosed space is an indicator of how well the air satisfies the following *(quantifiable)* conditions":

- Thermal conditions of the air (i.e., the dry-bulb temperature, relative humidity, and velocity) must be adequate to provide thermal acceptability for the occupants as defined by the American Society of Heating, Refrigerating, and Air Conditioning Engineers *ASHRAE Standard 55-1981* (1981a).

- Effects of mean radiant temperature, thermal resistance of clothing, and the occupant's activity levels must be considered in this evaluation.

- The concentration of oxygen and carbon dioxide must be within acceptable ranges to allow normal functioning of the respiratory system.
- The concentration of gasses, vapors, and aerosols should be below levels that can have deleterious effects, or that can be perceived as objectionable by the occupant.

This definition addresses three important requirements needed to achieve control. First, it identifies the factors to be controlled: thermal sensation, respiration, and contamination. Second, it suggests that a quantification can be described in terms of a subjective scale. Third, and maybe most important, it implies that simultaneous control of all of the relevant factors is required if satisfactory responses from the occupants are to be achieved.

## CONTROL STRATEGIES

Environmental control may be described in terms of five factors that influence human response: spatial, lighting, acoustic, thermal, and air quality. Four of these factors (lighting, acoustic, thermal, and air quality) may be directly related to the sensory receptors, and the fifth factor, spatiality, interacts with each of the other four.

Each functional area within a building requires special consideration of the spatial factors that may influence day-to-day activity of the occupants, the initial costs of the facility, and the operating costs associated with providing acceptable environmental control, maintenance, repairs, and housekeeping. Minimum spatial requirements for new construction and major modifications are specified in accepted standards (DeChiara and Callender, 1980).

To provide comfortable (acceptable) visual environments for building occupants, control of task lighting and general lighting is required. In addition to lighting level and uniformity, visual acceptability also requires control of the quality of light (i.e., the spectral characteristics). For detailed information refer to the Illuminating Engineering Society (IES) *Handbooks* (1981).

Noise associated with mechanical equipment (e.g., heating, ventilating, and air-conditioning [HVAC] systems, portable vacuum cleaners) must be suppressed, if acoustic comfort (acceptability) is to be achieved within the occupied spaces. Two types of noise must be controlled: transmission noise through the building structure and airborne noise. Waring's 1970 acoustic handbook and the ASHRAE *Handbook of Fundamentals* (1985) give detailed information for noise and vibration control.

To provide acceptable or comfortable thermal environments for the well-being of building occupants, energy-efficient and economic control of the heat exchange rates between the occupants and the environment is a major objective. See *ASHRAE Standards 55-1981* (1981a) and *90A-1980* (1980), and the *ASHRAE Handbook of Fundamentals* (1985) for further information.

To provide acceptable air quality for the occupants, control of gasses, vapors, inert and biologic particulates, and radionuclides within the environment is required. As indicated by the technical definition of indoor air quality stated earlier, simultaneous control is required for the following:

- The thermal quality of the environment. Not only do changes in the thermal environment affect the occupant's response, but the thermodynamic changes also affect the reactions of other contaminants within the environment.
- The concentrations of $O_2$ and $CO_2$ in the environment, caused by the respiration of the occupants.
- The concentrations of contaminants in the environment, caused by transmission of them from outdoors or generations of them indoors.

## Control Loops

Control of the indoor environment can be achieved by either *open-loop* or *closed-loop* control strategies. Both methods are commonly used for thermal control, but closed-loop or feedback control strategies are seldom used for luminous, acoustic, or air quality control. Figure 6.1 schematically shows the processes required in open-loop and closed-loop control systems. In both cases, a desired condition, R (e.g., dry-bulb temperature, lighting level, or gaseous concentration level) is controlled by manipulating the controlled device, M,

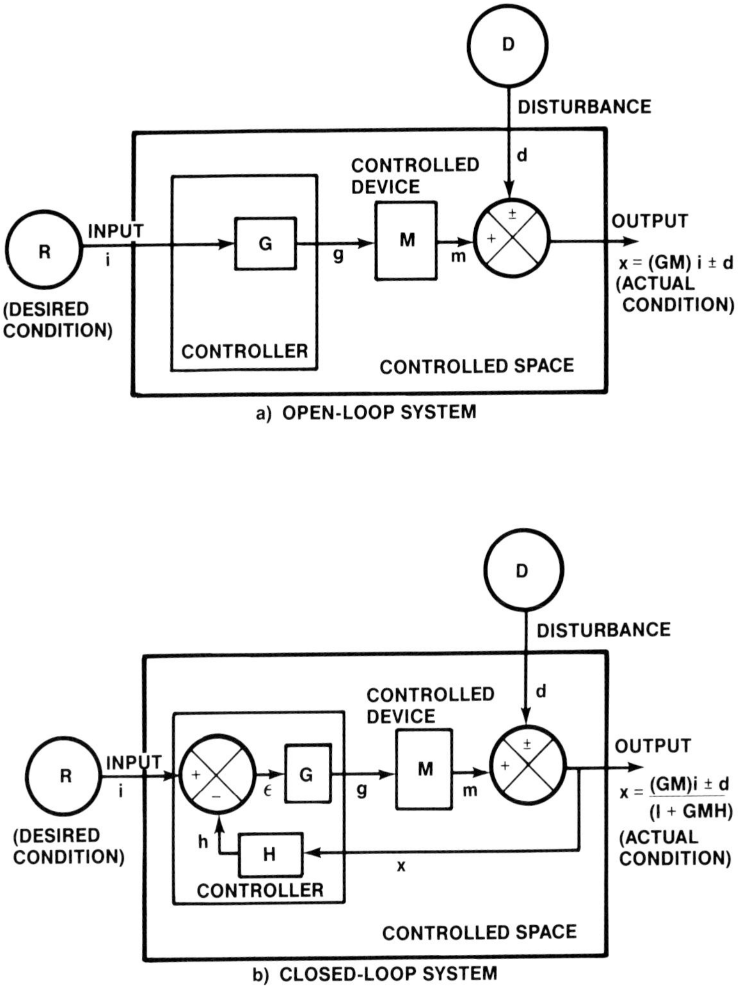


**Figure 6.1.** Schematic representations of (a) open-loop control system, and (b) closed-loop control system.

thereby adjusting the amount of the controlled variable, m (e.g., supply air temperature or flow rate, or the electric power) in response to a disturbance, D (e.g., thermal or lighting load, or generation rate of contamination) which acts on the system through signal d. With open-loop control, the actual condition within the occupied space, x (e.g., room dry-bulb temperature, lighting level, or gaseous concentration) will change in direct proportion to the magnitude of the changes in the controlled variable and the system disturbance. Unless this system is manually adjusted, large differences between the actual and desired conditions, x − R, can result. With closed-loop control, the condition within the occupied space is "sensed" (e.g., temperature sensor) and a "feedback signal," h, from the feedback element, H, of the controller, is automatically compared to the reference signal, i, which is representative of the desired condition, R. The difference between these signals, $\epsilon$ (known as the error signal), modifies the controlled variable, m, and thus tends to minimize the changes in the actual condition, x, when disturbances occur.

Although closed-loop systems for thermal control have been in existence for more than 100 years, reliance on open-loop systems for air quality control prevails in most indoor environments.

## Methods of Control

Three methods of air quality control can be identified: source control, removal control, and dilution control. A simple one-compartment model that is useful in describing these three methods of control is shown in Figure 6.2. In steady state, the contaminant mass balance for the model shown in Figure 6.2 may be expressed as:

$$\Delta C = \frac{\dot{N} - \dot{E}}{\dot{V}_o} \qquad 6.1$$

where

$\Delta C = C_i - C_o$ = difference between the uniformly mixed indoor air concentration, $C_i$, and the outdoor air concentration, $C_o$

$\dot{N} = \dot{Q} - \dot{S}$ = net generation rate of the contaminant which is equal to the source strength, $\dot{Q}$ (i.e., gross generation rate) minus the sink strength, $\dot{S}$ (i.e., settling or sorption rate)

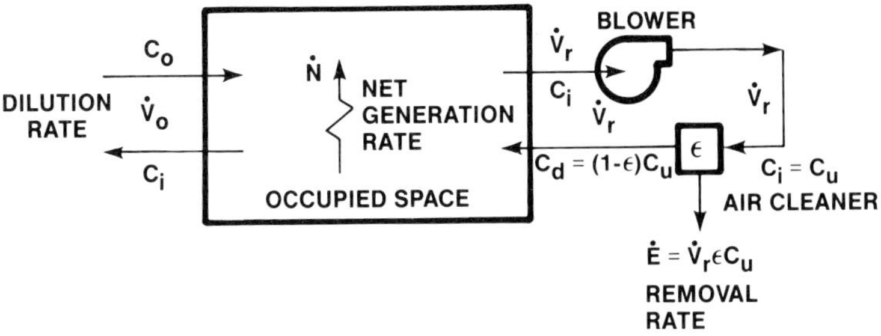


**Figure 6.2.** One-compartment, uniformly mixed, steady-state model for indoor air quality.

$\dot{E} = \epsilon\ \dot{V}_r C_i$ = removal rate of a contaminant in the air cleaner
$\epsilon$ = efficiency of the air cleaner rated in terms of the contaminant removed
$\dot{V}_r$ = volumetric flow rate of recirculated air
$C_i = C_u$ = concentration of the contaminant, upstream of the air cleaner
$\dot{V}_o$ = volumetric flow rate of outdoor air for dilution control (i.e., room ventilation rate).

In this model, the dilution rate, $\dot{V}_o$, represents infiltration, natural ventilation, or mechanical ventilation with outdoor air. The removal rate, $\dot{E}$, represents fan-filter modules now available as consumer products, or filtered 100 percent recirculated air commonly used in residential forced air systems. For cases where filters are located in other parts of systems, similar expressions for $\dot{E}$ can be derived (Woods et al., 1986).

### *Source Control*

Because the intent of the source control method, which pertains to $\dot{N}$ in Equation 6.1, is to minimize the presence of the contaminant within the occupied space, closed-loop control is not effective. Three methods of open-loop control are isolation, containment, and local exhaust.

***Isolation*** A source of contaminants may be isolated from the occupied space by product substitution or by prohibition. Examples of product substitution are the use of "low-emitting formaldehyde" particle boards and plywood, or the installation of electric ignition systems to replace standing pilots in furnaces and boilers. An example of prohibition is the restriction of smoking by occupants to certain areas within the building.

***Containment*** A source may be prevented from entering the occupied space by containing it within its own microenvironment with paints or other barriers which can be applied to building materials. Examples include the containment of radon out-gassing by applying epoxy paints or polyethylene vapor barriers to masonry products. Another example is the use of face masks and gowns by hospital surgical teams.

***Local Exhaust*** A source may be restricted or prevented from entering the occupied space by the use of hoods (e.g., laboratory fume hoods, biologic safety cabinets), and exhaust fans (e.g., toilet exhausts).

### Removal Control

The removal control method, which pertains to $\dot{E}$ in Equation 6.1, is often used as an alternative to, or in addition to, dilution control to reduce indoor concentrations by means of air cleaning devices. It is the only practical method available when it is necessary to control the environment at concentrations below those of the outdoor air. In its simplest forms, removal control of particulates and gaseous contaminants can be considered to comprise two mechanisms: passive removal and active removal.

***Passive Removal*** Airborne particles may be removed from the environment by several mechanisms, some of which are not well understood within occupied spaces. These include particle settling, ion diffusion charging, thermophoresis, photophoresis, and coalescence (Hesketh, 1979; Woods et al., 1985). Passive removal of gasses and vapors may also occur by these processes. Evidence is beginning to develop to indicate that some gasses, such as ozone, sulphur dioxide, nitrogen dioxide, carbon monoxide, and carbon dioxide, may be absorbed on building surfaces, furniture, and furnishings within buildings. These mechanisms may have adverse effects such as corrosion and deterioration of materials within the occupied spaces.

***Active Removal*** Air cleaning devices for active removal may be classified as particle removal devices which include media filters and electronic air cleaners, and as gas and vapor removal devices which contain sorbents, such as activated charcoal or activated alumina.

The collection efficiency, $\epsilon$, of an air cleaning device is usually expressed as a dimensionless fraction which is determined as the complement of the penetration, $P$, of the contaminant through the device:

$$\epsilon = 1 - P \qquad 6.2$$

where

$P = C_d/C_u$
$C_d$ = concentration of the contaminant in the airstream leaving the air cleaning device
$C_u$ = concentration of the contaminant in the airstream entering the cleaning device.

Active removal control methods are employed for both particulate and gaseous contaminants and are almost always open-loop control because appropriate sensors for closed-loop control are not yet cost-effective.

## *Dilution Control*

Dilution is probably the most common method to control indoor air quality in nonindustrial facilities. In some cases, dilution control, $\dot{V}_o$, may be the most energy-intensive and costly of the control methods available today. At other times, dilution control can provide energy savings (e.g., use of an economizer cycle) while improving indoor air quality control.

Dilution control is a means of reducing the concentrations of contaminants in the occupied space by exchanging the room air with air that contains less concentration of the contaminant. This dilution air is usually introduced from outdoors, but may be supplied from other occupied spaces and used for pressurization control (*ASHRAE Standard 62-1981,* 1981). Dilution control may be applied independently or in combination with removal control as shown in Figure 6.2. When these control methods are employed, the presence of a contaminant source, $\dot{N}$, is implied. In most cases where dilution control is employed, the concentration of the contaminant is assumed to be uniform throughout the environment. Thus, the occupants are usually exposed to the contaminant whenever these methods are used.

For some gaseous contaminants with low molecular weights (i.e., $\leq 50$), dilution is the only practical method of control available today. One of the most important of these gasses is $CO_2$, which requires dilution air to maintain an acceptable concentration in the environment. When the dilution rate is sufficient to provide acceptable levels of $CO_2$ in the occupied space (i.e., $<1{,}000$ ppm), the depletion of $O_2$ due to respiration is not significant.

Three methods of dilution control are infiltration, natural ventilation, and mechanical ventilation. Only open-loop control is available for infiltration and natural ventilation. However, closed-loop control can be achieved with mechanical ventilation.

***Infiltration*** Infiltration is usually an unwanted leakage of outdoor air through cracks, joints, and connections in the building envelope. In the past, infiltration has been considered as one method of introducing outdoor air into the occupied space for dilution control. However, several problems exist with this method, especially in the hospital environment:

1. No control exists over the quality of the outdoor air introduced by infiltration. Gaseous and particulate (i.e., viable and nonviable) contaminants may exist in higher concentrations in the infiltration air than may be allowed in the occupied space, especially in critical areas such as hospital operating rooms, laboratories, and other sensitive areas bounded by outside walls.
2. Air exchange rates estimated from infiltration calculations usually assume uniform distribution between adjacent occupied spaces and uniform mixing within the occupied space of concern. Neither is correct. If infiltration rates are significant in a building, the dispersion of contaminants between zones within the building will be strongly coupled to the wind velocity (i.e., speed and direction) around the building. And, within a particular zone, the penetration and mixing of the infiltra-

tion air will be a function of the frequency of the turbulent intensity of the wind on the walls and windows of the room (Teng, 1981).

3. Air exchange rates are usually estimated for winter design conditions. Because the indoor-outdoor temperature and pressure differences are maximized at these conditions, the resultant infiltration rate and energy consumption to heat this air will be maximal. However, winter design conditions occur only 2.5 percent of the year. Thus, at milder conditions, infiltration rates will be less, and dilution control by infiltration will be less effective than calculated for design conditions.
4. Infiltration through cracks, joints, and connections in the building envelope can accelerate soiling, corrosion, and deterioration of the building materials and furnishings within the occupied spaces. Thus, operating costs can be adversely affected.
5. Drafts caused by infiltration can cause thermal discomfort, especially for susceptible occupants.

***Natural Ventilation*** Operable windows can provide some dilution control, but their effectiveness depends on the location of the windows in the room, other means of cross-ventilation, and the outdoor environmental conditions (Teng, 1981). Closing windows tightly can minimize infiltration, but natural ventilation has similar limitations as those for infiltration. No control exists over the quality of the outdoor air introduced through the windows. Gaseous and particulates (i.e., viable and nonviable) contaminants may exist in higher concentrations than may be allowed in the occuped space. Moreover, estimates of ventilation rates through windows usually assume uniform distribution between different zones and uniform mixing within a particular zone. Again, neither is correct. Door closures and other barriers can result in nonuniform distribution of natural ventilation between different zones. And, within a particular zone, the penetration and mixing of the air from the window will be a function of the frequency of the turbulent intensity of the wind at the entrances of the window (Teng, 1981).

***Mechanical Ventilation*** For the simple case of no air recirculation for the occupied space (i.e., 100 percent outdoor air) and no contaminant removal control (i.e., $\dot{E} = 0$), Equation 6.1 indicates that the concentration indoors, $C_i$, varies inversely with the dilution air flow rate, $\dot{V}_o$. This relationship is the basis for the ventilation rates commonly specified in ventilation standards (*ASHRAE Standard 62-1981,* 1981; *Guidelines for construction and equipment of hospital and medical facilities,* 1984).

Forced air systems vary considerably: some may employ 100 percent recirculated air, some may be required to supply 100 percent outdoor air, and some may use thermostatically controlled mixed-air control systems.

Thermostatically controlled mixed-air systems, an example of which is shown in Figure 6.3, provide open-loop air quality control and are of particular concern because of their energy implications. Desires or demands for energy savings cause set-points of the mixed-air controllers to be reset to higher values, deactivation of the thermostatic function of these systems, manual adjustment to minimum amounts of ventilation, or complete deactivation of the systems. Unfortunately, these courses of action are usually counterproductive. Thermostatically controlled mixed-air systems, with either temperature or enthalpy control (i.e., economizer systems), probably were designed to provide supply air conditions to meet cooling requirements imposed by thermal loads. Thus, the amount of outdoor air introduced by these systems should meet or exceed the minimum required for dilution control. During these periods, the refrigeration equipment may remain deactivated or operate under part-load conditions. In this way, improved indoor air quality and energy savings can be achieved.

Conversely, an increase in the set-point of the mixed-air temperature controller results in significant reductions in the percentages of outdoor air available for ventilation. For example, as shown in Figure 6.4, a 10 °F (5.5 °C) increase in mixed-air temperature set-point results in approximately a 60 percent reduction in available outdoor air when the outdoor temperature is below 55 °F (13 °C). Morever, at a 55 °F set-point, a minimum of 15 percent outdoor air will be provided at outdoor temperatures as low as −40 °F (−40 °C); at 65 °F (18 °C) set-point, the outdoor temperatures will have to exceed 26 °F (−3 °C) to obtain more than 15 percent outdoor air, and outdoor air percentages will be decreased to as low as 6 percent during cold winter conditions. Also the capability of dehumidification control

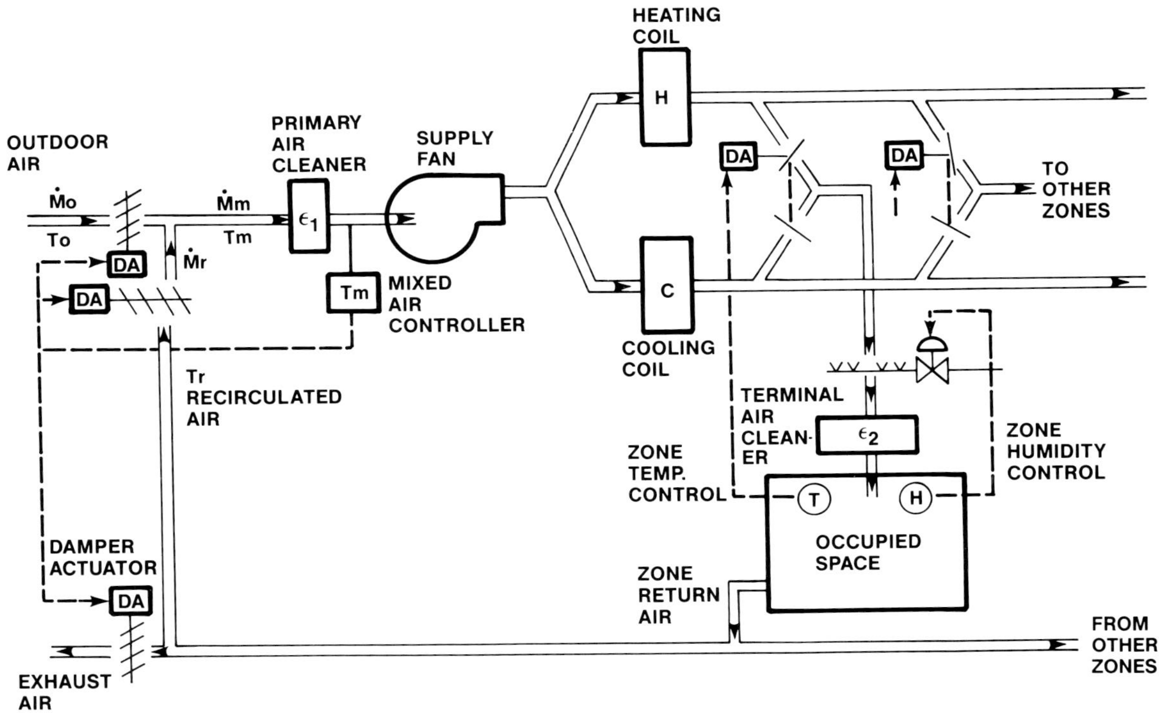


**Figure 6.3.** Schematic representation of a typical mixed-air control system.

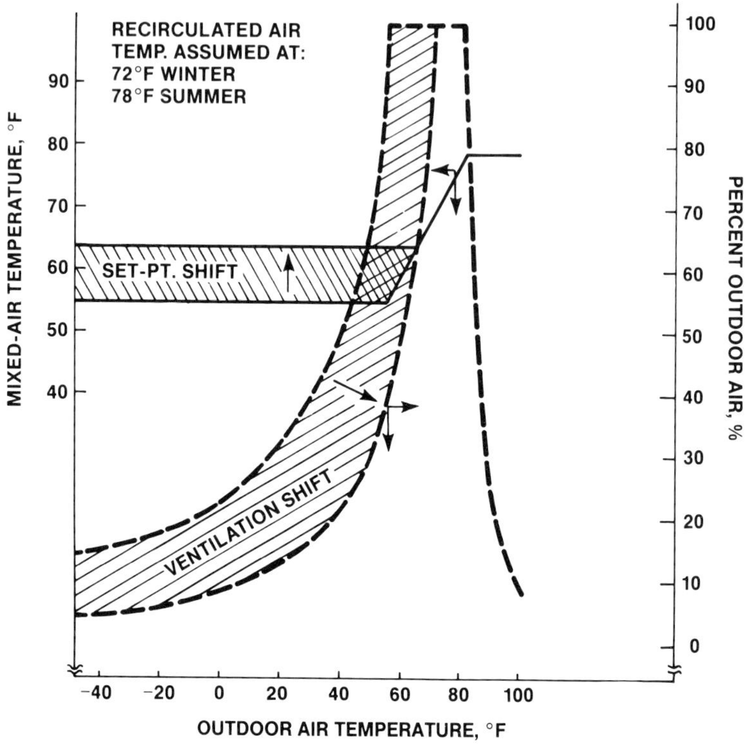


**Figure 6.4.** Relationships of mixed-air temperature and percentage of outdoor air for ventilation as functions of outdoor air temperature.

will be diminished by increasing the mixed-air set-point temperature.

Pressurization control is a special case of mechanical ventilation. It is used primarily to prevent cross-contamination between rooms or zones within the facility. Until the current version of the "Hill-Burton Standards" was published, the standard method of specifying pressurization control was provision of positive or negative pressure to a particular zone (*General standards of construction and equipment*, 1974; *Minimum requirements of construction and equipment*, 1974). However, because of the difficulty of measuring the small pressure differentials between these zones, "pressurization" has most recently been specified in terms of airflow direction (i.e., "in" or "out") at the zone interfaces (*Guidelines for construction and equipment,* 1984). Nevertheless, the importance of this control, direction of air movement or pressurization between zones, cannot be overemphasized.

One effect of pressurization control is especially stressed here. Mechanical ventilation systems are sometimes deactivated during reduced occupancy periods. If the major sources of contamination within the functional area are the occupants, and contagion is not a problem, the deactivation may not degrade the indoor air quality for the remaining occupants. On the other hand, if the sources of contamination are processes or materials that are independent of the occupancy density, deleterious effects to the remaining occupants can result. Therefore, it is of paramount importance to accurately assess the impact of deenergizing systems before these actions are taken.

## AIR DISTRIBUTION

Of the three methods of indoor air quality control (source, dilution, and removal control), only source control can eliminate exposure of the contaminant; the other two methods inherently require mixture of the contaminant with the indoor air before the control methods are applied. The engineering definition of ventilation (the process of supplying and removing air by natural or mechanical means to and from any space, *ASHRAE Standard 62-1981,* 1981), includes the methods of dilution and removal control, but excludes source control. Thus, the ability of the ventilation system to control the concentrations of contaminants within acceptable levels at the exposure site of the occupants in each functional area is highly dependent on the air distribution patterns within and between the occupied spaces.

In some functional areas, natural ventilation may be the primary method of dilution control. In most functional areas, however, the primary method of control is mechanical ventilation, which may employ a combination of dilution and removal control strategies. Whether mechanical or natural ventilation or a combination is employed, the effectiveness of the system for air quality control is dependent upon two system characteristics: the room air exchange rate, and the uniformity of the airflow patterns (i.e., uniform mixing) within the room.

If the room air distribution is not sufficient to dilute or remove contaminants from the location of most likely (critical) exposure, the effectiveness of the system will be impaired (e.g., excessive effects of increased energy consumption, nonuniform mixing in the occupied space, and drafty or uncomfortable subjective responses). Thus, the air distribution patterns within the room may be as important to the effectiveness of the ventilation system as the room air exchange rate.

## Room Air Exchange Rates

At least four pathways can be identified by which the air in a room may be exchanged:

- *Infiltration.* Air leakage through cracks, joints, and interstices in the walls, floors, and roofs of the building.
- *Natural ventilation.* Air exchange through opened windows, outside doors, and other controllable openings.
- *Interzonal transport.* Air exchange through inside doors and other openings.
- *Mechanical ventilation.* Air exchange through central air-handling systems.

When a mechanical ventilation system is the only method of dilution control, the supply airflow rate to the occupied space can be determined directly by measuring the flow rates from each of the supply and return terminal devices (diffusers, grilles, registers) in the room or zone. Although the supply and return airflow rates may provide sufficient information to assess the thermal performance of the system, they are insufficient to assess the air quality performance of the system because (1) the percentage of outdoor air in the supply air is unknown, (2) the infiltration and natural ventilation rates are unknown, (3) the interzonal airflow rates are unknown, or (4) the degrees of uniform mixing or stratification with the room or zone are unknown.

Methods of indirectly determining the air exchange rate within a space or zone have been developed. The two most common methods are the pressurization test and the tracer gas decay test (*ASTM Standard E 741-80,* 1980; Harrje et al., 1979). Although the pressurization test is valuable in locating sources of infiltration, it is impractical to use when dynamic factors (e.g., mixed-air control, natural ventilation, interzonal air exchanges, occupancy patterns) must also be evaluated. For this reason, the tracer gas decay test now generally is accepted as the preferred procedure for estimating the air exchange (i.e., dilution) rate within a zone. It should be noted, however, that this method provides no information regarding the uniform mixing or stratification of the air within the zone.

## Within-Room Air Distribution

The room air distribution system must be responsive to the thermal loads in the space, the indoor air quality requirements, and the acoustic room criteria. To meet all of these criteria simultaneously one must carefully select and place the supply and return air terminals.

### *Thermal Acceptability*

Acceptable thermal conditions may be defined as those that comply with *ASHRAE Standard 55-1981* (1981a) at the location of the occupants (near their microenvironments). The effectiveness of distributing the supply air to the occupants' locations may be evaluated in terms of the air distribution performance index (ADPI) (Nevins, 1976). This concept, shown in Figure 6.5, is based on the ability of the supply air to remove sensible cooling loads (i.e., heat gains) from the occupied space. Although it was originally intended as an evaluator for the selection and location of supply air terminal units, it can also serve as a reasonable index for evaluating the uniformity of the thermal conditions of the air throughout the room for either heating or cooling. For purposes of providing an evaluator of air movement to provide acceptable thermal conditions within an occupied room, a minimum ADPI of 75 percent has been proposed (Woods, 1984).

### *Air Quality Acceptability*

Acceptable air quality conditions may be defined as those that comply with *ASHRAE Standard 62-1981* (1981b) at the location of the

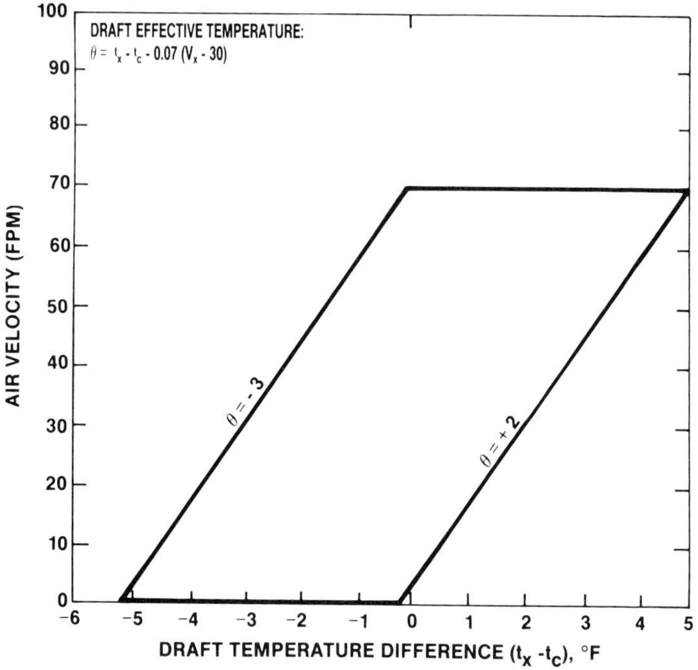


**Figure 6.5.** Air distribution performance index (ADPI) is the percentage of total points measured in an occupied space that meet the criteria: $-3 \leq \Theta \leq +2$ °F, and $0 \leq V_x \leq 70$ fpm. In this figure, $t_x$ and $V_x$ are the dry-bulb temperature and air velocity at a location x, and $t_c$ is "control" or average dry-bulb temperature of the occupied space. (Adapted from Nevins, 1976.)

occupants. Two procedures for providing acceptable air quality are specified in that standard: a "ventilation rate procedure" and an "air quality procedure." These procedures are intended to create acceptable conditions at the occupants' locations, but explicit methods for evaluating compliance have not been specified for either procedure. The ADPI can be used to evaluate the thermal uniformity of air mixing in the occupied spaces, but as previously indicated, it is insufficient as an overall evaluator of the room air distribution. For example, the ADPI does not provide for an evaluation of the amount of supply air that can bypass the occupied space because of short-circuiting of air from the supply to the return air terminal devices. The common practice of locating both supply and return air devices in the ceiling, or on opposing high side walls, has been shown to result in less than 50 percent of the supply air reaching the occupants before it is contaminated. However, the determination of "within-room ventilation efficiency" can serve to evaluate the distribution of the supply air to the occupants (Janssen et al., 1982). As shown in Figures 6.6 and 6.7, the within-room ventilation efficiency, $\eta_v$, can be expressed as a function of the percent of recirculated air, r, and a stratification factor, s, which has been defined as the ratio of the difference between the initial and steady-state decay rates, $(I_0 - I_\infty)$, divided by the initial decay rate, $I_0$. Of importance with the within-room ventilation efficiency, the stratification factor can be associated with the location of the supply and return air terminal devices, and the recirculation percentage can be associated with the ventilation control system.

For purposes of providing an evaluator of air movement for acceptable air quality within an occupied room, a minimum within-room ventilation efficiency of 80 percent has been proposed (Woods, 1984).

## Between-Room Air Distribution

Interzonal transport of gaseous and particulate airborne contamination is one of the most important aspects of indoor air quality. How-

**Figure 6.6.** Two-compartment model of a room with stratification of the indoor air. (After Janssen et al., 1982.)

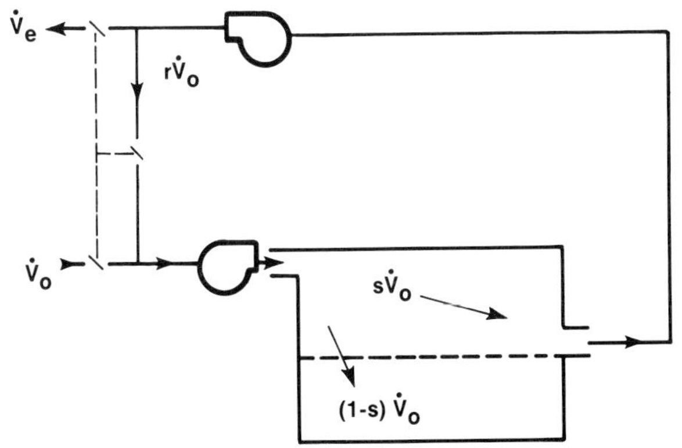

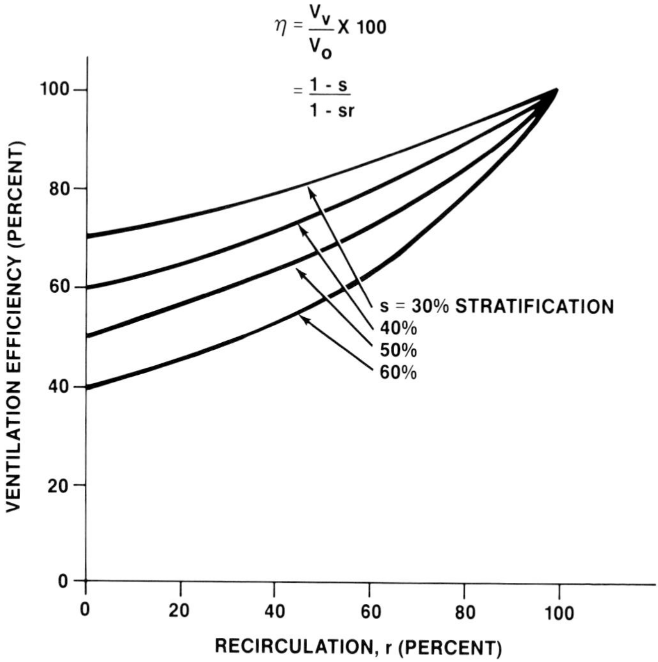


**Figure 6.7.** Ventilation efficiency as a function of recirculation percentage in a room with stratification of indoor air. (After Janssen et al., 1982.)

ever, air distribution between rooms is one of the least-controlled factors in HVAC systems. Except for special facilities, such as microbiologic laboratories in which recombinant DNA research is conducted, direct feedback control methods of pressurization control usually are not employed. Rather, indirect methods are relied upon, such as designing a 10 percent excess of supply or return air for positive or negative pressurization of a room with respect to its surrounding spaces. This indirect method of pressurization is often inadequate for acceptable indoor air quality in facilities such as hospitals, for the following reasons:

1. Pressurization provides no assurance that air movement in both directions across the pressure boundary will not occur. For example, bidirectional flow through doorways has been demonstrated (Luciano, 1977).

2. Pressurization of a room or zone may not be characterized by a single value. For example, four classifications for normal asepsis (i.e., clean, clean-contaminated, contaminated, and dirty) have been described by the American College of Surgeons. Furthermore, required pressure differences across different boundaries of a room or zone may not be the same.
3. Partial pressure gradients of gaseous and vaporous contaminants may allow diffusion of the contaminants to occur in opposition to convection or advection currents of air movement.
4. Cross-contamination can occur through common (i.e., zoned) recirculation systems, although pressurization between zones exists.
5. Dynamic imbalances in pressurization can occur in zones due to operation of variable air volume systems or to deactivation of systems (*Guidelines for construction and equipment,* 1984).

To assess the effectiveness of pressurization control between rooms or zones, two procedures, based on tracer gas technology, have been proposed: the ventilation effectiveness procedure and the relative exposure index procedure (Maldonado and Woods, 1983). These procedures are based on the determination of the integrated average concentration of a tracer gas, $C_i$, in zone i of a multicompartmental model as shown in Figure 6.8. Of particular importance to note in these procedures, the rate of tracer gas decay does not represent infiltration alone. Rather the decay represents the total "room ventilation rate," that is, removal by passive and active means, and dilution by the supply air, by natural ventilation and infiltration, and by interzonal air transport.

### *Ventilation Effectiveness*

The ventilation effectiveness ($VE$) procedure may be used to compare the occupant exposures to a contaminant in several rooms or areas, $C_i$, with exposure in a reference room or area, $C_R$, when the location of a specific contaminant is unknown or not critical.

$$VE = \left. \frac{\int_0^\infty C_R \, dt}{\int_0^\infty C_i \, dt} \right| \quad C_i(0) = \text{uniform}$$

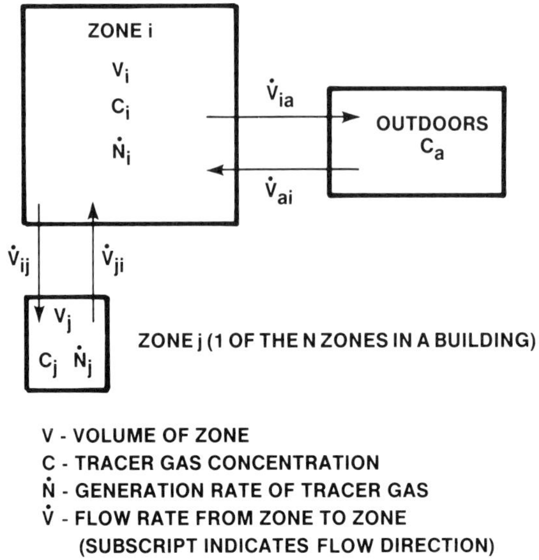


**Figure 6.8.** Multicompartment model of indoor air quality in an occupied space as affected by outdoor air and other zones within the building. (Adapted from Maldonado and Woods, 1983.)

In this procedure, the tracer gas is introduced into all rooms at the same initial concentration, $C_i(0)$, and allowed to decay for a sufficient period (a few hours) to obtain reliable data. Results obtained by this method in a three-bedroom house are shown in Figures 6.9 and 6.10 for cases in which the central supply air fan was energized and deenergized, respectively. In these figures, the areas under the curves represent the occupant exposure and the slopes of the curves represent the room air exchange rates, $hr^{-1}$. Note that this procedure assumes uniform mixing within rooms but not between rooms. These results also indicate that, although uniform mixing between rooms may exist when the supply fan is energized (Figure 6.9), significant differences may develop during light-load conditions when thermostatic control may cause the forced air system to be deenergized for extended periods (Figure 6.10). This procedure should be especially effective in zones served by variable air volume systems, and in areas where it may be desirable to deactivate the HVAC systems during unoccupied periods.

### *Relative Exposure Index*

The relative exposure index (*REI*) may be used to compare the occupant exposures to a contaminant in several rooms or areas with exposure in a reference room or area when the location of a specific contaminant is suspected:

$$REI = \left. \frac{\int_0^\infty C_i\,dt}{\int_0^\infty C_R\,dt} \right| \quad C_i(0) = \text{local}$$

In this procedure, the tracer gas is introduced into the room in which the suspected contaminant source exists, $C_i(0)$, and allowed to

**Figure 6.9.** Ventilation effectiveness of twelve locations in a three-bedroom house. Results shown were obtained after all zones were equalized at the initial tracer gas ($SF_6$, sulfur hexafluoride) concentration; the central fan was energized continuously during the decay period. (From Maldonado and Woods, 1983.)

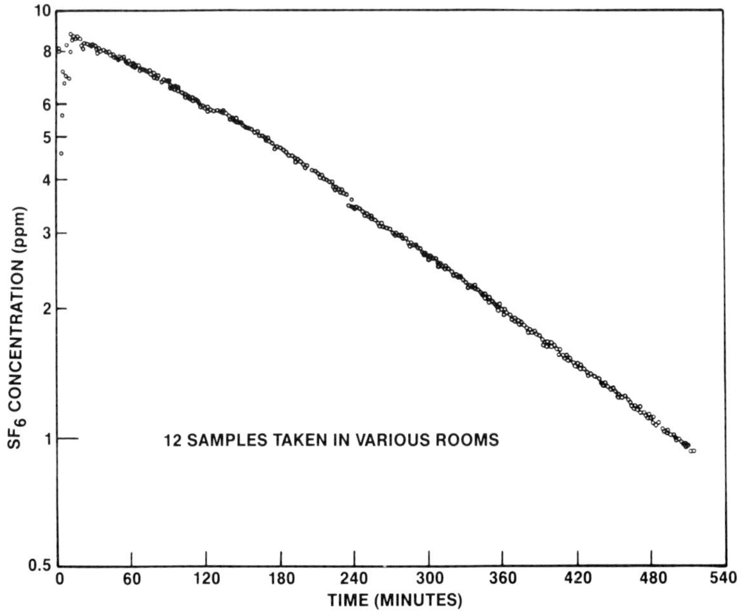

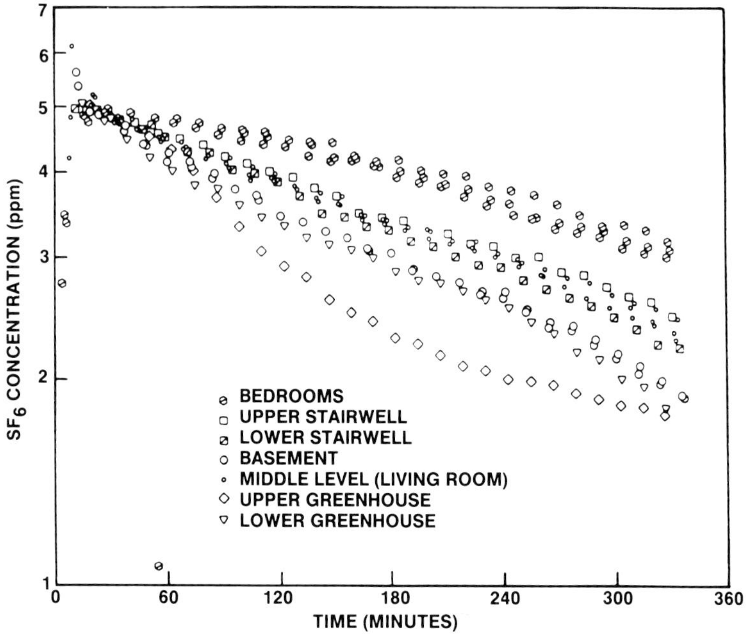


**Figure 6.10.** Ventilation effectiveness of seven locations in a three-bedroom house. Results shown were obtained after all zones were equalized at the initial tracer gas concentration; the central fan was deenergized continuously during the decay period. (From Maldonado and Woods, 1983.)

decay for a sufficient period to obtain reliable data. Results of challenging the three-bedroom house with a tracer gas in the living room are shown in Figure 6.11. Note that with the supply fan deenergized the concentrations in all three bedrooms exceeded the concentration in the living room after about five hours, although the bedroom doors remained closed during this test. In this figure, the areas under the curves represent the occupant exposure and the slopes of the curves represent the room air exchange rates, $hr^{-1}$, with the assumption that the room air concentrations are uniformly mixed. This procedure should be especially effective in zones where pressurization control may be critical or which contain known contaminant sources (e.g., copy machines, laboratory areas).

## ENHANCED CONTROL

Source, dilution, and removal control each provide methods of reducing indoor concentrations of contaminants, but unless a means of *sensing the indoor air quality* is also provided, feedback (closed-loop) control cannot be achieved. The analogy between mass and thermal balances again is useful. Open-loop control for space heating has been used since humans first used fire to warm themselves, but closed-loop thermal control was not available until the thermostat was invented in the late nineteenth century (Billington and Roberts, 1982). Closed-loop control of indoor air quality seems to be on a parallel course through history, but is lagging behind thermal control

**Figure 6.11.** Relative exposure index of seven locations in a three-bedroom house. Results shown were obtained after tracer gas was introduced into the living room; the central fan was deenergized continuously during the decay period. (From Maldonado and Woods, 1983.)

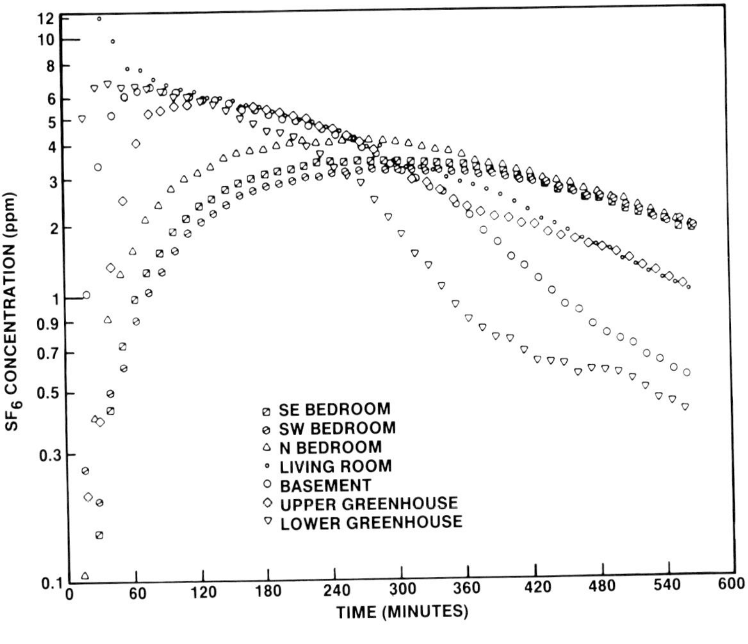

by about 100 years. Sensors for indoor air quality factors are now becoming available and methods of closed-loop control are being demonstrated (Geerts et al., 1985; Janssen et al., 1982; Suomi, 1985).

The analogy also serves in considering the values at which the air quality controllers should be set (i.e., reference R in Figure 6.1). For thermal comfort, factors such as "predicted mean vote" (PMV), "percentage of people dissatisfied" (PPD), and "standard effective temperature" (SET*) have resulted from years of research on responses from thousands of subjects and serve as a solid scientific basis for objectively selecting the thermostatic set-points (*ASHRAE Standard 55-1981,* 1981a; Fanger, 1973; Rohles, 1973). Conversely, few results from research on responses of subjects to indoor contaminants exist upon which standards can be set for control. As a result, *ASHRAE Standard 62-1981* (1981b) provides the following guidance:

> Various indoor activities may give rise to odors of unacceptable intensity or character, or to airborne materials that irritate the eyes, nose, or throat. In the absence of objective means to assess the acceptability of such contaminants, the judgment of acceptability must necessarily derive from subjective evaluations of impartial observers. The air can be considered acceptably free of annoying contaminants if 80% of a panel of at least 20 untrained observers deems the air to be not objectionable under representative conditions of use and occupancy.

## Closed-Loop Control

A schematic of a closed-loop variable ventilation control system is shown in Figure 6.12. This was a constant air volume system with terminal reheat for four zones. As this system was for a junior high school in Minnesota, a summer economizer cycle for the mixed-air dampers was not installed, thus 100 percent outdoor air was available during summer operation. During mild weather conditions, the control signal from the thermostat in the zone with the warmest temperature controlled the percentage of outdoor air delivered to the zones, and the amount of cooling provided by the direct expansion (DX) refrigeration system. When cooling was not required in any zone, the outdoor air and exhaust dampers could close and the recirculated air damper could open if the $CO_2$ concentrations were below the set-point of the $CO_2$ controller. However, if the $CO_2$ concentra-

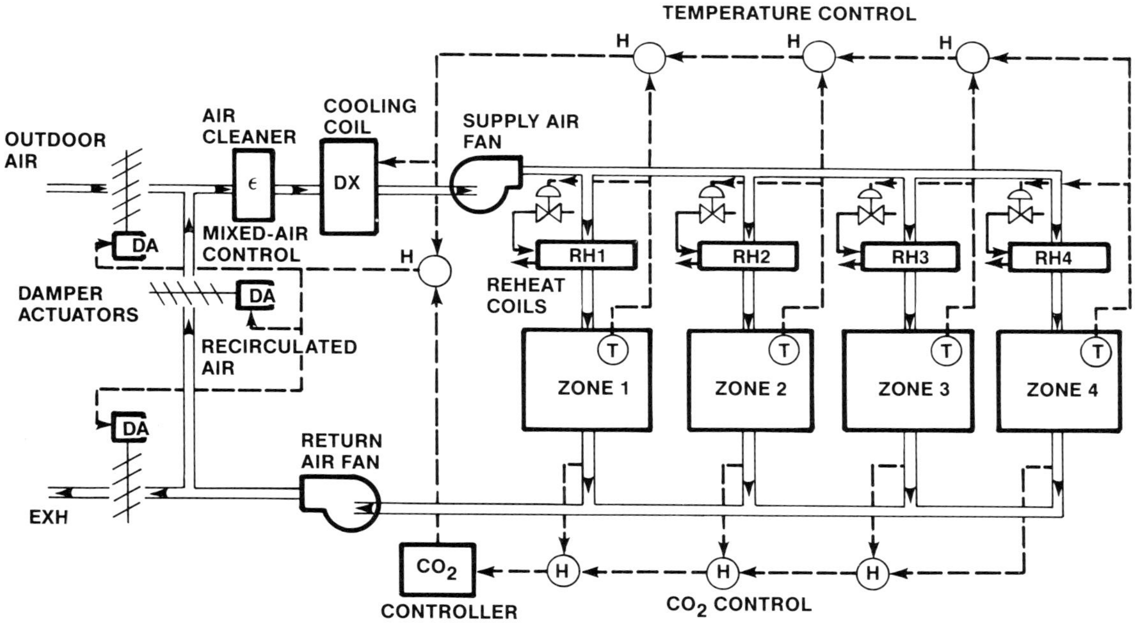


**Figure 6.12.** Schematic representation of $CO_2$ closed-loop variable ventilation control. (After Janssen et al., 1982.)

tions in any zone exceeded the set-point of the controller, the thermal control signal to the dampers was overridden and outdoor air was supplied in proportion to the zonal $CO_2$ concentrations.

## CONCLUSIONS

Indoor air quality depends on the concentration of the physical factors in the enclosed space and directly affects respiratory ventilation and occupant exposure to microorganisms. In a broad sense, control of the indoor environment can be achieved by either open-loop or closed-loop control strategies. Room ventilation is a common method of indirectly (open-loop) controlling indoor air quality by dilution and removal techniques. Sensors and control strategies need to be developed for closed-loop control of indoor air quality before optimization of total environmental control can occur.

Three methods of air quality control can be identified: source control, removal control, and dilution control. Source control can be implemented through isolation, containment, and local exhaust. Removal control via air cleaning devices is usually the only method available when it is necessary to control the environment at concentrations below those of the outdoor air. Dilution control is a means of reducing the concentrations of contaminants in the environment by exchanging the room air with air of less concentration of the contaminant (usually outdoor air). Generally, dilution control is employed in combination with removal control.

Of the three methods, source control is the only way to prevent exposure to a contaminant. With removal and dilution control, exposure to the contaminant is assumed.

The within-room air distribution is just as important as the amount of make-up (outdoor) air provided. Short-circuiting of the air from supply to the return air devices often occurs within a room. Then the supply air, which is required for dilution control, may not effectively ventilate the occupied spaces. The within-room ventilation efficiency is one parameter used to quantify within-room mixing of the make-up air and it must be considered more carefully if cost-effective control of indoor air is to be achieved.

A conclusion that may be reached from this discussion is that systems are capable, today, of providing acceptable indoor air quality in a cost-effective manner if care is taken in controlling the environmental conditions. If rigorous control and system maintenance are employed, acceptable environmental conditions, energy-efficiency, and attractive economic operations are likely results. In the future, as new sensors and methods of control become available, closed-loop optimization of environmental control will become practical.

## REFERENCES

*ASHRAE handbook of fundamentals.* 1985. Atlanta: American Society of Heating, Refrigerating, and Air Conditioning Engineers.

*ASHRAE Standard 90A-1980. Energy conservation in new building design.* 1980. Atlanta: American Society of Heating, Refrigerating, and Air Conditioning Engineers.

*ASHRAE Standard 55-1981. Thermal environmental conditions for human occupancy.* 1981a. Atlanta: American Society of Heating, Refrigerating, and Air Conditioning Engineers.

*ASHRAE Standard 62-1981. Ventilation for acceptable indoor air quality.* 1981b. Atlanta: American Society of Heating, Refrigerating, and Air Conditioning Engineers.

*ASTM Standard E 741-80: Standard practice for measuring air leakage rate by the tracer dilution method.* 1980. Philadelphia: American Society for Testing Materials.

Billington, N. S., and Roberts, B. M. 1982. *Building services engineering.* New York: Pergamon Press.

Constitution of the World Health Organization. 1946. *Official Record of the World Health Organization* 2:100.

DeChiara, J., and Callender, J. 1980. *Time saver standards for building types.* 2d ed. New York: McGraw-Hill.

Douglas, R. W., and Frank, S. 1972. *A history of glassmaking.* Henley-on-Thames, U.K.: G. T. Foulis.

Fanger, P. O. 1973. *Thermal comfort.* New York: McGraw-Hill, p. 15.

Foster, J. M. 1982. *Development of criteria and procedures for solving window design problems.* Master's thesis, Iowa State University, pp. 4–22.

Geerts, J. A.; Grindel, A.; Hardi, W.; and Schiltkencht, H. 1985. Durch luftqualitaetskriterien bestimmte frischluftmenger. *CLIMA 2000,* vol. 4, *Indoor climate,* P. O. Fanger, ed. Copenhagen: VVS Kongres-VVS Messe.

*General standards of construction and equipment for hospital and medical facilities.* 1968. Washington, D.C.: U.S. Public Health Service, Publication No. 930-14-7. Revised February 1969.

*Guidelines for construction and equipment of hospital and medical facilities.* 1984. Rockford, Md.: U.S. Department of Health and Human Services, Public Health Service, Health Resources and Services Administration, Publication No. (HRSA) 84-14500.

Harrje, D. T.; Dutt, G. S.; and Beyea, J. E. 1979. Locating and eliminating obscure but major energy losses in residential housing. Part 2. *ASHRAE Trans.* 85:521–34.

Hesketh, H. E. 1979. *Air pollution control.* Ann Arbor, Mich.: Ann Arbor Science Publishing.

*IES lighting handbook, application volume.* 1981. New York: Illuminating Engineering Society of North America.

*IES lighting handbook, reference volume.* 1981. New York: Illuminating Engineering Society of North America.

Janssen, J. E.; Hill, T. J.; Woods, J. E.; and Maldonado, E.A.B. 1982. Ventilation for control of indoor air quality: A case study. *Environment International.* 8:487–96.

Klauss, A. K.; Tull, R. H.; Roots, L. M.; and Pfafflin, J. R. 1970. History of the changing concepts in ventilation requirements. *ASHRAE Journal* 12(6):51–55.

Leeds, L. W. 1868. Quoted from a letter by Benjamin Franklin to Dr. Ingenhaus, Physician to the Emperor at Vienna. In *Lectures on ventilation at Franklin Institute, 1866–67.* New York: John Wiley and Sons, pp. 8–9.

Luciano, J. R. 1977. *Air contamination control in hospitals.* New York: Plenum Press.

Maldonado, E.A.B., and Woods, J. E. 1983. A method to select locations for indoor air quality sampling. *Building and Environment* 18(4):171–80.

*Minimum requirements of construction and equipment for hospital and medical facilities.* 1974. Rockford, Md.: U.S. Department of Health, Education, and Welfare, Public Health Service, Health Resources Administration, Publication No. (HRA) 74-4000.

Nevins, R. G. 1976. *Air diffusion dynamics.* Birmingham, N.J.: Business News Publishing Company.

Rohles, F. H. 1973. Rational temperature indices of man's thermal environment and their use with a 2-node model of his temperature regulation. *Fed. Proc.* 32(5):1572–82.

Suomi, U. 1985. Controlling the outdoor air intake by the use of contaminant monitoring. *CLIMA 2000,* vol. 4, *Indoor climate,* P. O. Fanger, ed. Copenhagen: VVS Kongres-VVS Messe.

Teng, M. H. 1981. *Control of indoor air quality by use of operable windows.* Master's thesis, Iowa State University.

Warring, R. H. 1970. *Handbook of noise and vibration control.* Morde: U.K. Trade and Technical Press.

Winslow, C.E.A., and Herrington, L. P. 1949. *Temperature and human life.* Princeton, N.J.: Princeton University Press.

Woods, J. E. 1984. Measurement of HVAC system performance. *Ann. Am. Conf. Gov. Ind. Hyg.* 10:77–92.

Woods, J. E.; Braymen, D. T.; Rasmussen, R. W.; Reynolds, G. L.; and Montag, G. M. 1985. Ventilation requirements in hospital operating rooms—Part 1: Control of airborne particles. Part 2. *ASHRAE Trans.* 92:396–424.

Woods, J. E.; Janssen, J. E.; and Krafthefer, B. C. 1986. Rationalization of equivalence between the ventilation rate and air quality procedures in ASHRAE Standard 62. Proceedings of ASHRAE IAQ '86, April 20–23, 1986, Atlanta.

Woods, J. E., and Maldonado, E.A.B. 1982. Development of a field method for assessing indoor air quality in single family residences. *Final report: Development of energy management program for buildings in Iowa—Fourth year.* Vol. 1. Sponsored by the Iowa Energy Policy Council, Des Moines. Iowa State University, ISU-ERI-Ames 82469, May 1982.

# 7

# Ultraviolet Irradiation and Laminar Airflow during Total Joint Replacement

J. DRENNAN LOWELL and SUSAN H. PIERSON

One of the most devastating complications of any surgery is a deep wound infection. Avoiding this complication has been a primary concern of surgeons since the days of Joseph Lister, but the problem has achieved renewed importance with the advent of total joint replacement surgery in the late 1960s and early 1970s.

The difference in outcome between a successful total joint replacement that alleviates the pain and disability of severe arthritis and a joint replacement complicated by wound sepsis is catastrophic for the patient, and monumental in terms of morbidity, mortality, hospitalization costs, and length of admission. Even in cases where deep wound infection may initially be treated with success, late recurrence of sepsis can necessitate removal of the prosthesis with disastrous functional results.

Total joint replacement presents a special problem in relation to wound sepsis since the blood supply to the joint may be poor to begin with secondary to disease or injury, particularly in the knee, ankle, and elbow, and it is further compromised by the surgery. As a result, achieving an adequate bactericidal level of antibiotic in the area may be a difficult task.

Weeks of intravenous antibiotic therapy and staggering costs are uniformly involved in dealing with the problem. Prolonged patient morbidity, and even death secondary to deep wound infection, in total joint replacement patients is not uncommon (D'Ambrosia et al., 1976). Hospital costs for treatment of deep wound sepsis following total hip replacement are estimated, at a minimum, to be $25,000 (Nelson et al., 1980).

Three routes of potential contamination of surgical wounds are generally recognized. The first, and foremost, is direct contamination. This problem was addressed early in the course of surgical history by the implementation of aseptic technique. Eventually, such refinements as disposable gloves, gowns, and drapes were also put into practice. The second route, contamination of wounds via endogenous routes, is often an issue in general and urologic surgery, where the gastrointestinal and genitourinary tracts must frequently be entered, but it is rarely a source of concern in orthopedic surgery, unless through dental manipulation or endotracheal intubation, a transient bacteremia is created. The third potential source, bacteria in the ambient air, is now being recognized as the single most important pathway for contamination in otherwise clean orthopedic surgery. Efforts to reduce this risk have been directed at the performance of efficient surgical procedures which decrease the amount of time the wound is actually open, improvements in the care with which tissues are handled so as to minimize damage to exposed surfaces, and last but most important, modification of the air environment of the surgical suite.

## LAMINAR AIRFLOW SYSTEMS

In the American aerospace industry during the early 1960s, laminar airflow systems, employing high-efficiency particulate air (HEPA) filters, were first introduced. John Charnley of Wrightington, England, was among the first to recognize the problem of bacterially contaminated operating room air and apply these clean air systems to medical practice. He developed a system of ultrafiltered, unidirectional linear airflow within an enclosure, and installed it in his operating theaters in 1961. The system employed multiple air changes per hour designed to cleanse the air within the enclosure of particulate matter and the bacteria that clung to it. This method reduced the number of viable bacterial colonies recovered on settle plates from eighty to zero. As a result, Charnley's incidence of deep wound infection dropped from 8.9 percent to 1.3 percent (Charnley et al., 1969).

Laminar airflow ventilation, as developed by Charnley, is also known as unidirectional flow. It involves the continuous introduction of filtered air at a uniform high velocity through the ceiling or walls of the operating room. The air exits at the opposite wall or floor via an exhaust system situated there. Ideally, laminar airflow systems offer an advantage over conventional operating theaters because they ventilate all areas of the room with air that is free of microorganisms. The air is also cleansed within seconds of any bacteria emitted by operating room personnel or equipment. Unidirectional laminar airflow theoretically prohibits airborne particles from settling onto the wound site or other surfaces because those particles are included in the moving airstream. In practice, laminar airflow wall systems only create laminar airflow for a distance of approximately 3 feet from the filter bank (Nelson et al., 1976). Beyond this point, the airflow becomes turbulent and that turbulence is enhanced when the airflow encounters any obstruction, such as the operating and instrument tables, and the members of the operating room staff themselves. It is conceivable that eddy currents form in the area of air over the operative site. In this case, the eddy currents would bring airborne contaminants from the surgeon's head and neck directly down into the wound. The optimal use of laminar airflow systems requires a complicated surgical procedure in which members of the surgical team wear gowns impervious to bacteria and helmets which are attached to exhaust systems to remove bacteria-laden expired air. Movement within the area of airflow must also be properly designed to minimize turbulence and the eddy effect.

The ability of laminar airflow systems to prevent contamination depends on the efficacy of the gown and the exhaust system (Bentley and Simmonds, 1976). The aspirator apparel is cumbersome and limits mobility. It causes visual distortion, and with the helmets in place, communication between members of the surgical team is often difficult. Though Charnley's results were impressive in terms of reduction of infection, other factors aside from his laminar airflow system should be considered. He continually refined his surgical technique and improved upon the enforcement of aseptic precautions. Many groups report higher infection rates without the use of laminar airflow systems, but others achieve infection rates comparable to Charnley's when unidirectional airflow systems were not in use (Mallison, 1976).

Other disadvantages to the unidirectional airflow systems are the cost of installation and the necessity of moving large volumes of air, which requires large motors, fans, and ducts. This results in high levels of noise and heat generation. In addition, utilization of space by ceiling or wall and floor filter banks and exhaust systems can prohibit the use of such rooms for other types of procedures.

## ULTRAVIOLET LIGHT SYSTEMS

It was Deryl Hart of Duke University who, early in the 1930s, recognized the value of sunlight in eliminating pathogenic bacteria and introduced ultraviolet lighting into the Duke operating suites. During the first five years of its use, the overall infection rate in clean cases dropped from 10 percent to 0.24 percent. The infection rate in orthopedic cases decreased from 16.5 percent to 0.74 percent (Hart, 1960). Overholt and Betts (1940) showed an improvement in postoperative infection rates after thoracoplasty, from 13.8 percent to 2.7 percent, in cases where ultraviolet light was used. The Massachusetts General Hospital reduced wound complications after neurosurgical procedures by approximately 90 percent with the use of ultraviolet light during those surgeries (Wright and Burke, 1969).

Nonetheless, the use of ultraviolet light to limit airborne bacteria was not widely accepted due in part to a study in 1964 by the National Academy of Sciences (Ad Hoc Committee, 1964), which reported only a modest improvement (from 3.8 percent to 2.9 percent) in sepsis rates with the use of ultraviolet lighting. The study has been criticized for procedural inadequacies related to the use of ultraviolet light, such as nonuniform lighting throughout the operating theater. The committee also did not consider the effect of humidity on the bactericidal action of ultraviolet light.

## PROPERTIES OF ULTRAVIOLET LIGHT

Ultraviolet lighting was first introduced into the operating suites at the Peter Bent Brigham and Robert Breck Brigham Hospitals in 1973. The construction of the new Brigham and Women's Hospital in July 1980 consolidated the orthopedic services of both hospitals and ultraviolet lighting was installed at that time in all of the orthopedic operating suites. Ultraviolet lighting is mounted on the ceilings to produce an intensity of irradiation at the operating table level in accordance with Hart's criteria (1960). This level of intensity is equal to 25–30 $\mu W/cm^2$. A wavelength of 2,650 angstroms on the electromagnetic spectrum provides the maximum bactericidal effect of ultraviolet light (Nagy, 1964) (see Figure 7.1). The mercury vapor lamp converts electrical input into the mercury resonance line (2,537 angstroms). Since almost 90 percent of the ultraviolet energy emitted from the bactericidal lamps is on this line, these lamps are highly efficient in destroying all types of viruses and vegetative bacteria. An intensity of 25–30 $\mu W/cm^2$ kills more than 95 percent of the common vegetative pathogens in less than three minutes. Bacterial spores and fungi are somewhat more resistant and require up to twenty minutes of ultraviolet irradiation. *Aspergillus* bacteria are the most resistant, and require sixty minutes of ultraviolet exposure (Hart et al., 1939).

## THE BRIGHAM EXPERIENCE

To establish the effectiveness of ultraviolet light in clearing the air of bacteria in the Brigham operative suites, several experiments were carried out. Nonpathogenic *Escherichia coli* bacteria were nebulized into half of the operating suites equipped with ultraviolet light. A Wells air centrifuge was used for volumetric sampling of air in those rooms, and trypticase soy agar was used as the recovery medium. Samples were obtained with and without the ultraviolet lamps illuminated. In those rooms without ultraviolet light, 930 organisms per 5 cu ft were recovered. In contrast, in rooms where ultraviolet lighting was used, no organisms were recovered. When the nebulizer was used to disperse nonpathogenic *Escherichia coli* into the operating rooms, illumination with ultraviolet light resulted in the removal of 100 percent of the organisms in one room, and 99.7 percent of the organisms in the other. Although a nonpathogenic strain of *E. coli* was used in the experiment, many of the common pathogens such as *Staphylococcus aureus, S. epidermidis, Proteus vulgaris, Pseudomonas aeruginosa, Streptococcus hemolyticus,* and *S. viridans* also

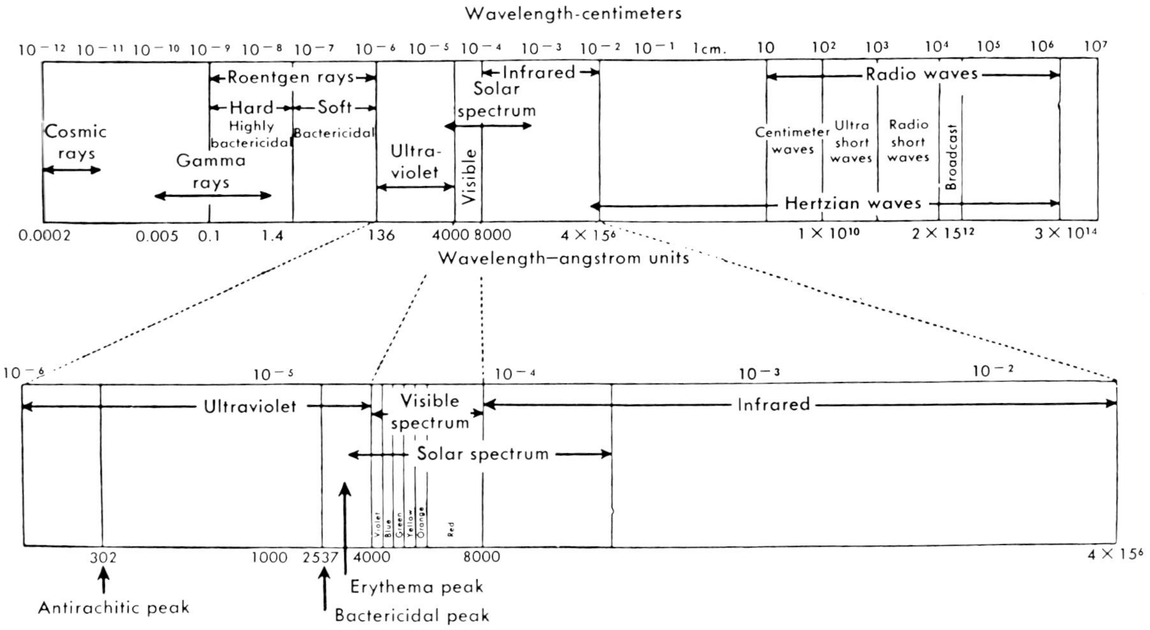


**Figure 7.1.** Ultraviolet portion of electromagnetic spectrum lies between 136 and 4,000 angstroms. (From Walter, C. W., The aseptic treatment of wounds, New York: Macmillan, 1948.)

exhibit the same susceptibility to the ultraviolet light (Lowell and Kundsin, 1977).

Bacteriologic assays of the air in the operating rooms during total hip procedures used fallout plates, volumetric air samples, and Rodac agar contact plates. Four to eight organisms were recovered per sq ft per minute in rooms without ultraviolet light (Figure 7.2). In rooms where ultraviolet light was used, only 0.2 organisms/sq ft/min were recovered, reflecting a 95 percent reduction in colony-forming units on the fallout plates (Figure 7.3).

When volumetric air samples were taken (Figure 7.4), 18–21 viable organisms/5 cu ft were recovered in operating rooms not illuminated by ultraviolet light. Adjacent to the operative wound in those same rooms, 9 organisms/5 cu ft of air were present. When ultraviolet lamps were in use, air samples taken from these rooms showed a maximum of 5 organisms/5 cu ft and many air samples recovered no organisms at all.

**Figure 7.2.** Without ultraviolet light. Bacteriologic assays of the air in operating rooms during total hip procedures using settling plates placed in all corners of the room and on the anesthetist's table show four to eight organisms settling on every square foot of surface per minute during the operation.

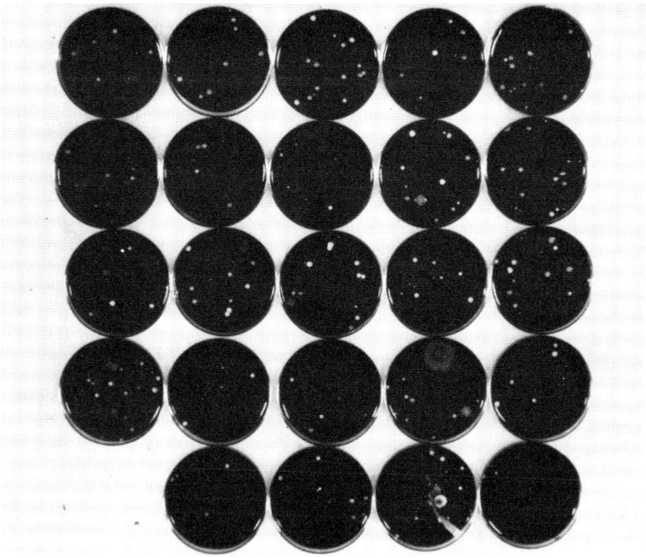

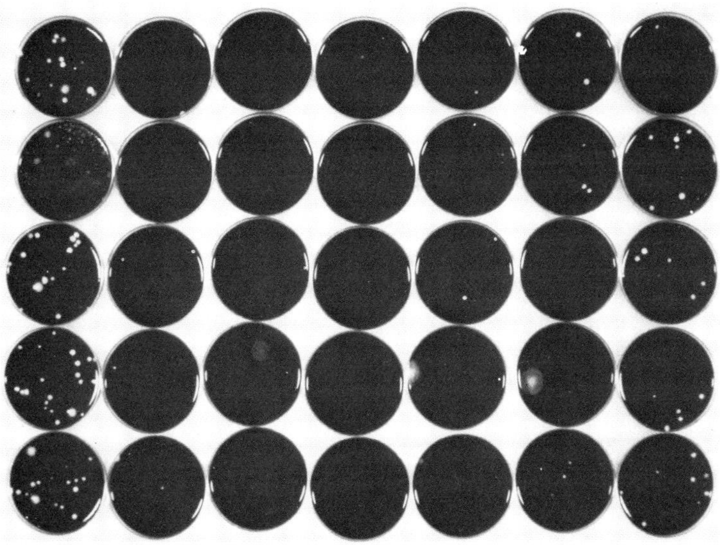

**Figure 7.3.** With ultraviolet light. The ultraviolet lamps were turned on after the patient was prepared and draped, and anesthesia was induced. They remained on for the next four and a half hours during a total hip arthroplasty. The final set of plates, obtained when the patient was transferred from the room and the cleaning of the room was under way, do not show the high counts that occurred during the first hour of surgery when there was greater occupancy. The next-to-last set of plates had fifteen minutes without ultraviolet irradiation.

The Rodac agar contact plates were used to assess the accumulation of viable organisms on such horizontal surfaces as the operating room lights and instrument tables. Bacterial counts at the start of procedures not illuminated by ultraviolet light rose from zero at the start of the surgeries, to 42 viable organisms/25 $cm^2$ by the time the wounds were closed (see Lowell, 1979). With ultraviolet irradiation, agar contact plate counts remained at zero from the beginning to the end of total hip replacement procedures. The floors of the unirradiated rooms contained organisms too numerous to count and included *Pseudomonas*. No viable organisms were recovered from the floors of the operating rooms irradiated with ultraviolet light. Mayo stands, the Bovie apparatus, and the top of the anesthesia cart were all rendered free of microorganisms in rooms where ultraviolet lighting was used.

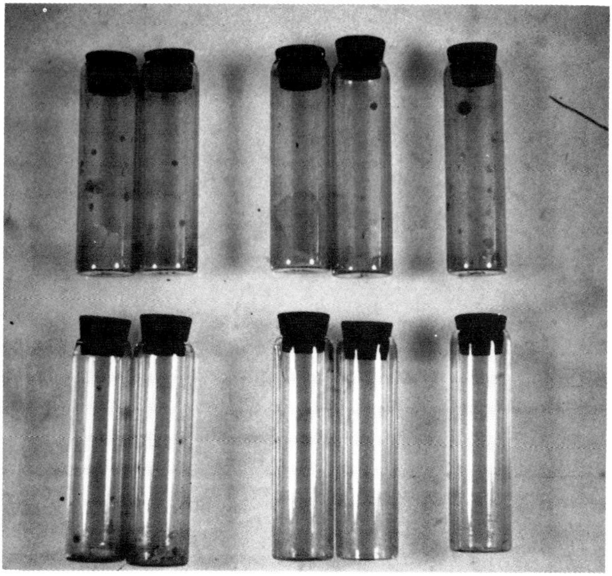

**Figure 7.4.** Volumetric air samples taken at the wound site using a Wells air centrifuge. The top row shows the eighteen to twenty-one organisms per 5 cu ft of air which were recovered in rooms without ultraviolet light. Air samples in the bottom row were taken from rooms irradiated with ultraviolet light. A maximum of 5 organisms per 5 cu ft of air were recovered and some of the samples recovered no organisms at all.

## PROCEDURES AND PRECAUTIONS

Because ultraviolet irradiation is immediately effective in destroying airborne microorganisms, the Brigham and Women's Hospital procedure calls for ultraviolet illumination to begin at the time the incision is made. The lights are turned off after the wound is closed. This protocol simplifies the logistics of bringing the patients into the room, transferring them to the operating table, and inducing anesthesia.

Each room at the Brigham and Women's Hospital is monitored for humidity levels, which are kept below 60 percent. This is done because it has been shown that the effectiveness of ultraviolet light is lost at humidities higher than this level (Figure 7.5). In fact, when the humidity reaches 80–90 percent, the bactericidal properties of ultraviolet irradiation are lost entirely (Dunkin and Puck, 1948). The intensity of ultraviolet irradiation is monitored during each procedure with a portable germicidal photometer, easily operated by nursing personnel within the operating rooms (Figure 7.6).

Additional measures taken at the Brigham and Women's Hospital to contain wound sepsis in the orthopedic department include disposable drapes and gowns impervious to bacteria even while wet, a carefully defined surgical scrub which lasts ten minutes, and the use of perioperative antibiotics. Patients who undergo a total joint arthroplasty at the Brigham and Women's Hospital routinely receive prophylactic antibiotics intravenously immediately before the operation, and for forty-eight hours afterward. Before 1974, oxacillin and streptomycin were given intramuscularly before, and for forty-eight hours after, the operation. Since 1974, first-generation cephalosporins have been the agents of choice. Currently, cephalothin, 1 g every four hours; cephapirin, 1 g every four hours; or cefazolin, 1 g every six hours, is given for forty-eight hours postoperatively (Poss et al., 1984).

**Figure 7.5.** Bactericidal power of ultraviolet radiation drops precipitously when the relative humidity exceeds 60 percent. (From Wells, W. F., Airborne contagion and air hygiene, Cambridge, Mass.: Harvard University Press, 1955.)

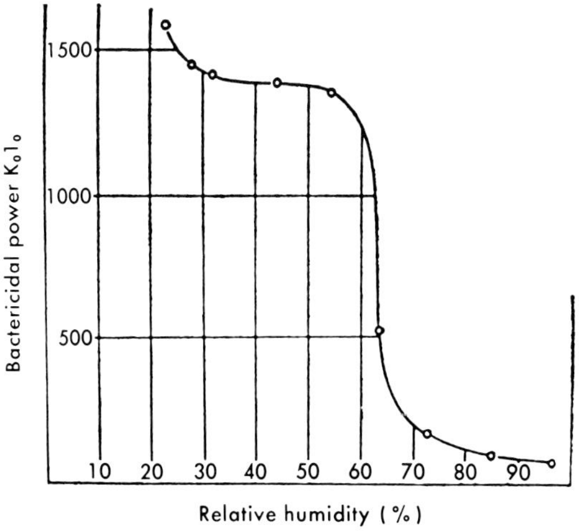

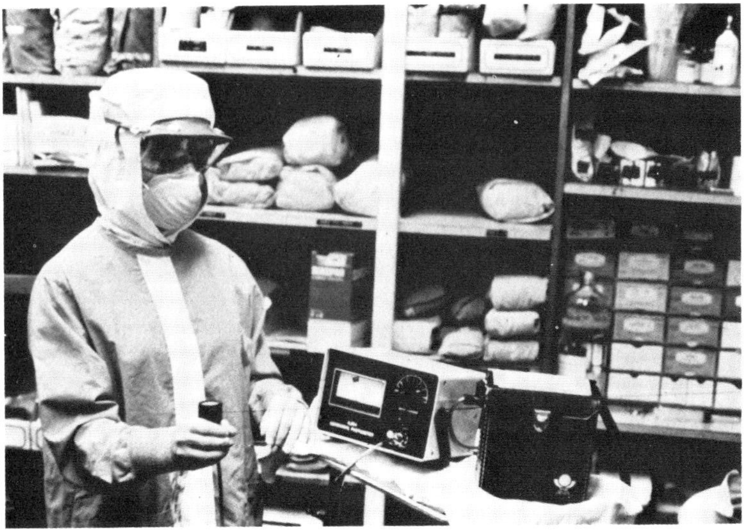

**Figure 7.6.** A photometer (IL254 by International Light, Newburyport, Mass.) is used to monitor the output of the ultraviolet lamps. Operating personnel wear eye shields and hoods, as well as protective creams on any exposed areas.

The risks to operating room personnel as a result of ultraviolet light has been a frequent topic for discussion. Since its inception in 1973 at the Brigham and since the 1930s at Duke University, no incidents of skin malignancy secondary to the use of ultraviolet light has ever been reported. As additional support, it has been shown experimentally that it is impossible to induce skin malignancy in mice using the same wavelength of ultraviolet light (2,357 angstroms) as that used during operative procedures for humans (Rusch et al., 1941). Hart and Sanger (1949) were unable to demonstrate any adverse effect of ultraviolet light on wound healing, and ultraviolet lights were not found to be drying to neural tissues during neurosurgical procedures where the lighting was used (Woodall et al., 1949). Nonetheless, standards at the Brigham and Women's Hospital for operating personnel require the use of eye shields, hoods, and protective creams on exposed skin surfaces while working in rooms illuminated with ultraviolet light.

## RESULTS

Since the 1980 update on septic total joints and the use of ultraviolet light (Lowell et al., 1980), a computerized data base has been implemented to better document the results of all total joint arthroplasties performed at the Brigham and Women's Hospital. This system included both prospective and retrospective components. Since July 1982 when the system was first implemented, data on all total hip and knee joint replacements performed at the hospital have been entered into the data base. The results and complications of those procedures, including deep wound sepsis, have been noted at six months postoperatively, and then at yearly intervals. Total elbow, shoulder, and ankle joint replacements have been followed up separately and future plans allow addition of these joints to the data base. Those total joint replacements performed before July 1982 have been reviewed retrospectively. Current information on joints done before 1982 is also entered prospectively as those patients return for annual follow-up visits. As a result, data are available for this review on all total joint replacements, with a minimum of six months follow up, done prior to December 31, 1985.

Compilation of these data reveals that more than 9,000 total joint arthroplasties were performed at the Brigham and Women's Hospital between 1970 and 1986. Updated data since ultraviolet light has been in use are compared with the preultraviolet experience in the following tables. Only primary total joint arthroplasties that subsequently became infected with deep sepsis were considered in this review. Primary surgeries, for the purposes of this review and in accordance with the total joint replacement registry data base, were defined as those joints without prior prosthetic implants. In some cases, particularly with the total knee replacements, a joint was included as a primary surgery although the joint had in fact been entered on a previous occasion. This situation would occur when a prior soft tissue procedure such as synovectomy or meniscectomy had been performed. However, all joints with prior implants, even when interim girdlestone procedures had been performed, were excluded from this review.

This decision was based on the fact that revision surgeries have an infection rate eight times higher than that of primary arthroplasties

(Poss et al., 1984). In the case of revision surgery, factors other than operating room environment, such as increased operating time in technically difficult procedures where extra dead space and scar tissue are present, and the possibility of occult infection, enter into the septic equation.

Before the installation of ultraviolet lights in 1973, 519 primary total hip replacements were performed. Since the use of ultraviolet light, 3,200 primary total hips have been replaced up to 31 December 1985. See Table 7.1 for the infection rates with and without irradiation.

The deep wound sepsis rate for total knee replacements with and without the use of ultraviolet light follows a similar course. Before 1973, 63 primary total knee replacements were performed. Since the use of ultraviolet light, 3,604 primary total knee arthroplasties have been done. See Table 7.2. When one separates the metal-to-metal hinged total knee arthroplasties from the metal-to-plastic total knee arthroplasties, the infection rate is even less for the majority of total knees done after 1973 (see Table 7.3). Before 1973, 63 primary and 5 revision total knee joints were implanted. Of these, 36 were of the metal-to-plastic design and the remaining thirty-two knees were of the hinged variety (Scott, 1982). Unfortunately, a breakdown of sep-

**Table 7.1** Infection Rates in Primary Total Hip Replacements

| | No. Operations | No. Infections (%) |
|---|---|---|
| Without ultraviolet light | 519 | 11 (2.12) |
| With ultraviolet light | 3,200 | 19 (0.594) |

$\chi^2 = 12.99$.
$p = .0003$.

**Table 7.2** Infection Rates in All Primary Total Knee Replacements

| | No. Operations | No. Infections (%) |
|---|---|---|
| Without ultraviolet light | 63 | 6 (9.52) |
| With ultraviolet light | 3,604 | 31 (0.86) |

$\chi^2 = 46.53$.
$p = .0001$.

**Table 7.3** Infection Rates in Primary Total Knee Replacements

| | No. Operations | No. Infections (%) |
|---|---|---|
| Metal-to-metal total knees (hinges) | 56 | 3 (5.36) |
| Metal-to-plastic total knees | 3,548 | 28 (0.789) |

$\chi^2 = 13.49$.
$p = .0002$.

sis in these two groups in order to compare them with the ultraviolet group is unavailable in our data base.

All of the total shoulder, elbow, and ankle replacements performed at the Brigham and Women's Hospital were done after the implementation of ultraviolet light. Table 7.4 indicates the infection rates between 1973 and 1986.

Table 7.5 evaluates the infection rates in the total number of all joint arthroplasties in the preultraviolet light era and since the use of ultraviolet light.

**Table 7.4** Infection Rates in Primary Total Shoulder, Elbow, and Ankle Replacements

| | No. Operations | No. Infections (%) |
|---|---|---|
| Total shoulder | 326 | 0 (0) |
| Total elbow | 289 | 7 (2.42) |
| Total ankle | 119 | 1 (0.84) |
| Combined | 734 | 8 (1.09) |

$\chi^2 = 8.42$.
$p = <.01$.

**Table 7.5** Infection Rate in Primary Total Joint Arthroplasties

| | No. Operations | No. Infections (%) |
|---|---|---|
| Without ultraviolet light | 582 | 17 (2.92) |
| With ultraviolet light | 7,541 | 58 (0.769) |

$\chi^2 = 27.35$.
$p = <.0001$.

If we compare overall sepsis rates among the total hip and total knee replacements alone and exclude total shoulder, elbow, and ankle arthroplasties, we can note a marked difference with the use of ultraviolet light (see Table 7.6).

When the data are evaluated by year, as in Table 7.7, we can see that for all primary total hip and total knee replacements done since ultraviolet light was instituted, the trend is variable from year to year in terms of rates of sepsis. In 1980, there was a higher than usual rate of sepsis for total hip replacement (2 percent). The reason for this is unclear, though this was the year the new operating suites at the

**Table 7.6** Infection Rate in Primary Total Hip and Knee Replacements

| | No. Operations | No. Infections (%) |
|---|---|---|
| Without ultraviolet light | 582 | 17 (2.92) |
| With ultraviolet light | 6,804 | 50 (0.735) |

$\chi^2 = 28.50$.
$p = <.0001$.

**Table 7.7** Rates of Deep Wound Infection in Primary Total Hip and Knee Replacements

| Year | No. Total Hips | No. Infections (%) | No. Total Knees | No. Infections (%) |
|---|---|---|---|---|
| 1973 | 192 | 3 (1.56) | 82 | 3 (3.45) |
| 1974 | 206 | 0 (0) | 190 | 1 (0.53) |
| 1975 | 190 | 1 (0.53) | 252 | 2 (0.79) |
| 1976 | 194 | 0 (0) | 292 | 3 (1.02) |
| 1977 | 208 | 2 (0.96) | 290 | 1 (0.34) |
| 1978 | 187 | 0 (0) | 314 | 6 (1.91) |
| 1979 | 192 | 1 (0.52) | 303 | 5 (1.65) |
| 1980 | 250 | 5 (2) | 297 | 3 (1.01) |
| 1981 | 311 | 1 (0.32) | 316 | 2 (0.63) |
| 1982 | 319 | 3 (0.94) | 264 | 3 (1.14) |
| 1983 | 302 | 1 (0.33) | 303 | 0 (0) |
| 1984 | 339 | 2 (0.59) | 357 | 2 (0.56) |
| 1985 | 310 | 0 (0) | 339 | 0 (0) |
| Mean | 246 | 1.5 (0.61) | 277 | 2.38 (0.86) |

**Table 7.8** Total Hip Infection Rates

| | No. Total Hips | No. Infections (%) |
|---|---|---|
| Regular operating room | 6,791 | 90 (1.3) |
| Ultrafiltered operating room | 2,754 | 17 (0.6) |
| Ultraviolet operating room | 3,180 | 19 (0.59) |

*From* Lowell, 1980.

Brigham and Women's Hospital were opened. At that time some initial difficulty with humidity and air-conditioning controls occurred as the new building went into operation.

According to a compilation of data in a previous study by Nelson (1977), patients who underwent a total hip procedure in a regular operating room, without ultraviolet light, but with perioperative antibiotics, had a deep wound infection rate higher than in rooms where ultrafiltered laminar airflow was employed ("clean rooms") along with perioperative intravenous antibiotics. In our ultraviolet-irradiated rooms where intravenous antibiotics were also used, the deep wound infection rate in total hips was 0.59 percent. This result compares very favorably with the vastly more expensive laminar airflow results (Table 7.8).

## CONCLUSIONS

The advantage of using ultraviolet light as a means of reducing bacterial contamination in the operating room is seen clearly by both the Brigham Hospital and the Duke University experience. In the follow-up study of more than 7,500 primary total joint arthroplasties since ultraviolet irradiation was introduced, the deep wound sepsis rate has dropped from 2.5 percent before that time, to an overall rate of 0.77 percent. By the end of 1985, the downward trend is statistically very significant and continues since the review in 1980 by Lowell and colleagues. This trend can be attributed to the use of ultraviolet irradiation, though other measures instituted over the years may also have some part to play. Prophylactic antibiotics, improvement in operative technique and efficiency, and changes in the surgical approach to the joint, as is the case with elbow replacements, also have had an impact on the sepsis rate. Overall, ultraviolet light seems to be one of the most consistent variables.

Total hip replacements continue to enjoy lower rates of deep wound sepsis compared with total knee replacements. In part this may be due to the fact that the blood supply to the knee is more tenuous than to the hip and more easily disrupted at surgery. The knee is also a more superficial joint and is more easily involved when wound dehiscence, superficial wound infection, or stitch abscess is present. The operating time is generally longer for knees than for hips, and this is a factor as well.

The sepsis rate for total knee replacements declines even further after the use of ultraviolet light if one excludes the metal-to-metal hinged arthroplasties from the total rate. Unfortunately, the data from the preultraviolet light era which looks separately at the metal-to-metal and metal-to-plastic total knee arthroplasties are not available, but a 1984 study at the Brigham and Women's Hospital (Poss et al., 1984) found the hinged total knee joints to be twenty times more likely to develop deep wound infection than the metal-to-plastic total knee joints. This notable difference is due to several factors other than ultraviolet light, including a metal synovitis which eventually occurs in all metal-to-metal joints and which renders phagocytes incapable of handling any bacteria within the joint.

Of the 582 primary total joint replacements without a history of previous joint invasion done before the use of ultraviolet light, there were 6 early infections. Early infections are those which occur within the first three months following surgery. Late infections occur more than three months postoperatively; 11 occurred in this group. In those total joint arthroplasties done after the use of ultraviolet light, there were 11 early infections and 47 late infections. Assuming early infections are more likely to be related to contamination in the perioperative period, 35 percent of deep wound infections were early infections when ultraviolet light was not used, whereas only 19 percent of infections in the group irradiated by ultraviolet light occurred in the early period. Late infections, some of which occurred as late as nine years postoperatively, are related to the hematogenous spread of infection, and all have occurred in the rheumatoid arthritics, who, in general, are an immunocompromised population.

It is of interest that no progressive downward trend by year is observed in the number of septic complications. One might attribute the decrease in sepsis to more efficient surgical procedures, newer prostheses, or changes in intravenous antibiotics, yet the data do not support that conclusion. Instead, a fairly variable rate of sepsis by year is related to larger groups of patients, longer follow-up studies of those individuals, and changes in surgical technique, such as a move away from the posterior approach at the elbow, which was associated with greater septic complications, to a posterolateral approach. Overall, the lower sepsis rate with the use of ultraviolet light remains fairly stable in comparison with previous studies, and speaks for the importance of continued use of this modality in environmental control.

The financial cost to the Brigham and Women's Hospital for the installation of the ultraviolet equipment in 1973 was approximately $1,500 per room; this included the cost of portable monitoring equipment and the rheostats used to control the lights. This is considerably less than what it would cost to install and operate air filtration systems. In addition, ultraviolet lamps occupy little space and do not interfere with the use of these rooms for cases other than total joint arthroplasty.

To date, only three cases of complications attributed to the use of ultraviolet light have been reported. All three involved conjunctivitis due to improper eye shielding by operating room personnel. No problems have been reported in the patients who have undergone procedures irradiated by ultraviolet light. Although the hazards that accompany the use of ultraviolet light are present, their risks are well defined and their avoidance by the use of appropriate precautions is relatively simple.

In view of the positive experience at the Brigham and Women's Hospital and other centers with the use of ultraviolet light, we recommend irradiation to any institution considering a system to reduce bacterial contamination in the operating room air. Its use in operative areas other than orthopedics needs further investigation, but ultraviolet irradiation appears to be a worthwhile consideration.

## REFERENCES

Ad Hoc Committee of the Committee on Trauma, Division of Medical Sciences, National Academy of Sciences—National Research Council. 1964. Postoperative wound infection: The influence of ultraviolet irradiation of the operating room and various other factors. *Ann. Surg.* (suppl.) 160:1.

Bentley, G., and Simmonds, A. B. 1976. Ultraclean operating theatres versus conventional theatres—a controlled clinical trial. In *Informal papers of a workshop on control of operating room airborne bacteria.* Comm. on Prosthetics Research and Development, Comm. on Prosthetic-Orthotic Education, Assembly of Life Sciences—National Research Council. National Acad. of Sciences, Washington, D.C. November 1976, p. 49.

Charnley, J., and Eftekhar, N. 1969. Postoperative infection in total joint prosthetic replacement arthroplasty of the hip joint with specific reference to the bacterial count of the operating room. *Brit. J. Surg.* 172:1019.

D'Ambrosia, R. D.; Shoji, H.; and Heater, R. 1976. Secondarily infected total joint replacements by hematogenous spread. *J. Bone Joint Surg.* 58A:450.

Dunklin, E. W., and Puck, T. T. 1948. The lethal effect of relative humidity on air borne bacteria. *J. Exper. Med.* 87:87.

Hart, D. 1960. Bactericidal ultraviolet light in the operating room. *JAMA* 172:1019.

Hart, D.; Devine, J. W.; and Martin, D. W. 1939. Bactericidal and fungicidal effect of ultraviolet radiation. *Arch. Surg.* 38:806.

Hart, D., and Sanger, P. W. 1949. Effect of wound healing of bactericidal ultraviolet radiation from a special unit. *Arch. Surg.* 38:797.

Lowell, J. D. 1979. The ultraviolet environment. *Orth. Rev.* 8:111.

Lowell, J. D., and Kundsin, R. B. 1977. Ultraviolet radiation: Its beneficial effect on the operating room environment and the incidence of deep wound infection after total hip and total knee arthroplasty. Am. Acad. Orth. Surgeons Instructional Course Lectures. St. Louis: C. V. Mosby.

Lowell, J. D.; Kundsin, R. B.; Schwartz, C. M.; and Pozin, D. 1980. Ultraviolet radiation and reduction of deep wound infection following hip and knee arthroplasty. *Ann. N.Y. Acad. Sci.* 53:285.

Mallison, G. F. 1976. Unidirectional airflow in hospital operating theatres. In *Informal papers of a workshop on control of operating room airborne bacteria.* Comm. on Prosthetics Research and Development, Comm. on Prosthetic-Orthotic Education, Assembly of Life Sciences—National Research Council. National Acad. of Sciences, Washington, D.C. November 1976, p. 209.

Nagy, R. 1964. Application and measurement of ultraviolet radiation. *Am. Ind. Hyg. Assoc.* 25:274.

Nelson, J. P. 1977. The operating room environment and its influence on deep wound infection. Proceedings of the Fifth Open Scientific Meeting of the Hip Society. St. Louis: C. V. Mosby, p. 129.

———. 1980. Musculoskeletal infection. *Surg. Clin. North Am.* 60:213.

Nelson, C. L.; Gavan, T. L.; and Schwartz, J. 1976. Clean air systems. In *Informal papers of a workshop on control of operating room airborne bacteria.* Comm. on Prosthetics Research and Development, Comm. on Prosthetic-Orthotic Education, Assembly of Life Sciences—National Research Council. National Acad. of Sciences, Washington, D.C. November 1976, p. 228.

Overholt, R. H., and Betts, R. H. 1940. A comparative report on infection on thoracoplasty wounds: Experience with ultraviolet radiation of operating room air. *J. Thor. Surg.* 9:520.

Poss, R. I.; Thomas, W. H.; Thornhill, T. S.; Ewald, F. C.; Batte, N. J.; and Sledge, C. B. 1984. Factors influencing the incidence and outcome of infection following total joint arthroplasty. *Clin. Orth. Rel. Res.* 162:117.

Rusch, H. P.; Kline, B. E.; and Bauman, C. A. 1941. Carcinogenesis by ultraviolet rays with reference to wave length and energy. *Arch. Pathol.* 31:135.

Scott, R. D. 1982. Duopatellar total knee replacement: The Brigham experience. *Orth. Clin. N. Am.* 13:89.

Woodhall, B.; Neill, R. G.; and Dratz, H. M. 1949. Ultraviolet as an adjunct in the control of post-operative neurosurgical infection: Clinical experience 1938–1948. *Ann. Surg.* 129:820.

Wright, R. L., and Burke, J. 1969. Effect of ultraviolet radiation on postoperative neurosurgical sepsis. *J. Neurosurg.* 31:533.

# 8

# Ultraviolet Air Disinfection for Control of Respiratory Contagion

RICHARD L. RILEY

In the early 1940s William F. Wells and his colleagues showed that the spread of measles in school children could be interrupted, under favorable circumstances, by disinfecting the air with ultraviolet light (Wells et al., 1942; Wells, 1955). Subsequent work, although less successful in controlling the spread of disease, led to a better understanding of the problems involved; that is, achieving adequate air disinfection within a given enclosed space, and prevention of airborne infection in the community. We shall deal in turn with both of these problems.

## AIR DISINFECTION WITHIN ENCLOSED SPACE

The goal is to prevent tiny ($<5\ \mu m$) infectious airborne particles (droplet nuclei) originating in the respiratory tract of an infected host from reaching the respiratory tract of a susceptible victim (Riley and O'Grady, 1961; Riley et al., 1962; Wells, 1955). Droplet nuclei have negligible settling tendency, disperse rapidly throughout the air of a room, and are carried wherever currents of air take them. Ultraviolet (UV) radiation in the wavelength range of 254 nm is germicidal for infectious droplet nuclei (Riley, 1972). The percentage of airborne organisms rendered nonviable depends on, among other factors, the intensity of UV radiation, the species of organism, and the relative humidity. Because the germicidal radiation is irritating to skin and eyes, it cannot be permitted to impinge on people in doses above the limit recommended by the National Institute for Occupational Safety and Health (NIOSH, 1972). The UV lighting must be confined, therefore, to the space between the top of people's heads and the ceiling. (Other types of application have been used in hospital and laboratory settings.) For overhead irradiation to disinfect air in the lower part of the room where people breathe, the upper air must be effectively sterilized and the air mixing must be adequate to dilute infectious particles in the lower air with uninfected upper air.

## Susceptibility to UV

Different organisms vary in their susceptibility to UV (Riley et al., 1976; Wells, 1955). To quantify these differences a chamber was designed in which aerosolized organisms were exposed to a known intensity of UV for a known period of time while passing through a narrow slot (Riley and Kaufman, 1972). Comparison of the number of organisms that could be cultured from the air leaving the chamber with the UV lights on and off yielded a quantitative estimate of susceptibility, $Z$, according to a formula proposed by Kethley (1973):

$$Z = \frac{ln\ N_o/N_{uv}}{\mu W \cdot sec \cdot cm^{-2}} \qquad 8.1$$

where

$ln$ = logarithm to the base $e$
$N_o$ = colony count without UV exposure
$N_{uv}$ = colony count with UV exposure
$\mu W \cdot sec \cdot cm^{-2}$ = UV dose.

The units of $Z$ can be understood by analogy with ventilation. Fresh air entering a room washes out stale air in a logarithmic fashion. When the volume of fresh air entering (and mixed air leaving) a room is equal to the volume of the room, one air change is said to have occurred, and 63 percent of the stale air has been washed out. Thirty-seven percent, or $1/e \cdot 100$, remains. Germicidal radiation reduces the concentration of viable airborne organisms in the air in a similar logarithmic fashion. Accordingly, when UV radiation reduces the concentration of viable airborne organisms by 63 percent, one equivalent air change is said to have occurred, and ln $N_o/N_{uv} = 1$. Thus, the value $Z$ is the number of equivalent air changes ($ln\ N_o/N_{uv}$) per given dose of UV ($\mu W \cdot sec \cdot cm^{-2}$). $Z$ can also be defined as the number of equivalent air changes per unit time ($ln\ N_o/N_{uv} \cdot sec^{-1}$) per given intensity, $I$, of UV ($\mu W \cdot cm^{-2}$).

Studies with the exposure chamber showed that *Escherichia coli* and *Serratia marcescens,* which have been used as test organisms because of their relative harmlessness, are highly susceptible to inactivation by UV; virulent *Mycobacterium tuberculosis,* bacille Calmette-Guérin (BCG), and *E. coli* bacteriophage ØX174 are intermediate; and *M. phlei,* phage f2, and the fungi *Aspergillus terreus* and *A. niger* are extremely resistant to inactivation by UV light (see Fig-

**Figure 8.1.** ● = $Z \cdot 10^4$. Susceptibility of aerosolized organisms to inactivation by UV radiation, as determined in exposure chamber. x = Eq AC/hr. Rate of inactivation of aerosolized organisms by overhead irradiation, as determined in a room of 200 sq ft floor area with a 30-watt UV tube ($\Delta K_{L30}$). See later section on effectiveness of UV in rooms.

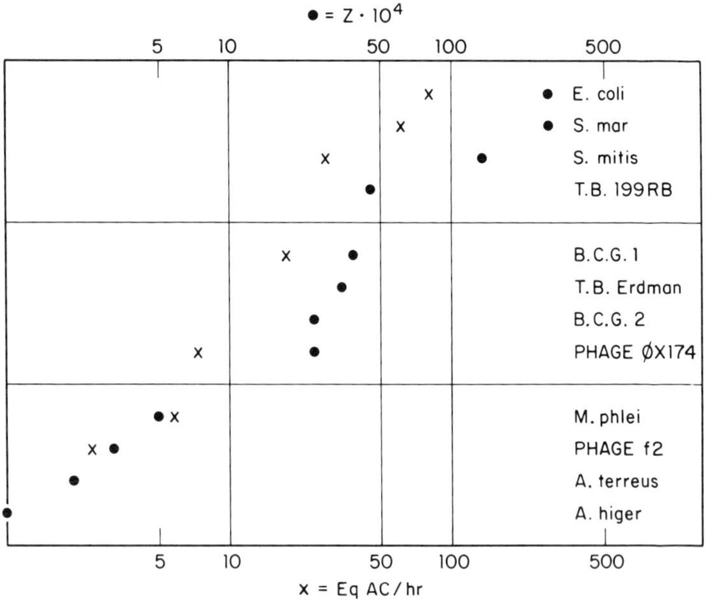

ure 8.1). Unfortunately, the respiratory viruses, such as measles, chickenpox, and the common cold viruses, are not represented because quantitative techniques for enumerating these virus particles were not available. Wells's early success in interrupting the spread of measles in the classroom with overhead UV light leads us to believe that airborne measles virus is at least as susceptible to inactivation with UV light as tubercle bacilli. The susceptibility value, $Z$, depends on many factors, including the age of the culture, the age of the aerosol, the composition of the suspending medium, the particle size, and the relative humidity. However, since the studies were carried out under similar conditions, the $Z$ values provide a useful basis for comparison. At relative humidities above 70 percent, $Z$ values decline precipitously, and UV light cannot be counted on for air disinfection (Riley and Kaufman, 1972).

## Air Mixing Between Upper and Lower Room

In deriving a mathematical expression to deal with air mixing, a number of simplifying assumptions were made (Riley, Permutt, 1971). Air in the upper and lower compartments, respectively, was considered well mixed but the concentration of viable organisms in each compartment could be different. Organisms were assumed to be introduced into the lower air at a constant rate. The boundary between upper and lower compartments was a horizontal plane between the upper irradiated air and the lower unirradiated air. The derived expression was as follows:

$$\frac{1}{\Delta K_{L_w}} = \frac{1}{\dot{V}/V_T}\left(\frac{V_L}{V_T}\right) + \frac{1}{\Delta K_{U_w}}\left(\frac{V_T}{V_U}\right) \qquad 8.2$$

where

$V_T$ = total room volume in cu ft
$V_L$ = volume of lower unirradiated air
$V_U$ = volume of upper irradiated air
$\Delta K_{L_w}$ = added rate of removal of organisms from lower air due to upper air UV, in equivalent air changes per hour (Eq AC/hr)
$\Delta K_{U_w}$ = added rate of removal of organisms from upper air due to UV, in Eq AC/hr
$\Delta K_{U_w}$ = $\ln N_o/N_{uv} \cdot \text{hr}^{-1}$
$\dot{V}/V_T$ = mixing rate between upper and lower air in Eq AC/hr.

A low value for $1/\Delta K_{L_w}$ (high rate of removal of organisms) depends on high values for $\dot{V}/V_T$ and $\Delta K_{U_w}$. Low values for the expressions on the right side of Equation 8.2 also depend on the values for the ratios $V_L/V_T$ and $V_T/V_U$. Good lower air disinfection thus requires good mixing between upper and lower compartments ($\dot{V}/V_T$), a high rate of disinfection of the upper compartment ($\Delta K_{U_w}$), and a large upper air space—the disinfection chamber ($V_U$) (Riley et al., 1971a).

## Calculation of Air Mixing ($\dot{V}/V_T$) and Mean Upper Air UV Intensity ($I$)

It is convenient at this point to combine Equations 8.1 and 8.2 even though this was not done at the time the experimental work was performed. Since

$$\begin{aligned} \ln N_o/N_{uv} \cdot \mathrm{hr}^{-1} &= \Delta K_{U_w} \\ \ln N_o/N_{uv} \cdot \mathrm{sec}^{-1} &= \Delta K_{U_w} \cdot 3{,}600^{-1} \\ \mu\mathrm{W} \cdot \mathrm{cm}^{-2} &= I \end{aligned}$$

substitution in Equation 8.1 yields

$$Z = \frac{\Delta K_{U_w}}{3{,}600\ I}$$

and

$$\Delta K_{U_w} = 3{,}600\ ZI \qquad 8.3$$

Substituting Equation 8.3 in Equation 8.2:

$$\frac{1}{\Delta K_{L_w}} = \frac{1}{\dot{V}/V_T}\left(\frac{V_L}{V_T}\right) + \frac{1}{3{,}600\ ZI}\left(\frac{V_T}{V_U}\right) \qquad 8.4$$

Many experiments were conducted in which the test organism, *S. marcescens,* was atomized into the air of a closed room with a floor area of approximately 200 sq ft (18.6 m$^2$) and a ceiling height of 12 ft (3.7 m) (Riley and Permutt, 1971). The rate of disappearance of viable organisms from the lower air due to fresh air infiltration and natural die-away was first determined with the UV light off ($K_{L_o}$).

This rate was subtracted from the disappearance rate with the UV light on to give the effect attributable to UV light ($\Delta K_{L_w}$). For the studies under consideration the UV tube was suspended from the ceiling in the middle of the room in a fixture that permitted unobstructed radiation above the 7.5-ft (2.29 m) level but cut out radiation below this level. Hence $V_L/V_T$ was 0.62, and $V_T/V_U$ was 2.67. To solve for $\dot{V}/V_T$ and $I$, $\Delta K_{L_w}$ was determined first with a 15-watt UV tube ($\Delta K_{L15}$) and then with a 30-watt tube ($\Delta K_{L30}$) that produced twice the intensity of germicidal radiation. The median results from many experiments carried out in this manner were $\Delta K_{L15} = 40$ Eq AC/hr; $\Delta K_{L30} = 60$ Eq AC/hr. Using these values, one can set up two statements of Equation 8.4:

$$1/40 = 0.62/(\dot{V}/V_T) + 2.67/(3{,}600Z \cdot I_{15}) \qquad 8.5$$

$$1/60 = 0.62/(\dot{V}/V_T) + 2.67/(3{,}600Z \cdot 2I_{15}) \qquad 8.6$$

where

$I_{15}$ = mean upper air UV intensity with 15-watt tube
$2I_{15}$ = mean upper air UV intensity with 30-watt tube

The value of $Z$ for *S. marcescens* ($Z_{SM}$) $= 220 \cdot 10^{-4}$ (Figure 8.1). Subtracting Equation 8.6 from Equation 8.5 yields

$$.0250 - .0167 = .0337/I_{15} - .0337/2I_{15}$$

$$I_{15} = 2.03\ \mu\mathrm{W \cdot cm^{-2}}$$

$$\dot{V}\ /V_T = 74\ \mathrm{AC/hr}$$

## Effectiveness of UV in Rooms ($\Delta K_{L_w}$) Versus Susceptibility to UV in Exposure Chamber ($Z$)

Theoretically, with the same intensity of UV, the rate of killing of organisms in the upper air should be directly related to the $Z$ value. The equivalent air changes in the lower air ($\Delta K_{L_w}$) should be less well correlated because of variations in mixing between upper and lower air. Unfortunately the room experiments were not all conducted with the same intensity of UV light or with the same style of fixture. The experiments with BCG-1 were carried out with a 17-watt UV tube in one case and with tubes totaling 46 watts in two cases. These results have been recalculated for 30 watts, using Equation 8.4 and the value 4.06 $\mu\mathrm{W \cdot cm^{-2}}$ ($2 \cdot I_{15}$) for mean upper air UV intensity ($I_{30}$). Thus, in

Figure 8.1 the x's represent the added equivalent air changes ($\Delta K_{L30}$) brought about by a 30-watt fixture in a room of approximately 200 sq ft (18.6 $m^2$) of floor area in which there was no mechanical ventilation or internal mixing of air other than that occurring naturally by convection. The x's paralleled the exposure chamber data (•'s) as closely as could be expected. The conformity of these two independent sets of experiments confirms the validity of the relative susceptibilities of the different organisms and gives an indication of the quantitative results to be expected from overhead irradiation with UV.

## Fixture Design

Two basic fixture designs are available for upper air irradiation: louvered wall fixtures and fixtures suspended from the ceiling.

Wall fixtures require accurately fabricated louvers that block downward radiation with minimal blockage of horizontal radiation. A carefully made and properly positioned parabolic reflector is also required to project a maximum amount of radiation into the upper air. If, when the fixture is installed, one can see the UV tube or its reflection between the louvers, downward radiation is probably excessive; if this is remedied by changing the angle of the louvers too much, horizontal radiation is blocked and upper air irradiation suffers.

The simplest suspended fixture is essentially an open tube, positioned horizontally and facing upward, with radiation below the horizontal blocked by wings or flanges on the tube holder. These wings extend upward and outward until they reach a horizontal plane not lower than the midline of the tube nor higher than the top of the tube. The fixture gains efficiency by radiating throughout 180 degrees. If there is too much reflection from the ceiling, upward radiation can be blocked by an adjustable strip of metal above the tube.

A third type of fixture with a vertical tube can be used in rooms with very high ceilings ($>12$ ft). The tube passes through holes in the center of disc-shaped louvers. This fixture has the advantage of radiating horizontally throughout all 360 degrees but the disadvantage of requiring accurately positioned louvers to block downward radiation.

Fixtures providing direct radiation or curtains of UV light have been used in hospital and laboratory settings. Protective clothing or strict discipline is required of personnel because the radiation exceeds recommended standards for exposure.

## Guiding Principles for Upper Air Irradiation

As implied by Equations 8.2 and 8.4, the UV fixture should be as low as possible, usually 7 or 7.5 ft above floor level. A high ceiling is desirable because it allows a large upper air disinfection chamber. A ceiling height of 9 ft or higher is desirable, but in many rooms and corridors the ceiling is as low as 8 ft. It then becomes impossible to use fixtures suspended from the ceiling. Wall fixtures, mounted at 7 ft, can be used although they, too, are inefficient when upper air space is limited.

One should aim at maximum UV ray length and equal distribution of radiation throughout the upper air space (Wells, 1944). The longer the UV rays, which project with maximum intensity at right angles to the tube, the greater the opportunity to intercept an infectious particle. Ordinarily, therefore, the fixture should be placed to radiate in the long dimension of the room, avoiding as far as possible such objects as illuminating fixtures, pipes, and ducts. These objects, as well as ceiling tiles, usually are highly reflective of UV light. Since prevailing standards permit only 0.2 $\mu W \cdot cm^{-2}$ of germicidal (254 nm) UV to impinge on people during an eight-hour period, it is essential to monitor a completed installation with a sensitive UV meter and to correct "hot spots" in the lower part of the room (Bromberger-Barnea et al., 1969; NIOSH, 1972). The correction can be accomplished by blocking upward radiation toward the reflecting surface or by reducing the reflectivity of the surface. The former approach is ordinarily more practical, although titanium dioxide-based paint is said to have low reflectance (NIOSH, 1972, Table X.7).

Mixing of air between the upper irradiated zone and the lower occupied zone of a room is facilitated by radiators and other heat sources that cause hot air to rise and displace an equal amount of air downward. Because of the very large area of the horizontal plane dividing upper from lower air, large exchanges can take place, causing air movement that is not noticeable to occupants of the room. In the winter months when the heat is on, convective mixing is ordinarily adequate for purposes of lower air disinfection. In buildings with central air conditioning, optimal mixing is obtained when hot air is introduced close to the floor and cold air through diffusers in the ceiling. If hot air is introduced through diffusers in the ceiling, the buoyant hot air may form a layer near the ceiling, and mixing may be inadequate (Riley et al., 1971b). Fans to supplement convective mixing are then needed. Slowly rotating large-bladed ceiling fans are ideal. If aimed toward the ceiling, they mix the air well without producing drafts in the lower part of the room.

## Wattage Required for UV Fixtures

Two studies bearing on the quantitative requirement for tuberculosis control help in determining the appropriate number, type, and wattage of UV fixtures.

The effectiveness of a single 30-watt louvered wall fixture in a single-bed hospital room was demonstrated at the Veterans Administration Hospital in Baltimore in March 1955 (Riley et al., 1957). Bovine tubercle bacilli were atomized into the ventilating system of a six-room ward which was isolated from the rest of the hospital. Twelve rabbits were placed in one of the rooms, the UV lights were activated, a portable fan was turned on to assure good air mixing, and atomization of culture fluid into the central supply duct began. The rabbits breathed the air with the UV lights on for two hours. Six animals were then removed, the UV lights turned off, and the atomizer restarted. The six remaining rabbits breathed the infected air for three hours. When killed about three weeks later, the six rabbits exposed in the absence of UV all showed infection with tuberculosis. An average of seven tubercles (range four to ten) was present in the five rabbits in which accurate counts could be made. None of the rabbits that breathed irradiated air showed any sign of infection. In this experiment the infected air was introduced through a diffuser in the ceiling so that the organisms were immediately exposed to high-intensity UV, whereas droplet nuclei from a patient would be introduced into the lower room air and would have to disperse to the upper air before being inactivated by UV light. In spite of this consideration, the effectiveness of a single 30-watt UV tube against an organism as resistant to destruction as the tubercle bacillus was impressive.

In 1975 three tests were made with BCG, which has the same $Z$ value as virulent tubercle bacilli (Figure 8.1; see Riley et al., 1976). The organisms were atomized into a room of approximately 200 sq ft of floor area, slightly larger than the single-bed hospital room used in the earlier study. This time mechanical samplers deposited infectious particles on artificial media. On two occasions two germicidal fixtures were used with a total of 46 watts. One of these tests, on a hot, humid day, yielded $\Delta K_{L46} = 19$ Eq AC/hr, and the other, on a cold, dry, windy day, yielded $\Delta K_{L46} = 33$ Eq AC/hr. A third test was performed under moderate, cool weather conditions and made use of a single 17-watt suspended fixture. This test yielded $\Delta K_{L17} = 10$ Eq AC/hr. The large discrepancy between the first two studies shows the importance of weather in an old leaky building. The third test, when recalculated to 46 watts using Equation 8.4, comes to 26 Eq AC/hr. This is halfway between the first two results and can be considered the average value. When recalculated for 30 watts, the average effect in the lower air, $\Delta K_{L30}$, comes to 19.3 Eq AC/hr. This is the equivalent of about four times normal ventilation, added to existing ventilation.

In a room that has a 200-sq-ft floor area, one 30-watt suspended UV fixture adds the equivalent of about 20 AC/hr (by calculation, 19.3); therefore we extrapolate from this finding and recommend, for larger rooms under conditions of normal occupancy, one 30-watt UV fixture for each 200 sq ft of floor area.

Under conditions of exceptional crowding, it is more reasonable to estimate the number of UV fixtures from the number of people to be protected rather than by floor area. The number of people protected by one 30-watt suspended UV fixture can be estimated since, in a room of 2,000 cu ft, 20 AC/hr corresponds to 40,000 cu ft/hr (20 × 2,000) or 667 cu ft/min. A common standard for classroom ventilation is 25 cu ft/min/person, and four times the standard ventilation is 100 cu ft/min/person. If we extrapolate from the findings in the small experimental room and consider that each 30-watt suspended fixture provides the equivalent of 667 cu ft/min, then each fixture adds the equivalent of four times the standard ventilation for six or seven people (667/100). The number of fixtures required can thus be estimated by dividing the number of people by 7. This calculation only applies in large rooms with relatively low ceilings, not exceeding, say, 12–14 ft in height. In auditoriums or large rooms with very high ceilings, upper air UV of given intensity, $I$, is much more effective because of the large upper air space, $V_U$ (see Equation 8.4), and fewer fixtures are needed.*

## Increased True Ventilation Versus Upper Air Irradiation

The choice of UV, as opposed to increasing true ventilation, as a means of ridding room air of infectious organisms is based on quantitative differences. Mass movement of air to flush out organisms becomes uncomfortable and very expensive at rates above 10 AC/hr. Average ventilation is in the 5 AC/hr range. By contrast, a UV fixture installation can render airborne tubercle bacilli nonviable at a rate equivalent to 20 AC/hr, yielding total ventilation equivalent to 25 AC/hr. More sensitive organisms can be eliminated at a still higher rate.

The advantage of UV light over true ventilation is lost in small spaces, such as sputum induction units that may be little bigger than telephone booths. Irradiation is relatively inefficient when ray length is short, and reflected radiation is difficult to control. Conversely, ventilation is more efficient than in larger spaces because unidirectional flow is easily accomplished with exhaust fans.

## Duct Irradiation Versus Upper Air Irradiation

In buildings with central air-conditioning, intense irradiation of air passing through central supply ducts can prevent respiratory organisms from being recirculated throughout the distribution of the system. This is technically easy and relatively inexpensive (Buttolph and Haynes, 1950).

In a measles epidemic in an elementary school with central air-conditioning, the index case produced twenty-eight secondary infections in fourteen different classrooms (Riley et al., 1978). The index case never shared the same room with most of the secondary cases,

*A sophisticated analysis of UV air sanitation, from the engineering point of view, was prepared by Buttolph and Haynes (1950) for the General Electric Company. The bacteriologic side of their studies was weak, as it was based on the effectiveness of UV light against organisms atomized into the air from diluted sputum. They did not study pathogens and had inadequate data on the relative susceptibilities of different organisms. In their sample calculations somewhat less upper air UV is recommended than we would now prescribe to control the spread of tuberculosis.

indicating that the airborne measles virus reached the different rooms through the ventilating system. The amount of recirculation depended on the outdoor temperature and was, for the three-day infectious period of the index case, 0 percent, 60 percent, and 71 percent. Filters removed about 12 percent of particles in the respirable range. Enough airborne virus recirculated to account for twenty-six of the twenty-eight secondary cases. The other two were in the same room as the index case. The use of UV irradiation in central supply ducts would probably have aborted this epidemic. It would not have prevented the infections in the same room as the index case, however, because of the uncontrolled virus produced within the room by the infectious child. Ultraviolet irradiation in central supply ducts would have been more cost-effective than UV fixtures in all the classrooms in this outbreak.

In the study at the Veterans Administration Hospital in Baltimore large guinea pig colonies were exposed in each of two chambers that received air from a tuberculosis ward (Riley et al., 1962). Air going to one chamber was irradiated in the supply duct. Over a two-year period, sixty-three guinea pigs were infected in the chamber that received unirradiated ward air while no animals were infected in the chamber receiving UV irradiated air. Both the hazard of breathing unirradiated ward air and the feasibility of disinfection in ducts were demonstrated.

In an outbreak of tuberculosis aboard the naval vessel *Richard E. Byrd* the ventilating systems serving two large bunking compartments were interconnected (Houk et al., 1968; Riley, 1982). The index case occupied the first compartment. The two groups had very little contact with each other at any time. The second group could only be infected by breathing contaminated air brought in through the interconnecting ducts. The rate of infection in the second group was comparable to that of the first group when dilution of infectious particles was taken into account. Infection of the second group could presumably have been prevented by irradiation of the air in the interconnecting duct.

In view of these experiences, a case can be made for irradiation in supply ducts in all buildings, airplanes, trains, ships, and busses where recirculated air is distributed throughout the system.

In buildings with recirculated air and with special hazards in individual rooms, it may be desirable to irradiate in central supply ducts to prevent diluted but widespread contamination and also in the rooms with special hazards.

When exhaust fans are used to control infectious hazards in small spaces, such as sputum induction booths or laboratory hoods, it may be necessary to disinfect the air in the exhaust duct before discharge to the outdoors. This precaution is needed when dangerous organisms are vented close to intake ducts or windows.

## UV for Prevention of Wound Infections

Surgeons were early in applying UV light to prevent wound infections (Hart, 1936; Overholt and Betts, 1940). Since that time Duke University has had extensive experience with UV lights in operating rooms (Goldner et al., 1980). Since 1973, the Brigham hospitals in Boston (Lowell et al., 1980) have used UV light. The entire operating room, including the operative site, is irradiated intensely with UV (25–30 $\mu W/cm^2$ at tabletop), and relative humidity is kept below 60 percent.

The high-intensity UV light controls organisms settling from the air and arising primarily from people in the operating room (Kundsin, 1980). Protective clothing is required for everyone in the operating room, with special care to protect the eyes from the irritant effects of UV light. When these exacting conditions are fulfilled, wound infections have been significantly reduced, as demonstrated in clean orthopedic operations such as joint replacements (Goldner et al., 1980; Lowell et al., 1980). The use of UV irradiation in operating rooms is dealt with in depth in Chapter 7.

## Calculations

The probability of escaping airborne infection, $P$, is equal to

$$e^{-Iqpt/Q}$$

where

$e$ = base of natural logarithms
$I$ = number of infectors (cases in the infectious stage)
$q$ = quanta (infectious doses) of infectious particles put into the air per unit time per infector

$p$ = pulmonary ventilation per susceptible person per unit time
$t$ = duration of exposure of susceptibles
$Q$ = fresh air ventilation, or equivalent ventilation due to UV, per unit time (Riley et al., 1978).

Increase in $I$, $q$, $p$, or $t$ decreases the probability of escaping infection, and increase in $Q$ increases the probability of escape. If the UV installation causes the equivalent of a five-fold increase in $Q$, the exponent is divided by 5 and the probability of escaping infection correspondingly increased. When, without UV light, the value of the exponent is more negative than $-8$, the effectiveness of the UV installation is overwhelmed, and with values less negative than $-0.3$, the probability of escaping infection is high even without UV light. There is thus a definable range in which overhead the UV fixture can have a significant effect on the transmission of airborne infection.

If exposure to airborne infection takes place in a single room or enclosed space, the number of new cases, $C$, equals the total number of susceptible people exposed, $S$, minus the number of susceptibles escaping infection ($S \cdot P$). Hence,

$$C = S\,(1 - e^{-Iqpt/Q}).$$

The values of all the unknowns except $q$ can be obtained or estimated. It is then possible to calculate $q$ and the resulting concentration of infectious particles in the air (Riley et al., 1978; Riley et al., 1962; Wells, 1955).

Over the four years of the study of a tuberculosis ward at the Veterans Administration Hospital in Baltimore, the average rate of introduction of quanta into the air was only 30/day or 1.25/hr, and the resulting concentration was 1 infectious particle in about 12,000 cu ft of air. By contrast, when a highly infectious patient with laryngeal tuberculosis was on the ward for three days, he produced 60 quanta of airborne tubercle bacilli per hour and during that period the concentration in the air was 1 quantum/200 cu ft of air. In an outbreak reported by Catanzaro, during 150 minutes of bronchoscopy and intubation of a tuberculous patient, 249 infectious airborne units were generated per hour, producing 1 quantum in each 69 cu ft of air (Catanzaro, 1982). In an outbreak in an office building studied by Nardell (1986), an average of 13 particles/hr was produced by the index case during 160 hr (4 weeks total duration), and there was 1 quantum of infection/6,580 cu ft of air. In the measles epidemic referred to earlier the index case produced an average of 93 quanta of airborne measles per minute or 5,480 quanta/hr (Riley et al., 1978). When diluted by ventilation, the concentration was 1 quantum/183 cu ft throughout the entire school. In the home room of the index case the concentration was 1 quantum/8.6 cu ft of air.

## PREVENTION OF AIRBORNE INFECTION IN THE COMMUNITY

A comprehensive discussion of efforts to control respiratory contagion by air disinfection was given by Wells (1955). The early studies had three overlapping objectives: to demonstrate the ability of UV irradiation to limit the spread of airborne infection in individual rooms; to trace channels of infection in the community; and, ultimately, to control the spread of airborne infection in the community. The first two objectives were accomplished; the third failed.

### Early Studies

The most successful study involved day schools in Swarthmore and Germantown, Pennsylvania. Overhead irradiation with UV was begun in 1937 and continued into 1947 (Wells et al., 1942). The level of control that the study achieved is demonstrated by comparison of measles attack rates in irradiated and unirradiated classrooms at the time of a major epidemic in 1941 (Figure 8.2). These particular schools were unusually favorable for a study of childhood diseases because exposures outside of school were minimal. Swarthmore and Germantown were small, well-to-do towns where children were transported to and from school by their parents and were relatively isolated from the community at large. Children's visits in other homes and attendance at parties and measles spread between siblings (home secondaries) were carefully investigated, and the probable locus of disease transmission appropriately allocated. In the absence of UV irradiation, higher attack rates would be expected in the primary classes where the percentage of susceptible children was higher. The opposite finding, when the primary classes were irradiated, is

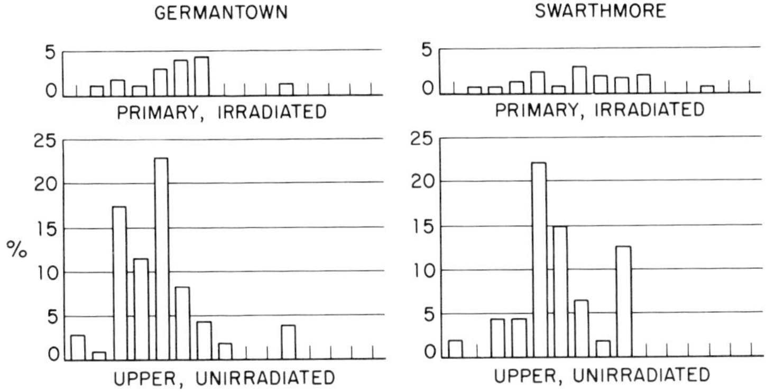


**Figure 8.2.** Measles epidemic, 1941, Germantown and Swarthmore, Pennsylvania. Ordinate: weekly attack rates, in percent of susceptible children (home secondaries excluded). Abscissa: time in weeks, beginning 17 February 1941. Above: primary classes with overhead UV irradiation. Below: upper classes, unirradiated. (After Wells, 1955.)

convincing evidence that air disinfection reduced the spread of measles. To do so, overhead irradiation clearly inactivated airborne measles virus in the classroom.

The New York State Department of Health undertook a study, expected to be comparable, in three large centralized schools in the Syracuse area of upstate New York (Perkins et al., 1947). In 1946 an epidemic of measles swept over the area. The unirradiated Mexico School showed a characteristic sharp outbreak. The irradiated Cato-Meridian School showed an endemic pattern, with infections spread out over time, but the total number of cases was not reduced. If the assumption is made that the slower rate of spread was due to control by UV irradiation in the school, the failure to reduce total numbers suggests that infections were occurring outside of school. Since 97 percent of pupils came to school by bus, the likelihood is that measles continued to spread at a relatively slow rate in the uncontrolled atmospheres of the buses. This was an early example of the way air disinfection of one atmosphere can point to outside channels of infection.

In Westchester County, New York, an attempt was made to demonstrate the feasibility of environmental control of epidemic contagion in a suburban community (Wells and Holla, 1950). In 1946, in the town of Pleasantville, schools, Sunday schools, churches, clubs, the theater, certain stores, and other places where children assembled, were irradiated with UV light. The study was designed to find out how far air disinfection must be extended to control childhood infections in the community. It became, in Wells's words, "a survey of the channels of commerce in contagion, using radiant disinfection of air as a tool of ecological analysis" (Wells, 1955). There was a shift in the places of infection away from the irradiated buildings, but endemic spread continued to occur, fed in part from surrounding communities and by commuters from New York City. The total incidence of childhood contagion was not greatly reduced as compared to Mt. Kisco, a neighboring town that served as control.

In 1954 the Air Hygiene Committee of the Medical Research Council of Great Britain reported on a three-year study in which half the schools in Southall, near London, were irradiated (MRC, 1954). Air disinfection reduced secondary attack rates in irradiated schools, but this effect was overwhelmed by infections acquired out of school. Childhood contagion was not controlled.

A by-product of the early epidemiological studies was the indirect evidence that the viruses of the childhood infections could be inactivated by overhead UV irradiation. This information has not to this day been obtained by direct measurements.

## Current UV Installations

In recent years the spread of airborne tuberculous infection in a government laboratory and in a municipal shelter for the homeless has led to UV installations that give promise of limiting infection among the relatively isolated population groups involved. In both cases, the likelihood of infection outside of the irradiated buildings is minimal, so the pitfalls of earlier community studies can be avoided.

In the government laboratory, fourteen people, previously tuberculin-negative, converted to positive between March and August 1983 (CDC, 1983). Members of the Division of Laboratory Training and Consultation of the Centers for Disease Control (CDC) were invited to investigate. After a careful study of the sixty-four-year-old building, they identified the probable route of infection. Air from a basement laboratory for processing sputum from tuberculosis patients was found to move to the floor above through an inadequately sealed pipe chase. On the floor above, six of sixteen previously tuberculin-negative personnel (37.5 percent) converted to positive. On the second floor above, one of nine previously tuberculin-negative employees (11.1 percent) converted to positive. When tracer particles (dioctylphthalate) were released into the air of the tuberculosis laboratory, they appeared on the floors above, and their concentration decreased from the first to the second floor by almost the same percentage as the decrease in tuberculin converters. The findings pointed strongly to the tuberculosis laboratory as the source of contamination and the pipe chase as the route by which airborne tubercle bacilli gained access to the upper floors. Seven other workers who converted to tuberculin-positive, bringing the total to fourteen, worked in other parts of the building but, with one exception, made visits to the laboratory wing. Several recommendations for improving safety were made by the CDC consultants, including installation of UV fixtures for overhead irradiation. In this case the source of infection and the population at risk were identified and the probability of infection outside the building was minimal. The limited objective of protecting this population from tuberculosis infection seems feasible.

Of 49 cases of tuberculosis appearing in shelters for the homeless in Boston, 22 had organisms that were resistant to isoniazid and streptomycin and were of the same phage type (Nardell et al., 1986). The 22 patients frequented the same large shelter. During fourteen months beginning in January 1984, 16 of 83 staff members showed conversion of the tuberculin test to positive. There were no conversions during a corresponding period before the epidemic. The sudden increase in cases whose organisms had identical characteristics and the sharp increase in tuberculin conversions in the staff members pointed to a highly infectious index case in the shelter. In the winter months as many as 700 homeless are taken into the shelter at night. Since the dormitories have only 350 beds, approximately half the guests are crowded into large ground-floor rooms. Fixtures for overhead irradiation with UV have been installed throughout the ground floor and will be extended to include the dormitories. Prevention of further spread of infection by air disinfection is handicapped by the fact that the guests sometimes stay in other shelters.

Furthermore, the intense crowding in the ground-floor rooms makes interruption of airborne transmission difficult. Results will be evaluated over a period of years by the rate of tuberculin conversion in the staff and by the number of cases with identical organisms occurring among the guests.

## Airborne Infection in Medical Facilities

The effect of tight buildings and recirculated air is occasionally documented when childhood diseases are transmitted in pediatricians' offices. In 1981 a twelve-year-old child with measles infected seven others (Bloch et al., 1985). Three of these were never in the same room as the source case, and one entered the office an hour after the source case had left. In a similar episode in 1982, three children, who arrived in a pediatrician's office sixty to seventy-five minutes after a child with measles had left, developed measles (Remington et al., 1985). In such offices, air disinfection should include both duct irradiation to eliminate recirculation of viable virus and overhead irradiation to protect children sharing the same room with an infectious case.

In a hospital outbreak of chickenpox (varicella) in 1980, eight children on a ward were infected even though the index case was under strict room isolation (Gustafson et al., 1982). Studies with a tracer gas ($SF_6$) showed that the isolation room, which was supposed to be under negative pressure with respect to the adjoining corridor, was in fact under positive pressure. Escaping airborne virus infected children in nearby rooms. The wayward movement of invisible airborne particles provides a strong argument for UV air disinfection in facilities housing infectious patients.

Recent developments have increased the need for air disinfection in hospitals. Patients who have acquired immune deficiency syndrome (AIDS) or are receiving immunosuppressive drugs have increased in number. They present a twofold hazard: they are exceptionally susceptible to infection, and, once infected, their inability to restrain the growth of the infecting organism makes them exceptionally infectious to others. Thus, both to prevent respiratory infection in these patients and to prevent transmission from them to others, disinfection of the air is needed. Also, the increased use of procedures involving the respiratory tract, such as bronchoscopy, tracheal suctioning, and stimulation of cough, add to the hazard of infection in hospitals because these procedures contaminate the air with respiratory organisms (Catanzaro, 1982).

## CONCLUSION

Occupants of a building can be given incomplete but significant protection from respiratory infection by UV air disinfection provided that (1) exposure to infection occurs predominantly in this building; (2) the ceilings are high enough to permit overhead irradiation with UV light; (3) the relative humidity in the building is less than 70 percent; and (4) the rate at which airborne pathogens are produced is not overwhelming. There is a particular need for air disinfection in medical facilities, shelters for the homeless, and other places housing sources of airborne infection. The construction of tighter buildings and the rising use of recirculation systems have exacerbated the problem of airborne infection and stepped up the need for control measures.

## APPENDIX

## INSTRUCTIONS FOR UV AIR DISINFECTION

### Consultant

Advice from a consultant is needed on two occasions when installing UV air disinfection. At the first visit detailed specifications and instructions for mounting each fixture should be provided, including type of fixture, number of fixtures, wattage, height from floor, and orientation. The exact position of each fixture should be indicated on a floor plan or sketch, and masking tape should be placed on the wall or ceiling to indicate how each fixture should be mounted.

An acceptance visit should be made by the consultant when the installation is completed. Adequacy of upper air irradiation and compliance with standards for exposure of people in the lower air should be confirmed by UV meter readings. If UV radiation in the lower air is excessive, the consultant should provide instructions for corrective measures.

## Supplier

Each fixture must have a "caution" label dealing with the hazard of direct exposure to UV radiation. The supplier should attach a label to each fixture indicating the UV tube identification number, the transformer specifications, the wattage at which the tube is operated, and the rated life of the tube. Space on the label should be left for "date turned on" and "replacement date."

## Installer

1. Mount fixtures as indicated by masking tape on wall or ceiling and by detailed instructions supplied by consultant.
2. Put UV tubes on circuits that are not connected with lighting circuits.
3. Do not install wall switches for UV tubes. They can be turned on and off using switches on the fixtures.
4. Leave 6 to 12 inches of slack in electric cord and suspending chains.
5. Never look at, or expose skin to, a UV source at close range.
6. Turn off UV tube before examining it for any purpose.

## Maintenance Personnel

1. Record "date turned on" and "replacement date" on labels on each UV fixture.
2. Leave UV tubes on continuously, day and night.
3. Turn off UV tube and inspect after one month. If outside of tube appears dusty, clean with a damp cloth. If tube appears clean, inspect again after three months. Required frequency of cleaning depends on the dustiness of the environment.
4. Replace UV tube and record new dates on label if an extensive deposit of mercury appears on inside of tube or if tube burns out or develops a pronounced flicker.
5. Change UV tubes at end of rated life, as indicated by "replacement date" on label.
6. Turn off UV tubes before examining for any purpose.

## UV Tubes in Air Ducts

Irradiation inside air ducts presents no hazard to the occupants of rooms and can therefore be as intense as is needed to kill organisms causing respiratory infection. Open, unshielded tubes should be installed in a straight section of duct. If duct is large enough, install tubes transversely so that they radiate a maximum distance in both directions in the duct. Safety devices should be installed to prevent maintenance personnel from opening access doors when tubes are on.

## REFERENCES

Bloch, A. B., W. A. Orenstein, W. M. Ewing, W. H. Spain, G. F. Mallison, K. L. Herrmann, and A. R. Hinman. 1985. Measles outbreak in a pediatric practice: Airborne transmission in an office setting. *Pediatrics* 75: 676–83.

Bromberger-Barnea, B., H. N. Bane, and R. L. Riley. 1969. A wide range ultraviolet exposure meter. *Am. Rev. Respiratory Disease* 99:279–81.

Buttolph, L. J., and H. Haynes. 1950. *Ultraviolet air sanitation.* LD-11. General Electric Engineering Division, Lamp Department, Cleveland.

Catanzaro, A. 1982. Nosocomial tuberculosis. *Am. Rev. Respiratory Disease* 125:559–62.

Centers for Disease Control (CDC). 1983. Report of consultative visit. Division of Laboratory Training and Consultation, Laboratory Program Office, Atlanta.

Goldner, J. L., M. Moggio, S. F. Beissinger, and D. E. McCollum. 1980. Ultraviolet light for the control of airborne bacteria in the operating room. In *Airborne contagion. Ann. N.Y. Acad. Sci.* 353:271–84.

Gustafson, T. L., G. B. Lavely, E. R. Brawner, R. H. Hutcheson, P. F. Wright, and W. Schaffner. 1982. An outbreak of airborne nosocomial varicella. *Pediatrics* 70:550–56.

Hart, D. 1936. Sterilization of the air in the operating room by special bactericidal radiant energy. *J. Thoracic Surg.* 6:45.

Houk, V. N., D. C. Kent, J. H. Baker, and K. Sorensen. 1968. The epidemiology of tuberculosis infection in a closed environment. *Archives of Environmental Health* 16:26.

Kethley, T. W. 1973. Feasibility study of germicidal UV lamps for air disinfection in simulated patient care rooms. Presented at American Public Health Association, Section of Environment, San Francisco, November 1973.

Kundsin, R. B. 1980. Documentation of airborne infection during surgery. In *Airborne contagion. Ann. N.Y. Acad. Sci.* 353:255–61.

Lowell, J. D., R. B. Kundsin, C. M. Schwartz, and D. Pozin. 1980. Ultraviolet radiation and reduction of deep wound infection following hip and knee arthroplasty. In *Airborne contagion. Ann. N.Y. Acad. Sci.* 353:285–93.

Medical Research Council (MRC). 1954. Air disinfection with ultraviolet irradiation: Its effect on illness among school children. Air Hygiene Committee. Special Report Series, no. 283. London: H.M. Stationery Office.

Nardell, E. A. 1986. Personal communication.

Nardell, E., B. McInnis, and B. Thomas. 1986. Exogenous reinfection with tuberculosis in a shelter for the homeless. *N. Engl. J. Med.* 315:1570–75.

National Institute for Occupational Safety and Health (NIOSH). 1972. *Occupational exposure to ultraviolet radiation.* Washington, D.C.: Government Printing Office.

Overholt, R. H., and R. H. Betts. 1940. A comparative report on infections of thoracoplasty wounds. *J. Thoracic Surg.* 9:520.

Perkins, J. E., A. M. Bahlke, and H. F. Silverman. 1947. Effect of ultraviolet irradiation of classrooms on the spread of measles in large rural central school. *Am. J. Public Health* 37:529–37.

Remington, P. L., W. M. Hall, I. H. Davis, A. Herald, and R. A. Gunn. 1985. Airborne transmission of measles in a physician's office. *JAMA* 253:1574–77.

Riley, E. C., G. Murphy, and R. L. Riley. 1978. Airborne spread of measles in a suburban elementary school. *Am. J. Epidemiology* 107:421–32.

Riley, R. L. 1972. Principles of UV air disinfection. Public Health Service, 00-2215. Reprinted by U.S. Department of Health, Education, and Welfare.

———. 1982. Disease transmission and contagion control. Koch Centennial Supplement. *Am. Rev. Respiratory Disease* 125(3, Part 2): 16–19.

Riley, R. L., and J. E. Kaufman. 1972. Effect of relative humidity on the inactivation of airborne Serratia marcescens by ultraviolet radiation. *Appl. Microbiology* 23:1113–20.

Riley, R. L., M. Knight, and G. Middlebrook. 1976. Ultraviolet susceptibility of B.C.G. and virulent tubercle bacilli. *Am. Rev. Respiratory Disease* 113:413–18.

Riley, R. L., C. C. Mills, F. O'Grady, L. U. Sultan, F. Wittestadt, and D. N. Shivpuri. 1962. Infectiousness of air from a tuberculosis ward: Ultraviolet irradiation of infected air; comparative infectiousness of different patients. *Am. Rev. Respiratory Disease* 85:511–25.

Riley, R. L., and F. O'Grady. 1961. *Airborne infection—transmission and control.* New York: Macmillan.

Riley, R. L., and S. Permutt. 1971. Room air disinfection by ultraviolet irradiation of upper air: Air mixing and germicidal effectiveness. *Arch. Environmental Health* 22:208–19.

Riley, R. L., S. Permutt, and J. E. Kaufman. 1971a. Convection, air mixing and ultraviolet air disinfection in rooms. *Arch. Environmental Health* 22:200–207.

———. 1971b. Room air disinfection by ultraviolet irradiation of upper air: Further analysis of convective air exchange. *Arch. Environmental Health* 23:35–39.

Riley, R. L., W. F. Wells, C. C. Mills, W. Nyka, and R. L. McLean. 1957. Air hygiene in tuberculosis: Quantitative studies of infectivity and control in a pilot ward. *Am. Rev. Tuberculosis and Pulmonary Disease* 75:420–31.

Wells, M. W., and W. A. Holla. 1950. Ventilation in flow of measles and chickenpox through community. Progress report, Jan. 1, 1946, to June 15, 1949. Airborne Infection Study, Westchester County Department of Health. *JAMA* 142:1337–44.

Wells, W. F. 1944. Ray length in sanitary ventilation by bacteriocidal irradiation of air. *Journal of the Franklin Institute* 238:185–93.

———. 1955. *Airborne contagion and air hygiene.* Cambridge: Harvard University Press.

Wells, W. F., M. W. Wells, and T. S. Wilder. 1942. The environmental control of epidemic contagion. I. An epidemiologic study of radiant disinfection of air in day schools. *Am. J. Hygiene* 35:97–121.

# 9

# Aspergillosis and Construction

ANDREW J. STREIFEL

Continuous advances in utilities such as communication and energy-efficient technology require updating of building services. Building managers must consider cost-effective construction to retrofit or replace existing buildings to accommodate this modern technology. Construction-related indoor mold aerosol pollution can create unhealthy conditions for sensitive individuals. The sources of indoor mold aerosols can originate from outdoor or indoor activity, which causes the disturbance of settled spores or the disruption of a locus of growth. The release of the indoor spore aerosols may be caused by activities ranging from construction to cleaning. Outdoor sources of indoor mold aerosols depend on proximity to such activities as construction or lawn mowing and the status of building penetrations by aerosolized mold and/or weather conditions. The source of an aerosol problem must be recognized and eliminated to protect the health and safety of the building occupants. Mold spores are common in air and are routinely breathed (Gregory, 1973). The presence of certain molds can cause hypersensitive reactions or infections in susceptible individuals (Solley and Hyatt, 1980). Detection and eradication of the indoor sources of mold aerosols requires environmental testing that uses air and surface microbial sampling methods.

The mechanisms for eliminating aerosols are not always obvious. Safety measures instituted to protect bone marrow transplant patients from nosocomial mycosis at the University of Minnesota during indoor and outdoor construction projects will be described in this chapter along with experiences at other institutions with similar concerns.

Indoor aerosols of microbes were described by Greene and colleagues (1962a and b). These studies described the relationship of normal hospital activities (cleaning, bed making, etc.) to microbial contamination levels in hospital air. Mold was recovered during air sampling and ranged from 5 to 43 percent of the total microorganisms collected at different locations in the University of Minnesota Hospital. Identification and the recovery frequency of airborne mold genus/species were not described in that study. Ambient conditions in the hospital building during 1962 required open window ventilation for comfort control. The study demonstrated that normal activity can affect mold air quality.

## HEALTH PROBLEMS ASSOCIATED WITH MOLD IN AIR

Nosocomial aspergillosis infections have been described in many institutions and continue to be a serious infection problem in certain patient groups (Aisner et al., 1976; Arnow et al., 1978; Gerson et al., 1984; Krasinski et al., 1985; Peterson et al., 1983; Sarubbi et al., 1982). Airborne molds that infect hospital patients are generally in the genus *Aspergillus.* The *Aspergillus* species most often associated with patient disease are *A. fumigatus* and *A. flavus.* The group of patients most susceptible to the airborne molds are patients with hematologic malignancies and bone marrow and organ transplants. Mycosis caused by filamentous fungi (mold) are extremely difficult to eradicate once the microbe has initiated mycelial proliferation in the patient's lung (Peterson et al., 1983).

Solomon and co-workers (1978), during a year-long indoor air sampling project at the University of Michigan clinical center, demonstrated air concentration variation of airborne *A. fumigatus.* Air concentrations of *A. fumigatus* were consistently less indoors than outdoors. However, on one sample day in January 1976, the indoor sample exceeded the outdoor sample. No explanation was given for this irregularity. During sampling in 1963 Noble and Clayton in England found a maximum of 2,400 colony-forming units (CFU)/m$^3$ of *A. fumigatus* in a hospital environment. This is the highest number of viable airbourne *A. fumigatus* reported in a hospital environment. Outdoor/indoor concentrations were not compared on that day. Wool blankets were found to be a source of *A. fumigatus.* However, high concentrations of aerosolized fungi were not observed during "blanket sweep" volumetric air sampling. Neither of these studies identified a source for these "unusual" indoor aerosols. The investigators recognized the serious nature of *A. fumigatus* in a hospital environment but they did not enlighten readers on how to prevent the generation/dissemination of the fungi. Nosocomial mycosis usually has been investigated retrospectively (Arnow et al., 1978; Krasinski et al., 1985; Lentino et al., 1982); hence difficulty exists when trying to "see" the reality of microbial aerosol generation. Bursts of aerosolized fungi can be evaluated if the air samples are taken during an aerosol event. Appropriate sampling methods are essential to assess an activity-related mold aerosol accurately. Basic microbiologic techniques are necessary for culture and genus level identification of the fungi recovered during air sampling evaluations.

## SAMPLING METHODS

Air sampling is not a means to control aerosols. Microbial air sampling can be instructive for determining the effectiveness of control measures instituted for minimizing dissemination of viable particles. Appropriate microbiologic techniques and the timing of the sample collection is essential for obtaining meaningful mold aerosol data. The association of nosocomial fungal disease and hospital construction has been described at several institutions (Aisner et al., 1976; Arnow et al., 1978; Krasinski et al., 1985; Lentino et al., 1982; Opal et al., 1986; Sarubbi et al., 1982). Investigators generally utilized limited air sampling resources to investigate the sources of the implicated airborne mold. Air sampling with settle plates is commonly used to determine fungal air quality because they are convenient. Utilizing the settle plate assumes that all air particles will settle at the same rate. The results of settle plate data are not quantitative. A single spore of *A. fumigatus* has been observed to settle at a terminal velocity of 0.03 cm/sec while larger particles, such as *Cladosporium,* settle at 0.3 cm/sec (Gregory, 1973). It can be assumed that settle plate data are biased to show primarily the larger particles rather than the buoyant smaller *Aspergillus*-sized spores which are approximately 2–4 $\mu$ in diameter.

Volumetric sampling utilizing a sieve cascade (Andersen, Atlanta) or slit impactor (Casella, London) and a selective growth media will provide the most meaningful sampling data when evaluating indoor mold air pollution. The inertial impaction of the particles on the growth media will arrest the majority of viable airborne particles pulled into the air sampler. Volumetric samplers have been used during aspergillosis investigations; however, air sampling is often retrospective to the implicated construction projects (Arnow et al., 1978; Lentino, 1982). Arnow and workers in 1978 detected a concentration of $>200$ CFU/$m^3$ of airborne *Aspergillus* and *Penicillium* species incubated at 37 °C (98.6 °F). The contaminated samples were taken after renovation directly below the construction site. Areas above and without the renovation had fungal concentrations generally $<70$ CFU/$m^3$. Arnow and colleagues postulated that settled dust and disturbance of ceiling tile were the source of the infection-causing contamination. They implied that dirt tracked in from the renovation was being disseminated throughout the hospital and may have been the source of the pathogenic fungi. The actual air sampling evaluated residual construction debris left over from the renovation rather than the actual aerosol experienced during that project. During a bathroom demolition in the University of Minnesota Hospital, air concentrations of airborne fungi (incubated at 37 °C) were found to be approximately $10^4/m^3$ (Streifel, 1987).

Low-volume samplers at 0.028 $m^3$/min (1 cu ft/min or $ft^3$/min) are essential for sampling in areas with expected high concentrations of airborne mold or if samples are incubated at room temperature. Higher incubation temperatures ($\geq$ 37 °C) are a selective means for determining fungal pathogens in air (Booth, 1971). The room temperature-incubated organisms exceed the 37 °C organisms by as much as 1 $\log_{10}$ depending on local activity and season. The increased numbers of recovered fungi may obscure the airborne pathogens if incubation is at room temperature. However, for indoor sampling in a highly filtered area or if the incubation temperature is $\geq$ 37 °C higher volumes ($>1$ cubic meter or $>1.0$ $m^3$) of air should be sampled in order to assure sufficient sample air volume. If a low-volume sampler is used for 10 min at 1 cu ft/min the likelihood of detecting 1 CFU/$m^3$ of *A. fumigatus* is diminished because there are

35.4 cu ft/m$^3$. Airborne mold content should be evaluated by utilizing various sample volumes to obtain a meaningful sample. Also, utilizing different incubation temperatures, room temperature and 37 °C, in a sampling protocol will provide a better overview of the total spore burden in ambient air. Reference samples should be obtained from outdoors and/or other areas not affected by the construction.

During active demolition of previously water-soaked areas, considerable viable/nonviable aerosols could be generated. Sampling with a low-volume multistage sieve impactor will separate different-sized particles and provide distinction of fungal types according to spore sizes. Identification of air samples is easier when samples have $<50$ CFU/100 × 15 mm plate. With a 400-hole sieve impactor air microbial concentrations from 19 to 400 CFU/plate are adjustable for multiple impaction using a positive hole correction (Andersen, 1958). This adjustment allows investigators to sample in areas with relatively high air concentrations. At high concentrations the differentiation of the colony types becomes tedious and incomplete because of multicolony growth at the impact points.

High-volume slit or sieve samplers are ideal in areas where low air concentrations are expected. When $>150$ CFUs are recovered on a 150 × 15 plate, the plates are difficult to evaluate. Care must be taken when using slit samplers because no statistical correction exists for a slit sampler. Sampling during construction is more difficult unless a variety of air sampling equipment is available. Variation of sample times allows for a bracketing of sample air volumes in order to collect a workable air sample. Volumetric air samplers offer a means to evaluate qualitative/quantitative parameters of viable air particles during indoor/outdoor construction projects. It is more important to develop consistent methods/protocols for controlling construction aerosols rather than air sampling protocols to evaluate the situations.

## OUTDOOR CONSTRUCTION

The location of construction projects either indoors or outdoors determines the specific methods needed for controlling the hazardous aerosols. Outside construction projects have been implicated in outbreaks of nosocomial infections caused by airborne fungi (Lentino et al., 1982; Sarubbi et al., 1982). Lentino and colleagues (1982) retrospectively found an outbreak of aspergillosis in renal transplant patients in a veterans hospital which occurred during a period of road and building construction. Environmental air sampling using volumetric samplers did not recover pathogens from the hospital air. The infectious agents *A. flavus* and *A. fumigatus* were recovered from dust in window air conditioners in patients' rooms. It was never determined whether the fungi were deposited in the air conditioner during construction and subsequently dislodged during maintenance or whether the mold grew and was dispersed into the patient room when the air conditioner was in use. The correlation between infection and construction was demonstrated retrospectively when the clinical isolates were found to increase during the construction period. Air sample data were not collected during construction; thus a concentration of airborne pathogens was never determined. Sarubbi and co-workers (1982) also described an increase of *A. flavus* clinical isolates during an outside construction project. These investigators evaluated airborne pathogen recovery rate differences using settle plate sampling at several hospital locations. Comparisons of areas in new and old buildings were made in the study. Various defects were noted in the air filtration system in the area with the greatest nosocomial infection problem. This evaluation demonstrated distinct differences in fungal air quality between the respective areas. An air concentration for fungi was never determined during the construction period. This experience should reinforce the importance of air handling system integrity/maintenance for providing basic protective measures.

Viable fungal spores are likely to be rafting on fast settling particles ($>10\ \mu$) or floating as small-sized spores in local air currents (Gregory, 1973). The smaller buoyant particles ($<5\ \mu$) are more likely to cause infection when they are breathed by sensitive individuals and deposited in the lung alveoli. The air concentration of fungi which causes infection has not been established. Infection-causing factors depend on individual immune system competence when the spores are breathed. A single spore could theoretically cause an infection in a compromised host. Therefore, any event that would increase airborne fungal content in the vicinity of sensitive individuals could be problematic. Obviously, it is important to recognize the events that

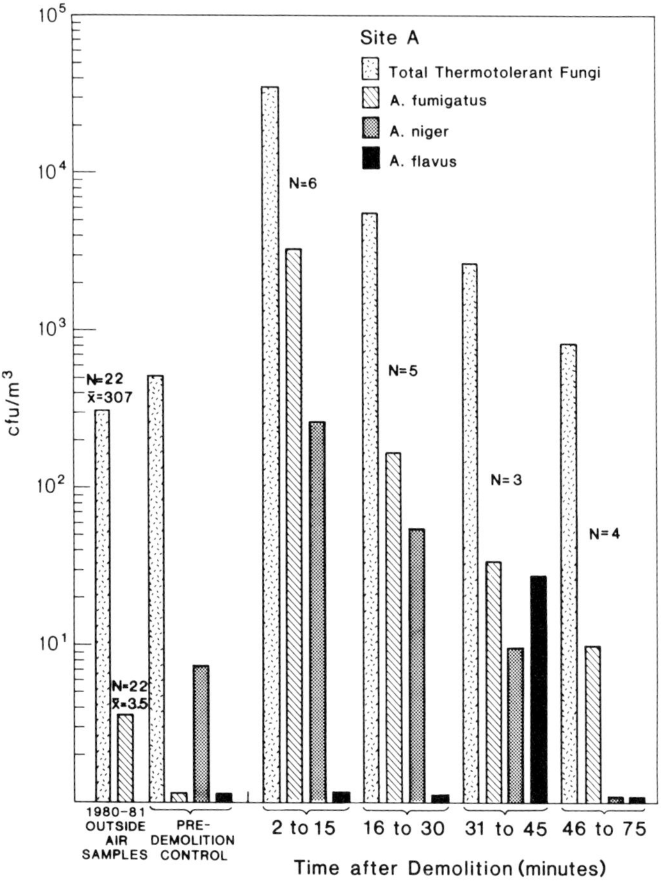


**Figure 9.1A and 9.1B.** Site A and Site B. Outside concentrations of 37 °C airborne fungi were determined at both sites predemolition and after demolition of a fifty-one-year-old building. Sieve cascade air samplers (@1.0 CFM) with inhib-

cause the generation of fungal aerosols in order to initiate precautionary measures.

During a demolition project at the University of Minnesota a building was explosively imploded adjacent to the University Hospital. Streifel and co-workers (1983) demonstrated a significant generation of a mold aerosol during the demolition of a fifty-one-year-old building. During the dispersion of the aerosolized debris, one

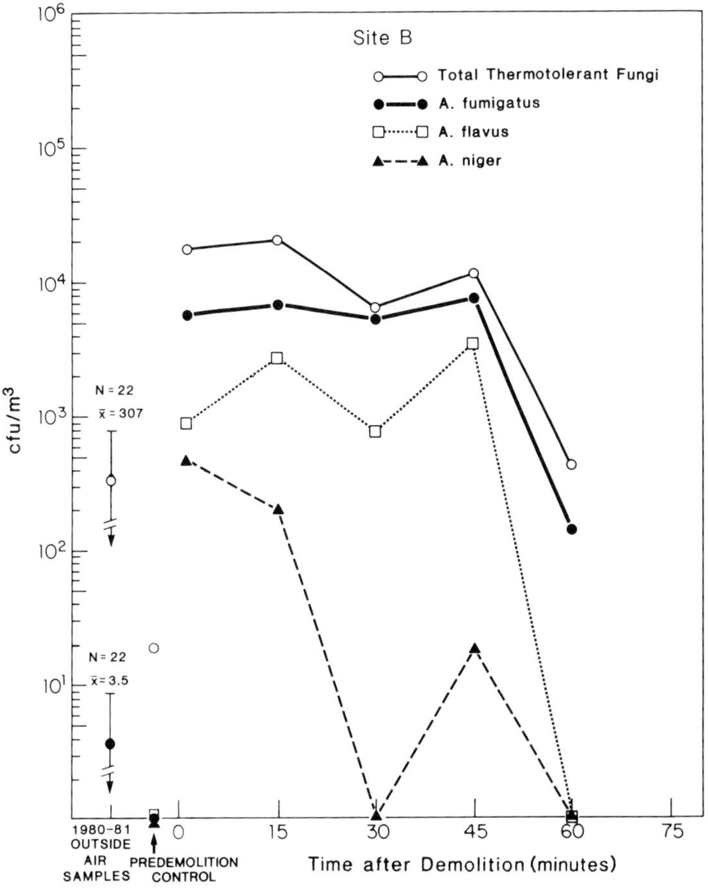


itory mold agar detected a large airborne cloud of aerosolized mold in both locations which dissipated with a wind shift. (Streifel et al., 1983.)

sample location recovered a significant cloud of *A. fumigatus* and *A. flavus* (Figure 9.1A) and other aerosolized fungi. The concentration of the main cloud of aerosolized debris at the primary sample site reached 840 *A. fumigatus* and 84 *A. flavus* CFU/m$^3$, respectively. At a nearby sample site (Figure 9.1B) the peripheral portion of the aerosolized debris had 1,000 and 5,000 CFU/m$^3$ of *A. flavus* and *A. fumigatus*, respectively. This cloud of pathogens dissipated over a period

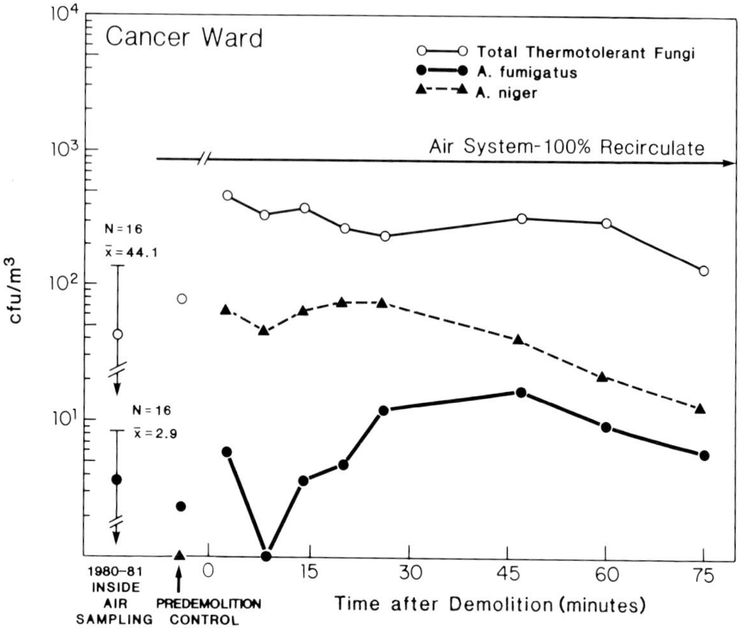


**Figure 9.2A and 9.2B.** A. Cancer ward. B. Bone marrow transplant ward. Inside concentrations of 37 °C airborne fungi were collected at these two indoor hospital locations predemolition and after demolition. High-volume slit (3.5 $m^3$/min)

of seventy-five minutes as a wind shift disrupted the local wind currents. This outdoor mold cloud was generated adjacent to the University of Minnesota Hospital while air sampling was being conducted indoors. An increase of indoor air mold concentration was noted during different air handling operational conditions (Figure 9.2). This event demonstrated building penetration of aerosolized mold during that demolition project. The mold-specific indoor samples were taken using slit samplers (Casella, London). All samples were incubated at 37 °C on inhibitory mold agar (Becton, Dickinson & Company). Results indicate a substantial increase of viable mold on outside samples by approximately 3 $\log_{10}$ immediately after the explosive demolition (Figure 9.1A). Within sixty minutes a gradual decrease to a predemolition concentration of total airborne fungi was noted. In patient areas immediately after the blast a dramatic air

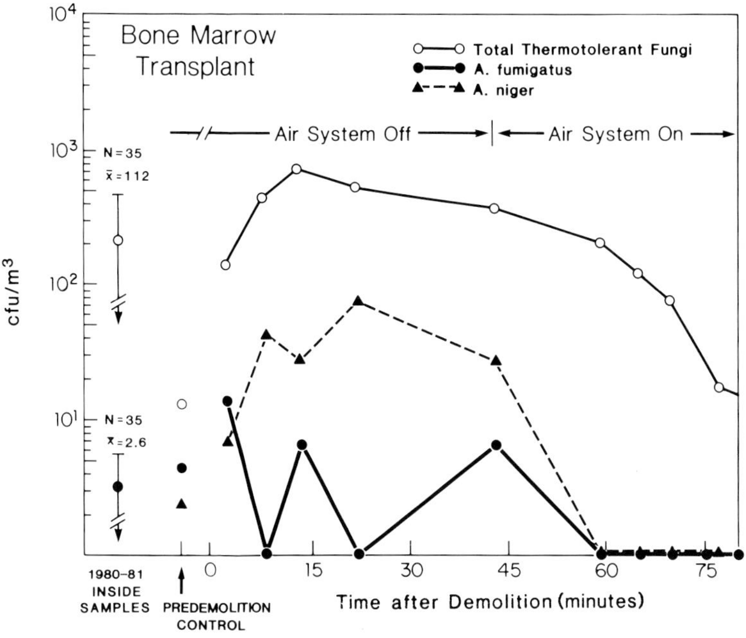


collected 5-min samples on inhibitory mold agar. A marked increase of airborne fungi was noted in all locations which dissipated with time or after the air handling system was restarted. (Streifel et al., 1983.)

concentration increase was also observed but the increases were not as substantial. Both indoor hospital areas increased approximately 1 $log_{10}$ above background predemolition samples. The level of *A. fumigatus* increased slowly on the cancer ward from about 5 CFU/$m^3$ to a peak of about 12 CFU/$m^3$ before decreasing over a 75 min sample period (Figure 9.2B). The slow increase of *A. fumigatus* indoors could have been caused by the penetration of the outdoor fungal spores during the dissipation of the peripheral spore cloud. *A flavus* did not appear on the culture plates. Slower-growing *A. flavus* colonies may have been obscured by other faster-growing fungi. Also, the outdoor samples were taken with multistaged sieve samplers which discriminated different-sized particles, thus allowing for the distinction of the two different-sized mold spores. This demolition evaluation illustrated construction-related fungal aerosol generation,

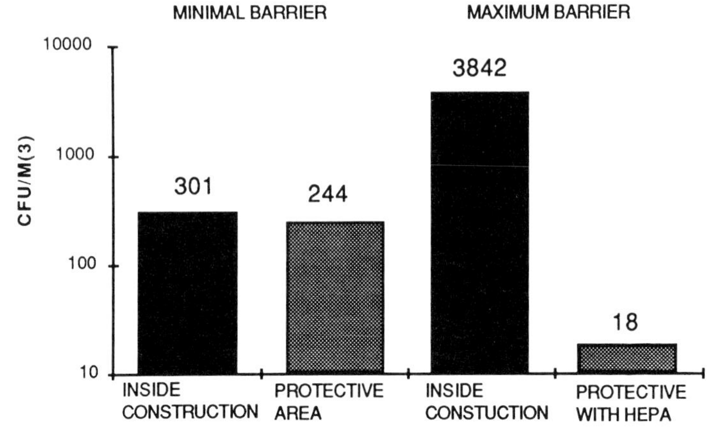


**Figure 9.3.** Construction barriers were evaluated during construction projects using volumetric air samplers. Minimum barriers consisted of plastic with wood frame and plastic flap doors. Maximum barriers include slab-to-slab insulated dry wall, sealed utilities, no doors, and airflow control.

mold cloud behavior, outdoor aerosol penetration into a building, and air handling system control measures (Figures 9.1, 9.2, and 9.3).

Outside construction aerosols are produced during structural demolition or while moving large amounts of dirt and debris. Traditional ball and crane demolition will produce construction aerosols over an extended period. The demolition Streifel and colleagues (1983) described produced a large short-term cloud of aerosolized particles which dissipated with the prevailing wind. University Hospital planners decided on an implosion for this building because long-term conventional demolition would affect sensitive patients and therapeutic radiology equipment. Rapid demolition simplified dust control after debris was on the ground. Implosive demolition allowed for a short-term maximum protection plan for the adjacent hospital buildings.

Building penetration by outdoor construction must be a common occurrence and could be minimized if construction and building maintenance personnel are reminded of control measures. Prevention of outdoor spore penetration requires adjusting the outdoor air building intakes, sealing windows, and controlling pedestrian egress.

The air handling system in buildings adjacent to known construction projects should be placed on minimum outside air intake and additional prefiltration should be provided. Spendlove (1975) described the means through which particle aerosols enter buildings. The list of penetrations includes windows, air intakes, cracks in the foundation, and doors. Preventing aerosol penetrations is difficult when construction is expected to last months or years. During major excavation or landscaping, wind direction will bias dust cloud movement. Air intake precautions must be considered if the building is a hospital with severely compromised patients. Construction roads should be sprayed with water to control dust. However, the proximity of outdoor construction to buildings housing sensitive individuals should dictate the extent of the required precautions. Sealing windows reduces outside aerosol influences; air filtration capability must be determined in older buildings because they often have minimum air filtration. Minimum filtration (approximately 40 percent on the American Society of Heating, Refrigeration, and Air Conditioning Engineers [ASHRAE] dust spot test) does not effectively remove particles $<5\ \mu$. Normally all buildings serve as a shelter, reducing exposure to outdoor microbes when major building penetrations are maintained. In unpublished studies (Streifel, 1987) of total room temperature indoor versus outdoor airborne fungal samples, even though a correlation exists between the influence of outside air variations on indoor minimum air filtered spore levels ($p =$ .84), the actual level of spores collected in each environment was significantly different ($p = .001$). Relatively minor precautions will prevent building penetration by different outdoor aerosols, thus reducing effects on indoor air pollution. Predetermination of occupant sensitivity requires preservation of indoor air quality; therefore, indoor generation of mold aerosols must also be controlled.

## INDOOR CONSTRUCTION

Indoor construction projects contribute to the deterioration of indoor air quality. Construction-related nosocomial infections were described in several hospitals by Opal and colleagues (1986) and Sarubbi and co-workers (1982). Experience with extensive renovation/construction at the University of Minnesota has helped to determine methods for the control of construction-related mold aerosols. The preparation of an indoor project site for construction could be the most hazardous factor in the generation of mold aerosols. Dust accumulators, such as ceiling tile, refrigerators, radiators, or carpeting, when removed prior to demolition/renovation could generate substantial mold aerosols. Depending on cleanliness, the disturbance of dirty equipment or material aerosolizes accumulated debris which includes opportunistic fungal spores. Accumulated dust removed from the surface of ceiling tile in the University of Minnesota Hospital was found to contain $10^3$ CFU/g of *A. fumigatus*. Removing this dust with a high-efficiency particulate air (HEPA)-filtered vacuum helped prevent this dust from being aerosolized. Other dust collected from mechanical systems such as heating units, exhaust vents, or refrigerator coils had concentrations ranging from $10^2$ to $10^3$ CFU/g. This dust can be removed by vacuuming or cleaning with a damp cloth. Care must be taken when vacuuming dust because aerosols are generated with standard unfiltered vacuum cleaners (Rhame et al., 1984). High-efficiency filtration on vacuums should be required when vacuuming is necessary in hospitals. Other routine maintenance procedures may also aerosolize microbes. For example, on 18 November 1983, during an eight-hour air sampling evaluation on the bone marrow transplant ward, the ceiling lights were cleaned. This procedure caused a detectable burst of *A. niger* which reached 90 CFU/m$^3$ compared with $<5$ CFU/m$^3$ from the same location during the previous six hours (Streifel, 1987). Because fungal aerosols are generated by a wide variety of procedures, protocols must be followed which protect sensitive individuals in the areas affected by maintenance/construction projects.

Demolition and/or construction will release a substantial number of viable and nonviable particles. Total air particles greater than 0.3 $\mu$ in construction areas, when measured using an optical particle counter, exceed particle counts of $1 \times 10^6$/cu ft. The human health effects of these particles vary with the type of debris being aerosolized. Aerosolized asbestos has been the focus of many hazardous material concerns when it is found in the construction environment, whereas mold is difficult to notice unless personnel recognize the water stains associated with mold growth or dust accumulations are evident. The focus on the viable particles during construction aerosols is now being evaluated by investigators.

The types of sensitizing particles aerosolized during construction depends on the phase of a scheduled project. For example, plasterboard taping and sanding produces large aerosol clouds of nonviable chalk particles; the demolition of water-damaged areas may generate viable fungal aerosols. The extent that viable particles are generated depends on the condition of the area and extent of work scheduled. Viable air sampling during plastering or painting has produced unremarkable results; however, during bathroom demolition a maximum of $1.8 \times 10^4$ CFU/$m^3$ of viable 37° C fungi was observed (Streifel, 1987). The presence of a wide variety of aerosolized particles during construction or renovation is normal. The proximity of a project and local control measures will determine the air quality of the nearby indoor environment.

Basic aerosol control measures such as sealing work areas, ventilation manipulation, and traffic control have been used in one institution (Opal et al., 1986). Control measures should be tailored to protect nearby occupants. The contractor who wins the bid for respective projects is responsible for preventing construction-related indoor air pollution. Because contractors work with a different fundamental motivation, the basic requirements for protecting occupants must be specified in the construction contract.

The determination of which protective measures are important often is made on the basis of experience gained while monitoring construction projects. For example, in November 1985 the University of Minnesota Hospital was preparing to open a new patient care facility. At that time construction projects were scheduled to connect the old occupied hospital building to the new hospital through a skyway/tunnel system. One skyway connection opened directly onto a critical care ward where an ongoing air sampling program was in place. Precautions for the construction project included slab-to-slab sealed barriers between the construction and patient areas, debris removal through nonpatient areas, and demolition methods specifically designed to reduce noise and dust. The workmen were requested to use small hammers rather than pneumatic jackhammers to implement demolition; water was sprayed on the debris to reduce dust. During the skyway demolition phase the "certified" sealed barrier was subverted when workers opened windows for relief from dusty conditions. Cold outside air (−10 °C, −23 °F) infiltrated through an open window into the demolition areas. This air infiltrated through unnoticed breaches in the barrier into the patient areas. As the infiltrated air mixed with construction aerosols, the spores floated in the air currents and were subsequently detected by the air sampling in the patient care area. During the demolition, air samples were taken on both sides of the construction barrier; the dirty side was sampled using two-stage sieve cascade impactors (Andersen at 1 cu ft/min). The samples were incubated at 37 °C on Inhibitory Mold Agar in order to detect pathogens capable of growth in humans. A high-volume slit (Casella at 25 cu ft/min) was used on the HEPA-filtered clean side of the barrier. A maximum of $1.8 \times 10^4$ CFU/$m^3$ of total fungi was collected on the demolition side of the barrier. At the same time samples from the clean side of the barrier, 80 CFU/$m^3$ total of fungi were noted. No pathogens were found on the clean side of the barrier. However, the pathogens *A. fumigatus* and *A. flavus* were found on the construction side of the barrier. Concurrent sampling from other locations within the clean area revealed a rise in total fungi during the period when the window was open. At normal 37 °C air, fungal concentrations were about 2.5 CFU/$m^3$ before construction. The dust-laden infiltrating air penetrated around electrical conduits and other difficult-to-seal spots on the pan-style ceiling slab. Due to a fire barrier wall at the end of the critical care unit, further penetration was prevented from reaching sampling locations on other patient wards. This information from the surveillance air samples was instrumental in stopping construction while the barriers were sealed and a large window fan was installed to exhaust the demolition dust. Once the additional precautions were instituted air quality samples from both sides of the barrier improved on subsequent sampling days. The improvement in air quality could also be attributed to a clean-up of the demolition debris. Greene (1962a) demonstrated marked improvement in microbial air quality after clean-up of a construction site.

Air quality control requires the removal of the fungal source. In the just-mentioned case, the demolition area had water-damaged wood in the pipe space behind the bathtub and sink in the bathroom. This had been an area with high humidity caused by condensation and occasional leaks; wood lath provided an ideal medium for fungal growth. Streifel and colleagues (1987) demonstrated that aerosols could be passively released from moldy wood. This release exceeded $5 \times 10^5$ CFU/hr. When fragments of this moldy wood were agitated in a controlled environment a short-term spore burst exceeded $6.3 \times 10^5$ CFU/$m^3$. Such unsuspected sources of fungi must be prevalent because water leaks in buildings are common. Recognition of these water-soaked areas and the protective measures necessary to contain the construction aerosols will benefit workers and occupants in and near construction areas.

Preventing the movement of indoor construction aerosol debris into "clean" areas requires maintenance of a substantial barrier and airflow control. Plastic barriers are vulnerable to damage. Conversely, slab-to-slab metal stud, taped sheetrock, and fiber-insulated barriers are superior but they are also prone to infiltration if not specifically evaluated. A comparison of minimum/maximum barriers (Figure 9.3) shows considerable difference of fungal aerosol control. Either type of barrier will provide adequate protection if infiltration holes are closed. Airflow should always be from clean areas to the dirty construction zone. Contractors and construction coordinators should maintain the effectiveness of the barriers by evaluating the barrier penetrations and maintaining airflow control. A simple smoke stick (Gastec: Sensidyne smoke tube) is a useful device for evaluating airflow direction. This device can provide a visual evaluation of air currents in the construction area (note that the material safety data sheet on these smoke sticks should be read before using in occupied areas).

Because indoor construction projects are so common, preventing the dissemination of aerosolized debris is not usually included in specified safety measures except in some enlightened institutions charged with treating immune-suppressed patients. The prolonged inhalation of sensitizing spores is probably common relative to the location of indoor construction or renovation. Preventive measures can be instituted without unreasonable inconvenience or expense; however, the consistent control of airflow during active demolition or during clean-up projects is more difficult to achieve. The degree of protection required depends on the building planner's judgment of potential sensitivity of the occupants. Even if the occupants are not initially sensitive they may become sensitized when construction dust is prevalent in work or patient care areas. Most construction aerosols do not cause infections, although many of the same aerosols are irritating to the individuals who inhale the suspended particles.

## CONSTRUCTION RECOMMENDATIONS

During outdoor demolition or dirt-moving construction projects the managers should consider the following recommendations.

1. The location of the project with respect to a building air intake should be considered. Covering the air intake and/or switching to a maximum recirculation of return air during active construction hours will prevent problems.
2. The integrity of the air filtration system should be maintained to minimize the penetration of construction aerosols into nearby buildings.
3. Building penetrations by aerosols should be avoided by excluding outside air, sealing windows, creating special worker exits for construction zones. Other building penetration points that are not so obvious should be sealed. This includes cracks around window and door frames.
4. The construction roads and demolition debris should be maintained properly to reduce dusty conditions.

Outdoor construction projects can contribute to an increase in indoor air pollution. The proximity of buildings to the site of the project determines the extent of the protection required. The feasibility of protection depends on normal operational situations in the building which could compromise protective measures. Thorough planning for protective measures will help to reduce the effects of outdoor conditions on the indoor environment.

During indoor construction, building airflow dynamics are often unpredictable because of airflow changes due to local weather conditions, open windows, outer wall demolition, or alteration of air handling service. The vigilance necessary for indoor projects varies with the perceived hazard to occupants. Ostensibly, the hospital environment is among the most sensitive areas requiring aerosol control measures during construction. Common practice should include the following measures.

1. Substantial barriers should be constructed to provide slab-to-slab seals to separate the construction zone from clean areas. Utility service should be made airtight. Plastic barrier integ-

rity is difficult to maintain; therefore, wallboard-reinforced barriers should be specified.

2. Airflow should be maintained from clean to dirty areas. Open windows subvert building ventilation specifications and airflow control. Window fans with substantial airflow will bias airflow and rid the building of construction aerosols.
3. Air balance in the construction zone should provide less supply than exhaust air to enhance clean to dirty airflow.
4. Workers and construction material must be prohibited from sensitive areas.
5. The application of the antifungal agent copper-8-quinolinolate was shown to be effective in decontaminating a construction environment during clean-up (Opal et al., 1986). Clean-up of the construction environment effectively reduces the air content of potentially hazardous particles from construction projects.
6. Airflow monitoring during the various stages of construction assures effectiveness of the airflow control measures.
7. Air sampling, while not required for construction monitoring, helps determine the effectiveness of the aerosol control measures.
8. Attention to the contractual specifications is essential for a safe environment for nearby occupants during construction activity.

## SUMMARY

In most instances the relationship between construction and disease is unknown. Occupants, either atopic or immune-suppressed, may develop a sensitivity to airborne particles. Infections by airborne *Aspergillus* fungi are rare in healthy individuals. However, unpredictable health effects may result when individuals inhale excessive numbers of airborne fungi or other material aerosolized during construction projects. The degree of sensitivity varies with the individual. Construction aerosols should be controlled whenever building occupants are potentially exposed. The methods described are reasonable; however, conscientious vigilance of controlled airflow is absolutely necessary for occupant safety especially in the hospital environment.

## REFERENCES

Andersen, A. 1958. New sampler for the collection, sizing, and enumeration of viable airborne particles. *Appl. Microbiology* 76:471–484.

Aisner, J.; Schimpff, S. C.; Bennett, J. E.; Young, V. M.; and Wiernik, P. H. 1976. Aspergillosis infection in cancer patients. *JAMA* 235:411–12.

Arnow, P. M.; Andersen, R. L.; Mainous, P. D.; and Smith, E. J. 1978. Pulmonary aspergillosis during hospital renovation. *Am. Rev. Respiratory Disease* 118:49–53.

Booth, C. 1971. *Method in microbiology.* Vol. 4. London: Academic Press, p. 393.

Gerson, S. L., et al. 1984. Prolonged granulocytopenia: Major risk factor for increased pulmonary aspergillosis in patients with acute leukemia. *Ann. Int. Med.* 100:345–51.

Greene, V. W.; Vesley, D.; Bond, R. G.; and Michaelson, G. S. 1962a. Microbiology contamination of hospital air. I. Quantitative studies. *Appl. Microbiology* 10:561–66.

———. 1962b. Microbiological contamination of hospital air. II. Qualitative studies. *Appl. Microbiology* 10:567–71.

Gregory, P. H. 1973. *Microbiology of the atmosphere.* 2d ed. New York: Wiley & Sons.

Krasinski, K.; Holzman, R. S.; Hanna, B.; Greco, A.; Graff, M.; and Bhogal, M. 1985. Nosocomial fungal infection during hospital renovation. *Infect. Control* 6:278–82.

Lentino, J. R.; Rosenkranz, M. A.; Michaels, J. A.; Kurup, V. P.; Rose, H. D.; and Rytel, M. W. 1982. Nosocomial aspergillosis: A retrospective review of airborne disease secondary to road construction and contaminated air conditioners. *Am. J. Epidemiology* 116:430–37.

Mullins, J.; Harvey, R.; and Seaton, A. 1976. Sources and incidence of airborne *Aspergillus fumigatus* (Fres). *Clin. Allergy* 6:209–17.

Noble, W. C., and Clayton, Y. M. 1963. Fungi in the air of hospital wards. *J. Gen. Microbiol.* 32:397–402.

Opal, S. M., et al., 1986. Efficacy of infection control measures during a nosocomial outbreak of disseminated aspergillosis associated with hospital construction. *J. Infectious Diseases* 153:634–37.

Peterson, P. K.; McGlave, P.; Ramsay, N.K.C.; Rhame, F.; Cohen, E.; Perry, G. S.; Goldman, A. I.; and Kersey, J. 1983. A prospective study of infectious diseases following bone marrow transplant: Emergence of aspergillus and cytomegalovirus as the major causes of mortality infection control. *Infection Control* 4:81–89.

Rhame, F. S.; Streifel, A. J.; Kersey, J. H.; and McGlave, P. B. 1984. Extrinsic risk factors for pneumonia in the patient at high risk of infection. *Am. J. Med.* 76(5A):42–52.

Sarubbi, F. A.; Kopf, H. B.; Wilson, B.; McGinnis, M. R.; and Rutala, W. A. 1982. Increased recovery of *Aspergillus flavus* from respiratory specimens during hospital construction. *Am. Rev. Respiratory Disease* 125:33–38.

Solley, G. O., and Hyatt, R. E. 1980. Hypersensitivity pneumonitis induced by Penicillium species. *J. Allergy Clin. Immun.* 65:65–70.

Solomon, W. R.; Berge, H. P.; and Boise, J. R. 1978. Airborne *Aspergillus fumigatus* levels outside and within a large clinical center. *J. Allergy Clin. Immun.* 62:56–60.

Spendlove, C. J. 1975. Penetration of structures by microbial aerosols. *Dev. Industr. Microbiol.* 16:427–436.

Streifel, A. J. 1987. Unpublished information, University of Minnesota.

Streifel, A. J.; Lauer, J. L.; Vesley, D.; Juni, B. D.; and Rhame, F. S. 1983. Aspergillus fumigatus and other thermotolerant fungi generated by hospital building demolition. *Appl. Environmental Microbiology* 46:375–378.

Streifel, A. J.; Stevens, P.; and Rhame, F. S. 1987. In-hospital source of Penicillium species spores. *J. Clin. Microbiology* 25:1–4.

# 10

# Legionellosis: Risk Associated with Building Design

JAMES C. FEELEY

Each year thousands of cases of legionellosis occur in the United States and in numerous other countries throughout the world. It is estimated that between 1 and 13 percent of all pneumonias seen in hospitals in the United States, Canada, the United Kingdom, and Germany are cases of legionellosis.

This illness should be of special interest to building owners, managers, and designers because outbreaks of legionellosis have been traced to flaws in building design and in faulty procedures used to start up systems such as cooling towers.

## THE DISEASE

Legionellosis is the umbrella name for two distinct types of illness, Legionnaires disease and Pontiac fever. Of the two, Legionnaires disease is the most severe. It causes a pneumonia and injury to numerous organs of the body. Hospitalization is essential and even when patients are given proper supportive and antimicrobial therapy, fatality can range from 5 to 80 percent depending on the health of the patient before illness. The highest fatality rates are among individuals who are either debilitated or immunosuppressed. Fortunately, only a small number of individuals (2–3 percent) develop illness after exposure to air containing legionellae. Symptoms usually become apparent in these individuals within four to ten days after exposure.

Pontiac fever is a flu-like illness. Recovery usually occurs within two to five days without hospitalization or antimicrobial therapy. Its attack rate (95 percent) is much higher, but its incubation period (thirty-six to forty-eight hours) is much shorter than Legionnaires disease.

Because legionellosis may be difficult to diagnose, many sporadic cases of this disease, especially Pontiac fever, are not reported to public health officials. In 1984 less than 1,000 cases were reported (Centers for Disease Control, 1986) even though between 25,000 and 50,000 cases are estimated to occur annually in the United States (Broome, 1984). Outbreak cases are more easily recognized and often are first reported by the local news media. To date nearly 50 outbreaks have been reported. Most have been traced to aerosols generated either from cooling towers or plumbing fixtures such as showers and faucets that were contaminated with legionellae.

## CAUSATIVE BACTERIA

These recently discovered diseases are caused by a group of small rod-shaped bacteria belonging to the genus *Legionella.* They stain gram-negatively, do not produce endospores (Brenner et al., 1984), and require special media containing the amino acid L-cysteine, a slightly acid pH, and low concentrations of iron for growth in the laboratory (Feeley et al., 1978). In contrast to their fastidious growth requirements in the laboratory, these organisms appear to be less specific in nutritional requirements in nature because they have been detected to grow, multiply, and survive in a wide variety of surface waters (Fliermans et al., 1981). Twenty-three species and more than forty serogroups of legionellae have been reported (Brenner et al., 1985). Several additional species and serogroups have already been discovered and will soon be reported. In addition, some strains of *Legionella,* such as serogroup 1 of *Legionella pneumophila,* can be further characterized by monoclonal subtyping (Joly et al., 1986), plasmid profiles (Brown et al., 1982), and isoenzyme electrophoresis patterns (Selander et al., 1985). These tests have been used in some investigations and have proved very helpful in identifying the environmental source of the *Legionella* that caused the outbreak (Garbe et al., 1985; Plouffe et al., 1983). This is accomplished by matching the bacteria isolated from the patients with bacteria isolated from the environment. The ecology of *Legionella* and the factors that enable it to cause human disease have not been completely determined. It must be emphasized that the mere presence of *Legionella* either in water or on a fixture does not mean that an outbreak of legionellosis will occur. Many buildings contain legionellae in their drinking water systems or cooling tower water with no cases of legionellosis having occurred among their occupants.

## OUTBREAKS TRACED TO DESIGN FLAWS

Although *Legionella pneumophila* was first identified in the 1976 outbreak of Legionnaires disease in Philadelphia (McDade et al., 1977), this investigation did not identify a building design flaw that could explain the outbreak (Fraser et al., 1977). Therefore, the 1968 Pontiac fever outbreak will be reviewed because it is an excellent example of an epidemic that was traced to building design flaws. The agent, *Legionella pneumophila* serogroup 1, which caused this outbreak remained unidentified for years until the investigation of the Philadelphia outbreak in which *Legionella* was detected and determined to be the cause. The outbreak of Pontiac fever began on Tuesday evening during the first week of July 1968 among employees of the Oakland County health department in Pontiac, Michigan (Glick et al., 1978). That evening 67 persons became ill with high fever, headache, muscle pain, and general feeling of discomfort. By Wednesday evening an additional 37 people had become ill. Ultimately, 95 of the 100 employees and 49 of 170 visitors became infected.

Because of the unusually high attack rate, Michigan state health authorities requested that the Centers for Disease Control (CDC) help in investigating the cause of the outbreak. Three CDC investigators entered the building on Saturday of the Fourth of July weekend and worked there during the rest of the weekend with the air-conditioning system turned off. They remained healthy and continued to work in the building the beginning of the following week with the air-conditioning operating. All three investigators became ill on Tuesday evening. They were replaced with three new investigators who also became ill thirty-six hours after they started work in the building with its air-conditioning operating. The building was closed to the public on 12 July.

The fact that the first three CDC investigators developed illness only after the air-conditioning system was turned on was of major significance in the investigation. It strongly suggested that the air-conditioning may have played some role in the outbreak. Consequently, this system was thoroughly inspected. It was established that cooling was achieved by a wet-heat-rejection-type system, an evaporative condenser, located in the basement of the building. Large volumes of outside air were mechanically sucked into ground-level intakes and exhausted on the roof after being blown over the heat exchange coils of the evaporative condenser. Cooling of the circulant contained within the cooling coils resulted from the evaporation of the water that was continuously being sprayed over the coils.

Two design flaws in the air-conditioning system were detected. Smoke and freon dispersant studies revealed that both would allow contamination of the conditioned air with the discharged exhaust air. The first flaw was detected on the roof, where the humid exhaust air from the evaporative condenser was vented within 2 meters of the conditioned air system's intake for outside make-up air. Smoke dispersal studies demonstrated that exhaust air could be easily sucked into the outside make-up air intake.

The second design flaw was in the arrangement and construction of the exhaust and intake duct systems. Cracks had developed in the walls of both systems. Because both duct systems were arranged side by side, water condensate in the exhaust duct was able to travel through the cracks into the duct of conditioned air system. Eventually contamination of the air with legionellae was documented when these bacteria were detected in water that had collected in the drain pans of the evaporative condenser and from the lungs of sentinel guinea pigs exposed either to the conditioned air at the time of the outbreak or to aerosols of the drain pan condensate generated in a CDC laboratory (Kaufmann et al., 1981).

The primary intervention measure that stopped the 1968 Pontiac fever outbreak and prevented future similar illness among occupants of and visitors to this building was the complete dismantlement and replacement of the implicated air-conditioning system with a properly designed one. After the Pontiac and Philadelphia legionellae outbreaks, several others occurred in which building design flaws contributed to air contaminated with *Legionella* which was sucked into buildings from cooling towers via air intakes (Dondero et al., 1980), through an improperly sealed chimney (Band et al., 1981), and open windows (Garbe et al., 1985), or entered into buildings via contaminated potable water systems (Best et al., 1983; Cielsielski et al., 1984) and their fixtures (Colburne et al., 1984; Cordes et al., 1981).

## PREVENTION

The best time to develop a strategy to reduce the chance or risk of an outbreak of legionellosis is when the building is first designed. This prevention strategy should contain measures designed to interrupt the chance of transmission of *Legionella* at as many links (sites) as possible in its transmission chain—namely, the reservoir, the amplifier, the disseminator, and the site of patient exposure. This will assure that if one measure fails, others will be available to safeguard against transmission. The plan should be implemented during construction. A scheduled preventive maintenance program should be designed to include an effective biocide water treatment against *Legionella*. This program should begin before the building is occupied and should be continued for the life of the building.

## RECOMMENDATIONS

The following list of recommendations should reduce the risk of an outbreak of legionellosis. However, it is emphasized that this list is not all-inclusive and its implementation is not a guarantee that a *Legionella* outbreak will not occur. The reader may wish to review the recommendations by professional organizations (American Society for Heating, Refrigeration, and Air Conditioning Engineers,

1988) and governmental agencies (Australian Department of Housing and Construction, 1986; Environmental Protection Agency, 1985).

## Air-Conditioning Systems

1. The installation of a dry-type of air cooling system should be considered for buildings such as hospitals housing individuals highly susceptible to legionellosis. However, it is emphasized that wet-heat-rejection-type systems, such as cooling towers, can be operated with minimum risk of *Legionella* transmission in high-risk areas as well as others, provided they are properly started up and well maintained with biocides effective against *Legionella.* The author believes that the continuous application of biocides with a mechanical pump or by use of slow-release compounds is preferable to intermittent addition of biocides in large amounts.
2. A cooling tower should be installed in a location that deters the cooling tower's drift from entering the air intakes of its own building and those of neighboring structures.
3. Air intakes and exhaust vents should not be installed in the immediate proximity of each other in order to prevent exhaust being sucked back into the building.
4. Air intakes should be located at least 100 meters from cooling towers to minimize cooling tower drift that enters buildings. If this is not possible, a protective shroud or a duct extension on the air intake should be installed so that air will be obtained from an area free of drift contamination. Also, installation of a high-efficiency particulate air (HEPA) filter in the air intake should be considered if these preventive measures are not feasible.
5. Windows in hospitals next to cooling towers should be sealed or prevented from opening when the tower is in operation.
6. Drain pans for draining the cooling coil condensate water should be designed to allow water to drain freely without collecting in the pan. Pans should be installed in such a manner so that future adjustments can be made to the drain pans and pipes to ensure that the water drains freely.

7. If humidification of the conditioned air is needed, it should be accomplished by a mechanism that injects cold water that has not been allowed to stand in a holding tank. This reduces the possibility of an outbreak of humidifier fever or legionellosis from microorganisms that might grow in stagnant water held in tanks.
8. Filters in the air-handling system should be changed frequently to prevent excessive accumulation of dust. This is especially necessary when the air passing over the filter has a relative humidity of 70 percent or greater. Under these conditions microorganisms will start to grow on the filters.

### Potable Water Systems

1. Hot water heaters should uniformly heat all the water that they contain above 60 °C (140 °F). However, water should not be excessively heated because of scalding potential to users. Water heaters that allow dead areas of lukewarm water should not be installed.
2. Use of long pipe runs and collection tanks that allow water to stagnate should be avoided because *Legionella* may be amplified in them.
3. Faucet aerators should be prohibited in hospital rooms housing patients having high risk to legionellosis because they can become colonized with legionellae as well as other microorganisms such as *Pseudomonas.*
4. Gaskets and like items made of materials that promote growth of *Legionella* should not be used.

## CONCLUSION

Building designers, owners, and managers should be aware that several outbreaks of legionellosis have resulted from flaws in building design. Faulty start-up procedures for cooling towers without effective biocide treatment have also caused outbreaks of legionellosis. These individuals should consider a prevention strategy to reduce the possibility of a legionellosis outbreak. This strategy should be formulated as the building is designed, implemented during construction, and continued throughout the life of the building.

## REFERENCES

American Society for Heating, Refrigeration, and Air Conditioning Engineers. 1988. Position paper on legionellosis. Atlanta.

Australian Department of Housing and Construction. 1986. Legionnaires' Disease Task Force Report. Dickson, Canberra.

Band, J. D.; LaVenture, M.; Davis, J. P.; Mallison, G. F.; Schell, W. L.; Skaliy, P.; Hayes, P. S.; Weiss, H.; Greenberg, D. J.; and Fraser, D. W. 1981. Epidemic Legionnaires' disease: Airborne transmission down a chimney. *JAMA* 254:2404–7.

Best, M.; Yu, V. L.; Stout, J.; Goetz, A.; Muder, R. R.; and Taylor, F. 1983. Legionellaceae in the hospital water supply—epidemiological link with disease and evaluation of a method on control on nosocomial Legionnaires' disease and Pittsburgh pneumonia. *Lancet* 2:307–10.

Brenner, D. J.; Feeley, J. C.; and Weaver, R. E. 1984. *Legionellaceae.* In *Bergey's manual of systematic bacteriology,* N. R. Krieg and J. G. Holt, eds. vol. 1. Baltimore: Williams & Wilkins, 279–88.

Brenner, D. J.; Steigerwalt, A. G.; Gorman, G. W.; Wilkinson, H. W.; Bibb, W. F.; Hackel, M.; Tyndall, R. L.; Campbell, J.; Feeley, J. C.; Thacker, W. L.; Skaliy, P.; Martin, W. T.; Brake, B. J.; Fields, B. S.; McEachern, H. V.; and Corcoran, L. K. 1985. Ten new species of legionella. *Int. J. Syst. Bacteriol.* 35:50–59.

Broome, C. V. 1984. Current issues in epidemiology of legionellosis. In *Legionella, Proceedings of the 2d international symposium,* C. Thornsberry, A. Balows, J. C. Feeley, and W. Jakubowski, eds. Washington, D.C.: American Society for Microbiology, pp. 205–9.

Brown, A.; Vickers, R. M.; Elder, E. M.; Lema, M.; and Garrity, G. M. 1982. Plasmid and surface antigen markers of endemic and epidemic *Legionella pneumophila* strains. *J. Clin. Microbiol.* 16:230–35.

Centers for Disease Control. 1986. *Annual summary 1984. Morbidity and mortality weekly report,* vol. 33, no. 54. Atlanta: Centers for Disease Control.

Cielsielski, C. A.; Blaser, M. J.; and Wang, W. 1984. Role of stagnation and obstruction of water flow in isolation of *Legionella pneumophila* from hospital plumbing. *Appl. Environ. Microbiol.* 49:984.

Colburne, J. W.; Pratt, D. J.; Smith, M. G.; Fisher-Hoch, S. P.; and Harper, D. 1984. Water fittings as sources of *Legionella pneumophila* in a hospital plumbing system. *Lancet* 1:210–13.

Cordes, L. G.; Wiesenthal, A. M.; and Gorman, G. W. 1981. Isolation of *Legionella pneumophila* from hospital showerheads. *Ann. Intern. Med.* 94:195.

Dondero, T. J. Jr.; Rendtorff, R. C.; Mallison, G. F.; Weeks, R. M.; Levy, J. S.; Wong, E. S.; and Schaffner, W. 1980. An outbreak of Legionnaires' disease associated with a contaminated air conditioning cooling tower. *N. Engl. J. Med.* 302:365–70.

Environmental Protection Agency, Office of Drinking Water. 1985. *Control of* Legionella *in plumbing systems, health advisory.* Washington, D.C.: U.S. Environmental Protection Agency.

Feeley, J. C.; Gorman, G. W.; Weaver, R. E.; Mackel, D. C.; and Smith, H. W. 1978. Primary isolation media for the Legionnaires' disease bacterium. *J. Clin. Microbiol.* 8:325–29.

Fliermans, C. B.; Cherry, W. B.; Orrison, L. H.; Smith, S. J.; Tison, D. L.; and Pope, D. H. 1981. Ecological distribution of *Legionella pneumophila. Appl. Environ. Microbiol.* 41:9–16.

Fraser, D. W.; Tsai, T. R. [sic]; Orenstein, W.; Parkin, W. E.; Beecham, H. J.; Sharrar, R. G.; Harris, J.; Mallison, G. F.; Martin, S. M.; McDade, J. E.; Sheppard, C. C.; and Brachman, P. S. 1977. Field investigation team: Legionnaires' disease: Description of an epidemic of pneumonia. *N. Engl. J. Med.* 297: 1189–97.

Garbe, P. L.; Davis, B. J.; Weisfeld, J. S.; Markowitz, L.; Miner, P.; Garrity, F.; Barbaree, J. M.; and Reingold, A. L. 1985. Nosocomial Legionnaires disease—epidemiologic demonstration of cooling towers as a source. *JAMA* 254:521–24.

Glick, T. H.; Gregg, M. B.; Berman, B.; Mallison, G.; Rhodes, W. W.; and Kassanoff, I. 1978. Pontiac fever: An epidemic of unknown etiology in a health department. 1. Clinical and epidemiologic aspects. *Am. J. Epidemiol.* 107:149–160.

Kaufmann, A. K.; McDade, J. E.; Patton, C. M.; Bennett, J. V.; Skaliy, P.; Feeley, J. C.; Anderson, D. C.; Potter, M. E.; Newhouse, V. F.; Gregg, M. B.; and Brachman, P. S. 1981. Pontiac fever: Demonstration of its mode of transmission. *Am. J. Epidemiol.* 114:337–74.

Joly, J. R.; McKinney, R. M.; Tobin, J. O.; Bibb, W. F.; Watkins, I. D.; and Ramsay, D. 1986. Development of a standardized subgrouping scheme for *Legionella pneumophila* serogroup 1 using monoclonal antibodies. *J. Clin. Microbiol.* 23:768–71.

McDade, J. E.; Shepard, C. C.; Fraser, D. W.; Tsai, T. R. [sic]; Redus, M. A.; Dowdle, W. R.; and the Laboratory Investigation Team. 1977.

Legionnaires' disease. Isolation of a bacterium and demonstration of its role in other respiratory disease. *N. Engl. J. Med.* 297:1197–1203.

Plouffe, J. F.; Para, M. F.; Maher, W. E.; Hackman, B.; and Webster, L. 1983. Subtypes of *Legionella pneumophila* serogroup 1 associated with different attack rates. *Lancet* 2:649–50.

Selander, R. K.; McKinney, R. M.; Whittam, T. S.; Bibb, W. F.; Brenner, D. J.; Nolte, F. S.; and Pattison, P. E. 1985. Genetic structure of a population of *Legionella pneumophila*. *J. Bacteriol.* 163:1021–37.

# 11

# Architecture and Commensal Vertebrate Pest Management

STEPHEN C. FRANTZ

Some readers might question the inclusion of the subject of vertebrate pest management in a volume concerned with architecture and microbial pollution. The following poem by John Updike (1977) should help to clarify the relevance and will broadly introduce this chapter.

Rats

A house has rotten places: cellar walls
where mud replaces mortar every rain,
the loosening board that begged for nails in vain,
the sawed-off stairs, and smelly nether halls
the rare repairman never looks behind
and if he did would, disconcerted, find
long spaces, lathed, where dead air grows a scum
of fuzz, and rubble deepens crumb by crumb.

Here they live. Hear them on their boulevards
beneath the attic flooring tread the shards
of panes from long ago, and Fiberglas
fallen to dust, and droppings, and dry clues

Note: The mention of commercial products in this chapter does not represent endorsement by the State of New York, the publisher, or the author.

to crimes no longer news. The villians pass
with scrabbly traffic-noise; their avenues
run parallel to chambers of our own
where we pretend we're clean and all alone.*

The basic thesis is that pest species which live in and around human structures (i.e., commensal or "synanthropic" pests) prefer inaccessible harborage, cause damage to people's belongings, disseminate a host of microorganisms and allergens, and are difficult to remove once established. Rapid urbanization (for much of the world), high population growth, and burgeoning marginal communities, taken together with opportunistic commensal pests, represent a significant public health concern (Kimm, 1986; National Research Council [NRC], 1980; Smith and Gratz, 1984). Furthermore, public health officials are becoming increasingly aware of the role of environmental and genetic factors and transmissible agents, especially viruses (e.g., cytomegalovirus, hepatitis B, Epstein-Barr virus, human parvovirus, and, more recently, human immunodeficiency virus), that have immediate and/or long-term effects on immunocompetency (Dodds, 1987). Hence, subsets of the population at large may exhibit an increased risk relative to such exposures which can be aggravated by more "typical" pathogenic agents including those associated with commensal vertebrates (and arthropods). More attention must be given to architectural intervention, simple or sophisticated, that is compatible with preventive public health. In short, "architects should be accountable to the people who inhabit their buildings" (Kundsin, 1986).

"Architecture is any shelter or enclosure, grand or mean, good or bad, erected at any time, for any social purpose, anywhere, and by any individual or group" (Chadirji, 1986). In contemporary production the processes of building have been segmented into design and implementation; performance task allocations have likewise been separated into designer, manager, and worker. Thus, for the purpose of my thesis, architectural intervention can be identified with the totality of building operations carried out by all of the performers (after Chadirji, 1986). Proper architectural intervention requires

*From *Tossing and Turning,* by John Updike. Copyright © 1977 by John Updike. Reprinted by permission of Alfred A. Knopf, Inc.

appropriate design and quality construction, with follow-up maintenance, in order to short-circuit the commensal pest/human/structure complex. Altering pest environments to make them intolerable for the animals concerned is often the best long-term solution (Areson, 1984; Davis and Jackson, 1981; McCabe, 1966).

This chapter focuses on physical/structural measures that deny pests access to basic life-supporting resources. However, the reader should be apprised that a holistic approach to pest management ("vector control") requires consideration of various interrelated measures including education, sanitation, trapping, and poisoning. For a review of holistic (integrated) pest management concepts, see Cohen (1985), Ebling (1978), Frantz and Davis (in press), Frishman (1982), NRC (1980), and Olkowski and Olkowski (1984). Of primary concern here is the prevention of commensal pest infestations in and on human structures through proper architectural intervention.

## COMMENSAL PESTS

### Definition

A pest (or nuisance) species in the broadest sense is virtually any animal that is not desired in a particular place at a particular time. The desirability or tolerance of a species depends upon the attitudes and perceptions of human residents and varies widely with cultural and socioeconomic differences (Flyger, Leedy, and Franklin, 1984; Kellert, 1976; O'Donnell and VanDruff, 1984). One person may detest tree squirrels and desire to eliminate all that visit his property; on the other hand, his neighbor may enjoy observing squirrels in his yard and may even provide food and shelter for them. However, inside the home (including attic or garage) squirrels can be quite destructive and would be labeled "pest" by most residents. Similar comparisons could be drawn for many animal species. In some parts of the world even common rats may be viewed and fed with pleasure by the public in the urban park habitat (Figure 11.1), while in nearby commercial food warehouses the same species is a significant pest (Figure 11.2).

Our limits of tolerance for a pest species are tempered by aesthetic, economic, and public health considerations depending upon the particular pest situation, the institutions involved, and sanitation and legal standards. When a pest population size can be correlated with

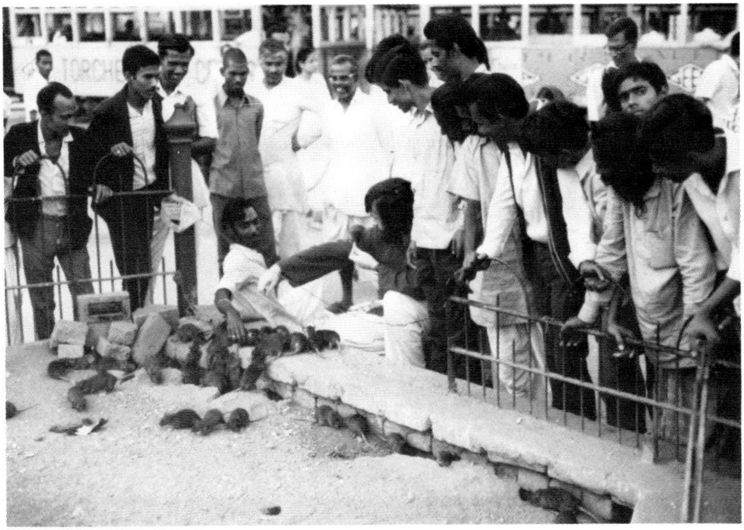

**Figure 11.1.** Feeding wild rats *(Bandicota bengalensis)* in a public park, Calcutta, India. (Photo by S. R. Frantz.)

**Figure 11.2.** Rats (*Bandicota bengalensis* and *B. indica*) eating rice intended for human use; note holes gnawed in bags and rat feces mixed with spilled grain on floor of food grain warehouse, Calcutta, India. (Unless indicated otherwise, all photos by S. C. Frantz.)

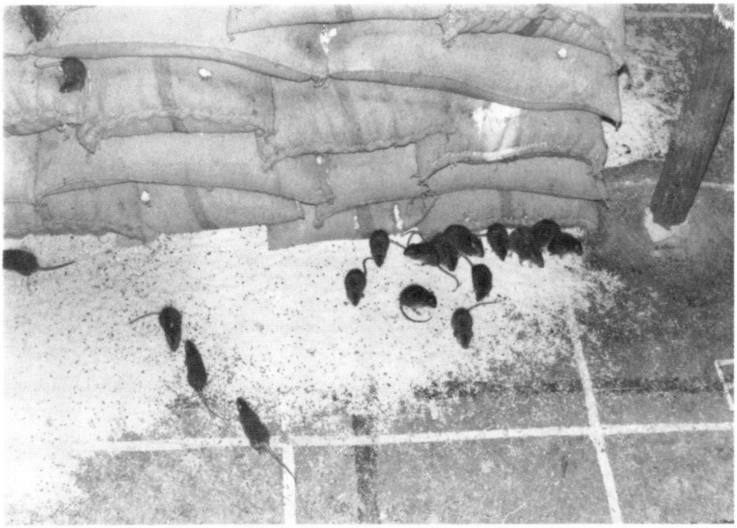

"injury" (i.e., intolerable depredating effect), some intervention is warranted. Obviously, there can be no set standard for all situations. A construction firm may not be alarmed by a rat infestation in a hospital under construction; however, the same infestation could not be permitted in the finished structure. The presence of a single bird inside a food processing plant can result in a costly citation from the U.S. Food and Drug Administration. Although many factors must be considered in outdoor situations, residents commonly define wildlife inside or on a building as a pest situation. Before initiating control, one should always consult the appropriate government authorities to ensure that the target species is not protected—especially with regard to bats and birds.

## SPECIES

A catalog of animals considered to be commensal pest species is beyond the scope of this presentation, but may be reviewed in various publications, including Ebling (1978), Herms and James (1965), Story and Moreland (1982), and NRC (1980). Some ubiquitous arthropod pests include cockroaches, flies, and mosquitoes. Among the most cosmopolitan vertebrate pests are rodents, bats, and birds. This discussion will focus on the latter vertebrate groups, which provide a diversity of problems in the pest/human/structure complex.

Vertebrate species vary widely in their geographic distribution and importance as pests. Commensal rats, mice, and bats are exemplary. The Norway rat *(Rattus norvegicus),* roof rat *(Rattus rattus),* and house mouse *(Mus musculus)* are worldwide household pests, but local distributions are disjointed (Brooks and Rowe, 1979; Davis and Jackson, 1981; Pratt and Brown, 1977). The Norway rat and house mouse are found throughout the United States; the roof rat is restricted to the South and the West Coast. In parts of India, the lesser bandicoot rat *(Bandicota bengalensis)* is the dominant commensal species and displaces *Rattus* (Deoras, 1963; Seal and Banerji, 1969). In Africa, the multimammate rat *(Mastomys natalensis)* is widely distributed south of the Sahara. Recent work has shown that there are at least two distinct genetic species of *Mastomys* (Monath and Johnson, 1986). One (thirty-two chromosomes) is found principally as a commensal animal (particularly when the roof rat is not present) in wet, forested areas. Another (thirty-eight chromosomes) predominates in the savannah bushland. Lassa virus infection occurs in both rats, but the ecologic adaptation of the thirty-two-chromosome *Mastomys* results in greater transmission of Lassa virus to humans in wet climate areas. As with the other vertebrate species considered here, their commensal habits provide the necessary link for zoonosis transmission and is a major cause for concern.

Two of the most widely distributed commensal bat species in the United States are the little brown bat *(Myotis lucifugus)* and the big brown bat *(Eptesicus fuscus)* (Barbour and Davis, 1969; Hill and Smith, 1984). Both species are found in buildings throughout the warm seasons. In the winter, *M. lucifugus* hibernates in caves and deep rock crevices. *E. fuscus* hibernates in similar niches but will also overwinter in houses, with erratic periods of winter activity. Compared with *M. lucifugus, E. fuscus* is larger and has a wider-opening jaw and larger teeth. In New York State, the prevalence of rabies in sick bats submitted for rabies diagnosis is generally greater in *E. fuscus* (5 percent) than in *M. lucifugus* (1 percent) (Frantz and Trimarchi, 1984). The prevalence of rabies also tends to be greater in random collections of naturally occurring populations of *E. fuscus.* This combination of factors results in the big brown bat being considered somewhat more significant than the little brown bat for rabies transmission in New York.

A structure may be occupied by one or more species that fulfill the pest role in different ways. Although Table 11.1 relates to conditions in the United States, the same species (rats, mice, pigeons, starlings, and sparrows) or closely related species (bats and squirrels) occur worldwide. Feral pigeons, common starlings, and house sparrows are the three most common bird pests in much of the world (Areson, 1984; Flyger, Leedy, and Franklin, 1984; Miller, 1975; Nuorteva, 1971; Woldow, 1972). Considerable overlap occurs in ecologic adaptation and crossover/multipest infestations are not uncommon. Sources of information regarding local pest species include government agencies (health, environment, wildlife), schools of public health, university zoology and entomology departments, and professional pest management firms. Note that architectural interventions directed against one vertebrate species may concomitantly prevent the development of other vertebrate and/or arthropod pest situations. In addition, such interventions are long-lasting; recrudescent infestations are not likely to occur in adequately maintained, sanitary buildings.

**Table 11.1** Deleterious Effects of Commensal Vertebrate Pests

| | | | Infestation of Occupied Buildings* | | | | Nuisance/Damage Complaints | | | | | | | | | |
|---|---|---|---|---|---|---|---|---|---|---|---|---|---|---|---|---|
| Species | US Distribution (Excl. Hawaii) | Primary Activity Period | Attic | Living Quarters | Base-ment | Exterior Shell** | Noise | Odor | Feces/ Urine† | Stored Food | Material Goods†† | Struc-tural Damage | Stain/ Deface Building | Ectopara-sites | Bites‡ | Ref.‡‡ |
| BATS | | | | | | | | | | | | | | | | |
| Little brown bat (*M. lucifugus*) | Northern, some southern | twilight, night | x | (x) | — | x | x | x | x | — | — | (x) | x | x | (x) | 2, 4, 5, 8, 12, 16, 19 |
| Big brown bat (*E. fuscus*) | Throughout, excl. parts of FL and TX | twilight, night | x | (x) | x | x | x | x | x | — | — | (x) | x | x | x | 2, 4, 8, 12, 15, 16, 19 |
| Mexican free-tailed bat (*Tadarida brasiliensis*) | Southern, some western | twilight, night | x | — | — | x | x | x | x | — | — | — | x | x | (x) | 2, 15, 16 |
| Yuma myotis (*Myotis yumamensis*) | Western | night | x | — | — | x | — | — | x | — | — | — | — | (x) | (x) | 2, 16 |
| Pallid bat (*Antrozous pallidus*) | Southwestern, some north-western | night | x | — | — | x | — | x | x | — | — | — | — | x | x | 2, 16 |
| RATS | | | | | | | | | | | | | | | | |
| Norway rat (*Rattus norvegicus*) | Throughout | night | (x) | x | x | x | x | x | x | x | x | x | — | x | x | 9, 11, 13, 24 |

| | | | | | | | | | | | | | | | | |
|---|---|---|---|---|---|---|---|---|---|---|---|---|---|---|---|---|
| Roof rat *(Rattus rattus)* | Southern, West Coast | night | x | x | (x) | x | x | x | x | x | x | x | — | x | x | 9, 11, 13, 24 |
| MICE | | | | | | | | | | | | | | | | |
| House mouse *(Mus musculus)* | Throughout | night or day | x | x | x | x | (x) | x | x | x | x | x | — | x | (x) | 9, 11, 13, 24 |
| TREE SQUIRRELS | | | | | | | | | | | | | | | | |
| Eastern gray squirrel *(Sciurus carolinensis)* | Mainly eastern, some western | day | x | (x) | — | x | x | — | x | — | (x) | x | — | x | (x) | 3, 5, 10, 16, 20, 22 |
| Western gray squirrel *(Sciurus griseus)* | West Coast | day | x | — | — | x | x | — | x | — | (x) | x | — | x | (x) | 3, 5, 16, 20 |
| Red squirrel *(Tamiasciurus hudsonicus)* | Northern, some southern and western | day | x | (x) | — | x | x | — | — | — | (x) | x | — | x | (x) | 3, 5, 16, 20, 22 |
| Douglas squirrel *(Tamiasciurus douglasii)* | Western | day | x | — | — | x | x | — | — | — | (x) | x | — | x | (x) | 16, 20 |
| Fox squirrel *(Sciurus niger)* | Eastern, central, some western | day | (x) | — | — | — | x | — | — | — | (x) | x | — | x | (x) | 16, 20, 22 |

**Table 11.1** Deleterious Effects of Commensal Vertebrate Pests (*Continued*)

| | | | Infestation of Occupied Buildings* | | | | Nuisance/Damage Complaints | | | | | | | | | |
|---|---|---|---|---|---|---|---|---|---|---|---|---|---|---|---|---|
| Species | US Distribution (Excl. Hawaii) | Primary Activity Period | Attic | Living Quarters | Base-ment | Exterior Shell** | Noise | Odor | Feces/ Urine† | Stored Food | Material Goods†† | Struc-tural Damage | Stain/ Deface Building | Ectopara-sites | Bites‡ | Ref.‡‡ |
| FLYING SQUIRRELS | | | | | | | | | | | | | | | | |
| Northern flying squirrel (*Glaucomys sabrinus*) | Northern, some southern and western | night | x | (x) | — | x | x | — | — | — | — | (x) | — | x | (x) | 3, 5, 10, 16, 20, 22 |
| Southern flying squirrel (*Glaucomys volans*) | Eastern, central, some western | night | x | (x) | — | x | x | — | — | — | — | (x) | — | x | (x) | 3, 5, 10, 16, 20, 22 |
| BIRDS | | | | | | | | | | | | | | | | |
| Feral pigeon (*Columba livia*) | Throughout | day | x | — | — | x | x | x | x | (x) | (x) | x | x | x | — | 1, 3, 6, 14, 16, 17, 18, 20, 23, 25 |

| | | | | | | | | | | | | | | | | |
|---|---|---|---|---|---|---|---|---|---|---|---|---|---|---|---|---|
| House (English) sparrow *(Passer domesticus)* | Throughout | day | x | (x) | — | x | x | x | x | (x) | (x) | x | x | x | — | 1, 3, 5, 6, 7, 14, 16, 17, 20, 23 |
| Common (European) starling *(Sturnus vulgaris)* | Throughout | day | x | (x) | — | x | x | x | x | (x) | (x) | x | x | x | — | 1, 3, 6, 14, 16, 17, 20, 21, 23 |

*Parentheses indicates not a primary effect, occasional.

**May include eaves, spaces between walls and floors, in and behind rain gutters, behind chimney.

†Accumulation, adulteration, contamination, etc.

††Damage due to chewing, gnawing, pecking, etc.

‡Of the vertebrate pest.

‡‡Numbers refer to these author/date citations; see references for full citation.

1. Areson (1984)
2. Barbour and Davis (1969)
3. Caslick and Decker (1981)
4. Constantine (1970)
5. Cooperative Extension (1979)
6. Ebling (1978)
7. Erz (1966)
8. Fenton (1983)
9. Fitzwater (1979)
10. Flyger et al. (1984)
11. Frantz and Davis (in press)
12. Frantz and Trimarchi (1984)
13. Frishman (1982)
14. Geis (1976a and b)
15. Greenhall (1982)
16. Hall and Kelson (1959)
17. Hartlage et al. (1984)
18. Johnsen (1982)
19. Kunz (1982)
20. Marsh and Howard (1982)
21. Miller (1975)
22. NPCA (1980)
23. Nuorteva (1971)
24. Pratt and Brown (1977)
25. Woldow (1972)

## General Habits

In order to apply preventive architectural interventions one must recognize what species represent problems not only geographically but *where* on or in a structure. Of the animals listed (Table 11.1) bats and birds are the only ones capable of true flight. Because of their increased mobility, they can be expected to infest somewhat different portions of structures than the other species. In fact, bats and birds both tend to prefer the higher, less-accessible areas of buildings—indoors and/or outdoors. Inadvertently, they occasionally wander into human living quarters but do not "roost" there.

Because of their colonial habits, aggregates of several hundred bats are not uncommon in attics (Figure 11.3) and roof areas. However, it should be noted that bats use nearly any secluded space provided by a building. Big brown bats also hibernate in basements, but this is generally not a summer roost site.

Birds usually seek exterior niches. Feral pigeons prefer roofs and

**Figure 11.3.** Portion of bat colony *(Myotis lucifugus)* roosting on roof beams in church attic, North Greenbush, N.Y.

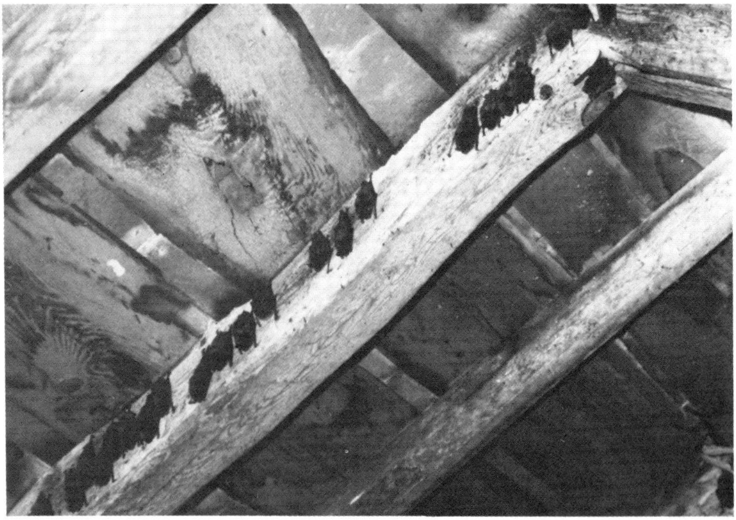

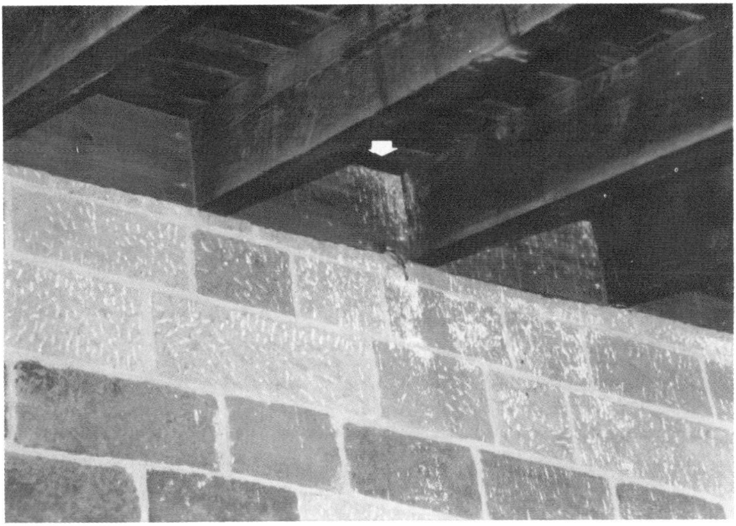

**Figure 11.4.** Birds *(Passer domesticus)* nesting in crevice of open eaves; note droppings on wall and at joists. National historic site, New York City.

high ledges. Common starlings nest in eaves, roofs, and other structures; window ledges are used in cold weather. House sparrows use any sort of cavity or hollow in buildings including eaves (Figure 11.4) and rain gutters.

Flying squirrels cannot fly, but do glide considerable distances to reach attics and eaves from nearby trees or other structures. Tree squirrels and roof rats also infest upper areas of buildings, gaining access via trees, ornamental shrubbery, cables and conduits, or nearby buildings from which they can jump or climb. Squirrels use attic areas, and also uninhabited cabins and cottages, for shelter and food storage especially during cold seasons.

The roof rat also infests other floors of buildings, but tends to prefer upper levels and roof areas (Figure 11.5) especially when more dominant species (e.g., Norway rat) are present elsewhere. House mice are also very good climbers and use most floors of buildings. The heavier, less nimble Norway rat (and lesser bandicoot rat) tends to stay on ground levels (Figure 11.6) and basements, but it also

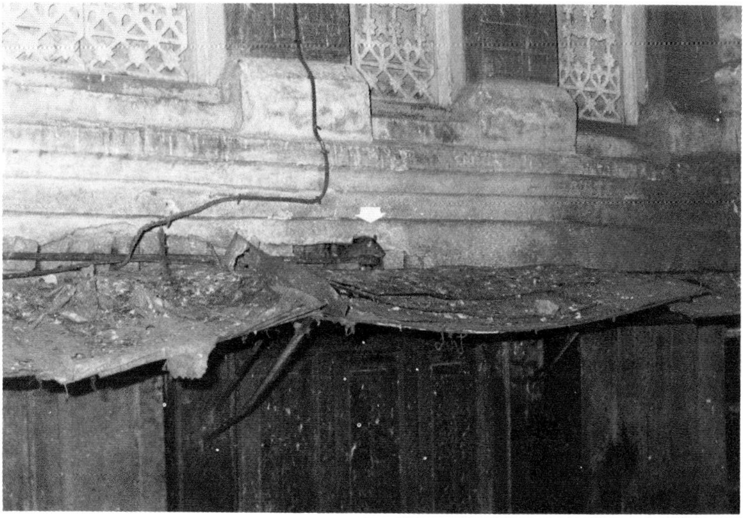

**Figure 11.5.** Rat (*Rattus rattus brunneus*—a type of "roof" rat), at hole in wall of second floor, feeds on bird droppings and other ejecta that accumulates on roof overhang and ledges. Residential/commercial building, Kathmandu, Nepal.

**Figure 11.6.** Rats *(Rattus norvegicus)* feed on garbage and enter opening around conduits in foundation wall of residential compound, Kuwait City, Kuwait.

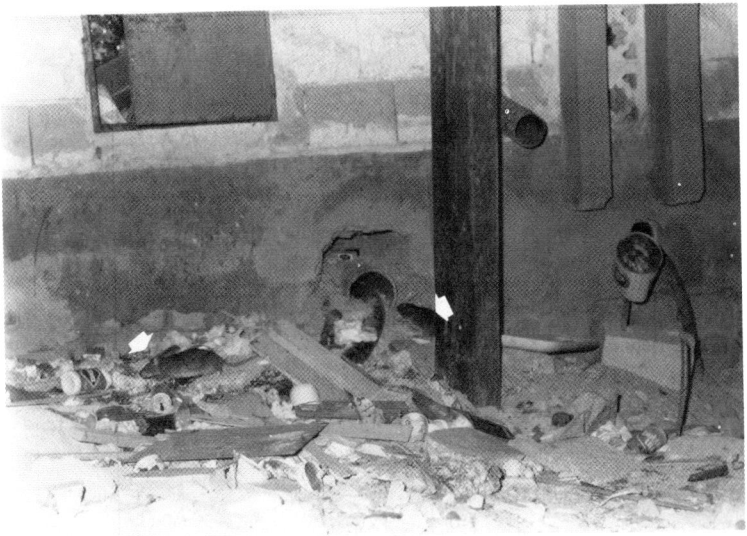

climbs stairs and crosses roofs. When necessary, both species show considerable agility in climbing pipes and wires to reach food or harborage.

## SIGNIFICANCE OF PROBLEM

### Infestation Level

Commensal pest situations are not isolated, unpredictable events that merely demonstrate the perversity of nature. They are a function of human design—industrial/agricultural production systems, ornamental landscapes, and architecture. Pests occur virtually everywhere, but their overall population densities tend to increase along the gradient of urbanization (NRC, 1980; O'Donnell and VanDruff, 1984; Tangley, 1986). This tendency can be attributed to common ecologic characteristics that favor them, to varying degrees, in human settlements. Two principal items are favorable architecture for shelter, breeding, and access to food; and abundant food and water resources in refuse, lawns or parks, stored food, and deliberate feeding. Urbanized areas also tend to be a few degrees warmer than the surrounding countryside; such areas also provide shelter from wind and have less species diversity and reduced natural predation. Sample data for rats and mice are described in the following paragraphs.

A 1974 government survey revealed that 3.6 percent of all occupied housing units in the United States and nearly 13 percent of units with structural defects showed some presence of vermin (NRC, 1980). Vermin ranked second among eighteen specific defects cited, and while all other defects declined over the next decade the units with vermin increased 17 percent. In Waterbury, Connecticut, a 1977 sample revealed nearly 40 percent of the households infested with vermin; mice (13–17 percent) and rats (3–5 percent) ranked second and third, respectively (Zahner et al., 1985). A 1982–83 World Health Organization (WHO) survey of twenty-six major urban areas worldwide found that 85 percent of the areas had vectorborne disease present or threatening (Smith and Gratz, 1984). Rats and mice, the only principal vertebrate pests reported, were problems in 73 percent of the cities surveyed. In a study in thirteen communities of metropolitan Syracuse, New York, 30.3 percent of upper-income

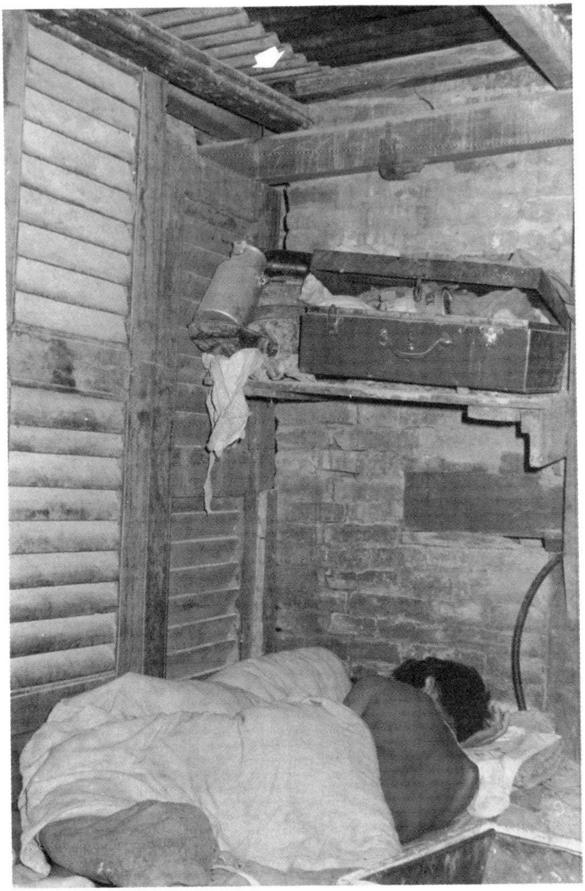

**Figure 11.7.** Rat *(R. r. brunneus)* rests on roof beams directly above sleeping workers. Grain mill cum residence, Kathmandu, Nepal.

households reported a vertebrate pest problem (O'Donnell and VanDruff, 1984).

Of species listed in Table 11.1, rats and mice have undoubtedly achieved the greatest degree of year-round commensalism and may actually cohabit with humans, especially in poorer-quality dwellings (Figure 11.7). Hopkins (1974) found that 16 percent of premises in degraded areas of twenty major cities in the United States in 1969 showed at least exterior rat infestation. Rodents, primarily rats and mice, currently comprise 17 percent of the total pest control market in the United States (Mix, 1986b).

Drummond (1973) reported an average of 1 percent of all urban properties in Britain to be infested with rats and/or mice at any moment in time. By comparison, a mean of 25.7 percent of properties (in more than 400 localities) were infested in Lower Saxony, West Germany. The mean rodent infestation level (before control measures) in premises throughout Budapest, Hungary, was estimated in 1970 to be 32.8 percent; in the city center 100 percent infestation was reported (Bajomi and Sasvari, 1986).

In some developing countries, infestation rates may be generally higher. Observations by Drummond (1974) indicated rat- and/or mice-infested properties as follows: roughly 90–100 percent in Bombay, India, and in Rangoon, Burma; 38.2 percent in Kowloon, Hong Kong. Frantz (1974) reported a mean of 70.0 percent (range = 50–87 percent) of properties in four Nepalese communities to be infested with rats, mice, and/or shrews. In a survey of eighteen districts of Kuwait, the rodent infestation rate averaged 70 percent (range = 38.2–93.8 percent) of premises surveyed prior to control (Rennison, 1981).

## Deleterious Effects

From the architectural viewpoint, it is clear that commensal vertebrate pests are very opportunistic (Table 11.1). Bats, rats, mice, squirrels, and birds collectively utilize niches that are indoors (dwellings, outbuildings, warehouses), semienclosed (loading docks, entrance foyers), partially sheltered (porches, carports, pavilions, highway underpasses), and open structural areas (window shutters, signs, ledges, windowsills). Once there, the mere presence of active animals in and on buildings can have numerous interrelated, deleterious (economic and aesthetic) effects, often intertwined with public health relationships (see Tables 11.1 and 11.2). Since people spend most of their time indoors, at least in some cultures (Leonard, 1986), exposure to deleterious effects is chronic and the public health impact may be exacerbated.

Reported problems with vertebrate infestations are discussed in the following paragraphs (notations are given in parentheses where limited species are involved).

**Table 11.2** Selected Zoonoses Associated with Commensal Vertebrates Pests*

| Zoonosis | Distribution | Transmission to Humans: Cat.** | Transmission to Humans: Route | Bats | Rats | Mice | Tree Squirrel | Flying Squirrel | Feral Pigeons | Common (European) Starlings | House (English) Sparrows | Ref.† |
|---|---|---|---|---|---|---|---|---|---|---|---|---|
| BACTERIAL | | | | | | | | | | | | |
| Leptospirosis (Weil's disease, hemorrhagic jaundice) | Worldwide | 1 | Infective rodent urine ingested or urine-contaminated food/water/soil contacts broken skin or mucosa | — | x | x | (x) | — | — | — | — | 2, 4, 15, 17, 27, 28 |
| Murine plague (pest, Black Death) | Worldwide (sporadic); urban in Africa, Burma, S. Vietnam | 2(1) | Infective flea bite; handling infective rodent tissues | — | x | — | (x) | — | — | — | — | 2, 9, 15, 27, 28, 29 |
| Psittacosis (ornithosis, parrot fever) | Worldwide | 1 | Inhalation of desiccated aerosolized bird feces | — | — | — | — | — | x | — | x | 2, 11, 17 |
| Rat bite fever (Haverhill fever and Sodoku) | Worldwide | 1 | Infective rat bite (risk of secondary infection and tetanus); ingestion of food contaminated with infective secretions | — | x | (x) | — | — | — | — | — | 2, 11, 22, 24, 27, 28 |

| | | | | | | | | | | | | |
|---|---|---|---|---|---|---|---|---|---|---|---|---|
| Salmonellosis | Worldwide | 1 | Direct and/or indirect fecal contamination of food/water | — | x | x | — | — | x | x | x | 7, 9, 15, 20, 27, 28 |
| Tickborne relapsing fever | Western USA and Canada; Central and South America | 2 | Bite of infective rodent tick;†† contamination of skin/wound with coxal fluid | — | x | — | x | — | — | — | — | 2, 9, 13, 16, 17 |
| Yersiniosis (pseudotuberculosis) | Worldwide | 1 | Infective fecal contamination of food/water | — | x | (x) | — | — | x | — | x | 6, 7, 9, 15, 27, 28 |
| RICKETTSIAL (BACTERIA) | | | | | | | | | | | | |
| Squirrel typhus (epidemic/ fleaborne t.) | Eastern USA | 2 | Probably infective flea bite; infective flea/feces contamination of bite wound or other broken skin; inhalation of desiccated, infective flea feces | — | — | — | — | x | — | — | — | 2, 3, 12, 17, 18, 19, 25 |
| Murine typhus (endemic t.) | Worldwide | 2 | Infective flea feces contaminate bite (flea) wound or other broken skin or mucosa, or are inhaled or ingested | — | x | x | (x) | — | — | — | — | 1, 2, 9, 26, 28 |

**Table 11.2** Selected Zoonoses Associated with Commensal Vertebrates Pests* *(Continued)*

| Zoonosis | Distribution | Transmission to Humans | | Bats | Rats | Mice | Tree Squirrel | Flying Squirrel | Feral Pigeons | Common (European) Starlings | House (English) Sparrows | Ref.† |
|---|---|---|---|---|---|---|---|---|---|---|---|---|
| | | Cat.** | Route | | | | | | | | | |
| Rickettsialpox (vesicular rickettsiosis) | North America, USSR, Korea, So. Africa | 2 | Bite of infective mite | — | — | x | — | — | — | — | — | 1, 2, 17 |
| HELMINTHIC | | | | | | | | | | | | |
| Hepatic capillariasis (capillariasis) | Americas, Hawaii, India, Turkey, Africa, Japan | 1 | Embryonated nematode eggs (released from decomposed rodent body) ingested in contaminated food/water/soil | — | x | x | x | — | — | — | — | 2, 10, 28 |
| Hymenolepis (mouse tapeworm) infection | Worldwide | 1 | Helminth eggs ingested with rodent fecal-contaminated grain and other foods; may involve ingestion of grain beetles | — | x | x | — | — | — | — | — | 17, 28 |
| MYCOTIC | | | | | | | | | | | | |
| Cryptococcosis (torulosis, European blastomycosis) | Worldwide (sporadic) | 1 | Inhalation of desiccated, aerosolized bird feces | — | — | — | — | — | x | — | — | 2, 9, 22 |

| | | | | | | | | | | | |
|---|---|---|---|---|---|---|---|---|---|---|---|
| Histoplasmosis | Worldwide | 1 | Inhalation of spores in desiccated, aerosolized feces; ingestion of contaminated food/soil | x | — | — | — | — | x | x | — | 2, 4, 6, 9, 14, 17, 22 |
| PROTOZOAN | | | | | | | | | | | | |
| Amebiasis (amebic dysentery) | Worldwide | 1 | Ingestion of food/ water contaminated with infective rodent feces | — | x | — | — | — | — | — | — | 2, 9, 16, 28 |
| American trypanosomiasis (Chagas disease) | Southern USA, Central and South America | 2 | Infective feces of conenose bugs (Reduviidae) contaminate bite (bug) wound, mucosa, or other broken skin | (x) | x | x | — | — | x | — | — | 2, 4, 9, 19, 23, 28 |
| VIRAL | | | | | | | | | | | | |
| Rabies | approx. worldwide | 1 | Bat bite: contamination of mucosa or broken skin with infective bat saliva or central nervous system tissue | x | — | — | — | — | — | — | — | 2, 4, 12, 17, 22 |
| St. Louis encephalitis | Americas, Caribbean | 2 | Infective mosquito bite | x | — | — | — | — | x | — | x | 2, 9, 17 |
| Western equine encephalitis | Americas | 2 | Infective mosquito bite | x | — | — | (x) | — | x | — | x | 6, 7, 9, 17 |

**Table 11.2** Selected Zoonoses Associated with Commensal Vertebrates Pests* (*Continued*)

| Zoonosis | Distribution | Transmission to Humans: Cat.** | Transmission to Humans: Route | Bats | Rats | Mice | Tree Squirrel | Flying Squirrel | Feral Pigeons | Common (European) Starlings | House (English) Sparrows | Ref.† |
|---|---|---|---|---|---|---|---|---|---|---|---|---|
| Lymphocytic-choriomeningitis | Worldwide | 1 | Ingestion of infective rodent urine, saliva, or feces directly or in contaminated food; inhalation of infective aerosolized urine or feces | — | (x) | x | — | — | — | — | — | 2, 6, 15, 17, 27 |
| Bolivian hemorrhagic fever (Machupo) | Bolivia | 1 | Ingestion of infective mouse urine | — | — | x | — | — | — | — | — | 2, 17, 29 |
| Lassa fever | West Africa | 1 | Ingestion of infective rodent urine or saliva | — | x | — | — | — | — | — | — | 2, 17, 28, 29 |

*Parentheses under pest species indicates incidental or probable minor role.

**Category 1 = direct or indirect transmission from vertebrate animal to humans; 2 = arthropod vector transmits causative agent from vertebrate animal to humans.

†Numbers refer to these author/date citations; see references for complete citation.

1. Azad (1986)
2. Benenson (1975)
3. CDC (1982)
4. Constantine (1970)
5. Courtsal (1983)
6. Davis et al., (1970)
7. Davis et al., (1971)
8. Dias and Dias (1982)
9. Ebling (1978)
10. Farhang-Azad (1977)
11. Fitzwater (1983)
12. Flyger et al., (1984)
13. Gelman (1961)
14. George and Penn (1986)
15. Gratz (1969)
16. Herms and James (1965)
17. Last (1986)
18. Lauer and Sonenshine (1978)
19. McDade et al., (1980)
20. Marsh and Howard (1982)
21. Moretti et al., (1980)
22. NRC (1980)
23. Olsen (1974)
24. Scott (1966)
25. Sonenshine et al., (1978)
26. Traub et al., (1978)
27. Velimirovic (1969)
28. Weber (1982)
29. WHO (1974)

††In western USA and western Canada = *Ornithodoros hermsi* (on tree squirrels and chipmunks); for Central and South America = *O. rudis* (on rats); both ticks readily feed on humans and are closely associated with commensal rodents, unlike most vectors for relapsing fever.

### *Noise*

Disturbing sounds may be heard from vocalizations (bat, rats/mice, birds); gnawing (rats/mice, squirrels); and scratching, crawling, or climbing in attics and eaves (all), in walls and between floors (bats, rodents), and on exterior ledges (birds).

### *Feces/Urine*

Excrement produces unpleasant odors as it ferments and decomposes in attics and voids; similar problems occur when animals die in out-of-reach areas. It has been suggested by Sterling (1985) that odors can act as stressors (a negative health effect) and thus increase one's susceptibility to other agents. Odor also attracts arthropods (e.g., cockroaches, dermestid beetles) which may subsequently invade other parts of a building.

Feces and urine raise the humidity of enclosed spaces, promote wood deterioration, and provide a medium for proliferation of microorganisms, some of which are pathogenic in humans. As a point of reference, in one study (Frantz and Davis, in press), Norway rats and roof rats averaged, respectively, 37 and 59 droppings per animal per day. The house mouse is reported to excrete 50 or more droppings daily (Rowe, 1981). A pair of rats voids approximately 5.7 L urine per year (Bullard and Shuyler, 1983).

Accumulation of excrement (Figure 11.8) fills spaces between floors and walls and/or collapses ceilings (bats) or rain gutters (birds). Also, it interferes with operation of doors, windows, and automatic fire/smoke detectors (birds). On floors, steps, and ladders, it creates safety hazards (bats, birds). Excrement may also adulterate stored food and other goods or commercial products, making them unusable. Contamination of food (Figure 11.2), food preparation surfaces (Figure 11.9), and equipment results in health hazards. Excrement accumulation causes staining of ceilings (bats, squirrels), soffits, and siding (bats, birds), producing generally unsightly and unsanitary conditions. High acid content speeds the deterioration of roof shingles and corrodes masonry (birds) and metal and polished or painted surfaces (bats, birds).

Bird droppings tend to cover and deface sides of buildings, windowsills, ledges, and statuary (Figures 11.4 and 11.5). Droppings and nesting material in rain gutters and on roofs may cause water to back

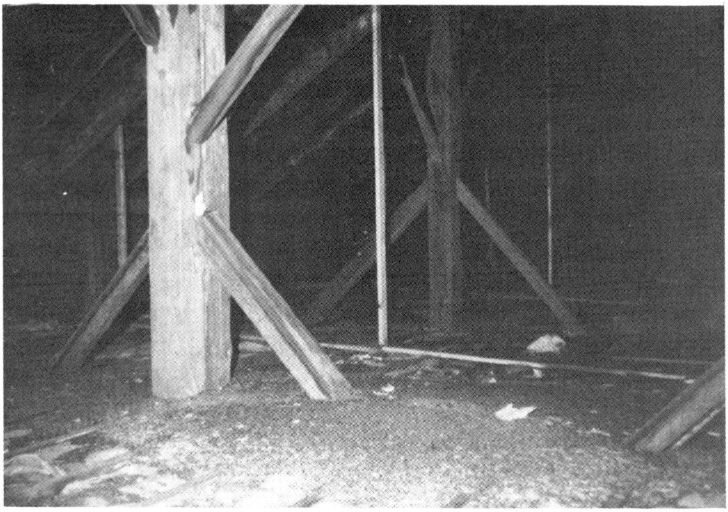

**Figure 11.8.** Heavy accumulation of bat guano on attic "floor" insulation of church, North Greenbush, N.Y.

**Figure 11.9.** Mouse fecal droppings and urine contaminate kitchen countertop in a residence, Hillsgrove, Penn.

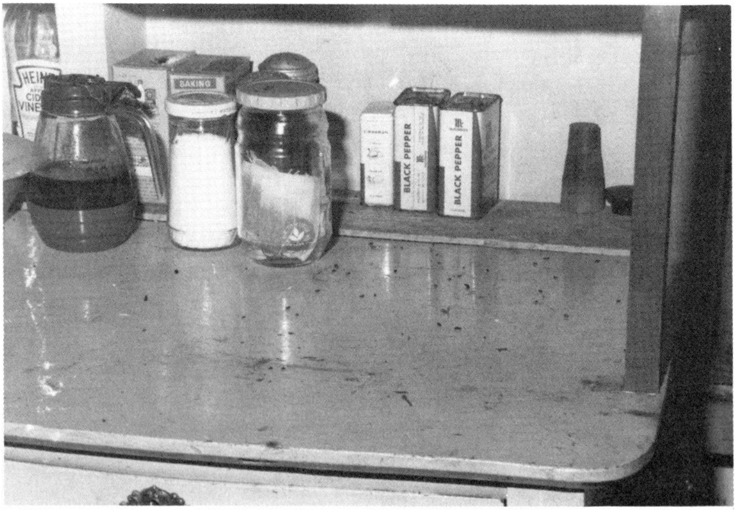

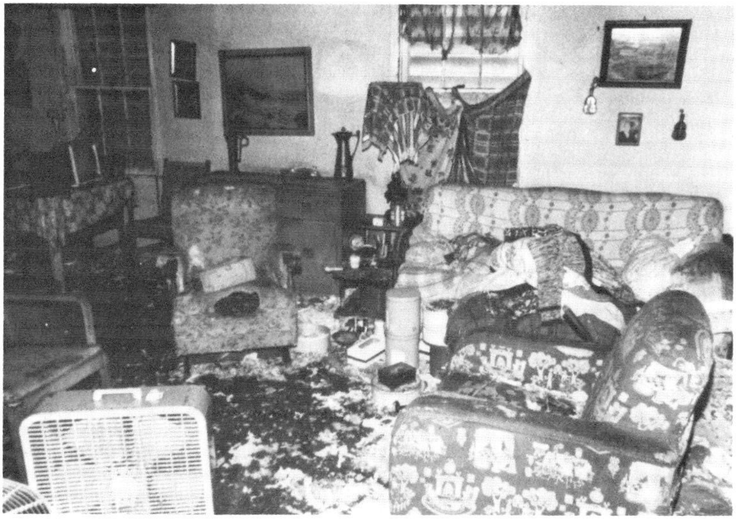

**Figure 11.10.** Residential interior destroyed by large infestation of roof rats. Residential bungalow, Miami. (Photo courtesy of A. Ros, Dade County Dept. of Public Health, Miami.)

up and subsequent roof leaks. Bats urinate and defecate in flight, causing multiple spotting and staining on sides of buildings, windows, patio furniture, and so on near their entrance holes.

### *Food*

Consumption and destruction of human food is most significant when rats and mice live in dwellings, food processing and handling establishments, warehouses, and granaries (Figure 11.2). Birds play important roles primarily at agricultural facilities, though warehouse infestations also occur.

### *Material Goods and Structural Damage*

Damage to material goods and structural integrity arise from animals' gnawing, chewing, pecking, scratching, or burrowing into packaged goods, clothing, furniture, walls, window and door frames, support beams, and so on (Figure 11.10). Holes made in walls, insulation, floors, and roofs reduce the energy-efficiency of buildings and provide entry for other vertebrate and arthropod pest species (rats/mice, squirrels). When insulation is chewed or pecked from electrical wires and telephone cables, it results in loss of power or communications; it may even cause fires (rats/mice, squirrels, birds).

Nesting material in and around light fixtures, heaters, and chimneys is a fire hazard (rats/mice, squirrels, birds). Birds and rats have been reported to bring smoldering cigarettes into their nests (Areson, 1984; Wolcott and Vincent, 1975). Nests built in air handling ducts, air intakes, or kitchen vent pipes (and even on windowsills and building ledges) may block the air flow (Figure 11.11) and/or rain down nesting material, excreta, and ectoparasites on the unfortunate residents. Such effluvium is rich in animal dander, insect fragments, and various microorganisms and can result in bioaerosols of public health significance (Burge, 1985; Olfert, 1986; Smith, 1985; Squires, 1986). Bullard (1983) reports that a rat naturally sheds its half-million body hairs twice per annum. Each of its droppings may also contain 100–200 hair fragments ingested by the rat during grooming. Hairs from these sources (as well as feathers from birds) may drift through a building on normal air currents or through forced-air heating, ventilating, and air-conditioning systems. Additionally, droplets emanating from commensal animals (mouth or nose during vocalization, coughing, and sneezing; or from the excretory system) can dry and form droplet nuclei (bacterial or viral residues) which can remain suspended in air for long periods of time (Feeley, 1985; Smith, 1985). Exposure to these various particulates is heightened in individuals who work directly under roost or nest sites of commensal vertebrate pests.

Air-conditioner coils can become plugged with bird feathers, rodent fur, and/or decomposing remains of animals that were chopped up by the fan blades. Bats are similarly destroyed in attic ventilation fans. When such events occur near or in air intake vents (or windows), biologic pollutants can be circulated throughout a structure.

### *Ectoparasites*

Some vertebrate pests' ectoparasites (mainly fleas, mites, and ticks) readily feed on humans and may function as zoonosis vectors. Humans are commonly bitten when in an area (e.g., attic) from which animals have recently departed or been removed. Hence,

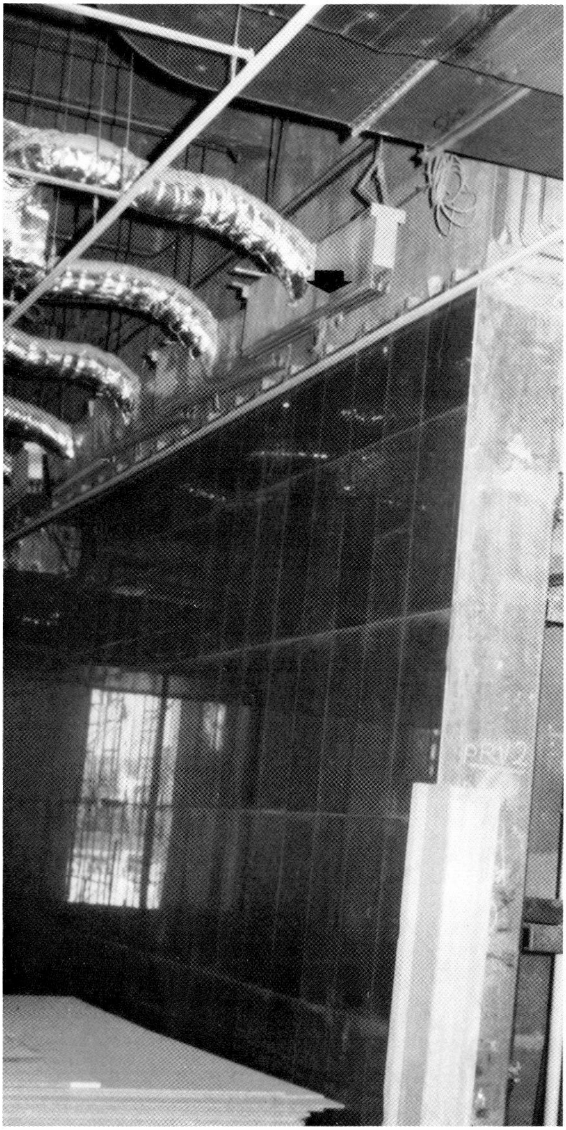

**Figure 11.11.** Bird nesting material hangs from air-conditioner outlet in new office complex (ground floor), Baghdad, Iraq.

insecticidal treatments for ectoparasites is an important adjunct to vertebrate pest management.

### *Bites and Other Hazards*

Bites from commensal vertebrates rarely occur unless the animal is cornered, startled, or carelessly handled. Some rats may seek out food-tainted humans (young or incapacitated) as part of their foraging activity (Scott, 1966). Bats in the furious state of rabies infection may bite other animals or people. When someone is working high on a ladder, windowsill, building ledge, or so on, an escaping bat, bird, or rodent may startle the person, resulting in a fall.

## Public Health Considerations

In 1980, it was estimated that annually in the United States alone, vertebrate and arthropod pests cause at least 100 to 300 deaths and 20,000 cases of disabling disease and injury (NRC, 1980). The actual toll would be considerably greater since the pathologies in question are often not recognized, diagnosed, or related directly to pest species. Additionally, many other people suffer pain, annoyance, disfigurement, emotional distress, or disabling conditions resulting from bites, stings (of arthropods), or physical reactions to pest species and their excreta, dander, hair, and decomposed bodies (Brooks and Rowe, 1979; Burge, 1984; Last, 1986; NRC, 1980; Olfert, 1986; Wolcott and Vincent, 1975). In one study (Zahner et al., 1985), rats in dwellings consistently were shown to have the greatest impact on residents' psychologic well-being. Unpleasant odors (e.g., from excreta accumulation) can function as stressors (Sterling, 1985). Another whole class of health problems could be cited if we also examined chronic effects of the pesticides used in attempts to control pests in and around buildings (Diamond and Grimsrud, 1984; NRC, 1980; Seligmann, 1982; Sterling, 1985). "We need to consider how to keep pesticides out of the environment in order to reduce building sickness," suggested R. Gold of the University of Nebraska (Mix, 1986a). Obviously, worldwide statistics for pest/public health issues would be staggering.

With a global perspective, Table 11.2 reviews selected zoonoses associated with some commensal bats, rodents, and birds. Zoonoses are infections or infectious diseases transmissible under natural conditions from vertebrate animals to humans or other vertebrates (Brooks and Rowe, 1979). The risk of exposure to humans increases when the animal source lives in close proximity on and in buildings. Details of each condition can be found in the references provided. Many of the zoonoses are worldwide in distribution or nearly so, (e.g., leptospirosis, salmonellosis, murine typhus, histoplasmosis) while others are quite limited (e.g., Bolivian hemorrhagic fever, squirrel typhus).

Some causative agents are transmitted directly from animals to humans via a bite (i.e., with rat bite fever and rabies). In other cases, the agent may be inhaled and/or ingested in dust, food, water, or soil contaminated with urine, feces, or other bodily secretions or residue of pests (i.e., with leptospirosis, psittacosis, salmonellosis, yersiniosis, hepatic capillariasis, hymenolepis infection, cryptococcosis, histoplasmosis, amebiasis, lymphocytic-choriomeningitis, Bolivian hemorrhagic fever, and Lassa fever—see Figures 11.12 and 11.13). Some zoonoses typically require an arthropod vector to carry the causative agent (via a bite, infective fecal- or crushed tissue-contamination of mucosa or broken skin) from animals to humans (as in bubonic plague, tickborne relapsing fever, squirrel typhus, murine typhus, rickettsialpox, American trypanosomiasis, St. Louis encephalitis, and western equine encephalitis). With some zoonoses, the vertebrate becomes ill (and dies) and thus provides some warning sign (e.g., murine plague, rabies). In others, there is no apparent infection in the maintenance species, hence no warning (e.g., leptospirosis, tickborne relapsing fever, histoplasmosis) with possible long-term exposure of humans in buildings.

The involvement of animals as a source of infection for humans depends upon numerous variables, including their numbers, their degree of commensalism and (where appropriate) the arthropod vector species that predominates in an area. Other factors include potential synergistic or antagonistic interrelationships between zoonotic agents either abetting or negating the probability of concurrent transmission. Some zoonoses in Table 11.2 are strongly associated with the vertebrates listed (e.g., psittacosis/pigeons; rat bite fever/rats; rickettsialpox/mice; Lassa fever/rats) and others may involve additional animals to those listed (e.g., salmonellosis, American trypanosomiasis, western equine encephalitis). It must also be noted that although feral pigeons, common starlings, and house sparrows

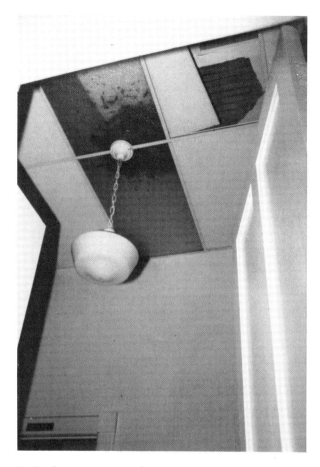

**Figure 11.12.** Bat guano accumulation on dropped ceiling filters down into office space below. Office building, Chatham Center, N.Y.

each represent one species, the other groups (e.g., bats, rats, squirrels) may involve numerous species. The following examples should help to clarify some of the complex relationships.

### *Murine Plague*

Historically, plague has had a major effect on human populations worldwide. An estimated one-fourth to one-third of the European

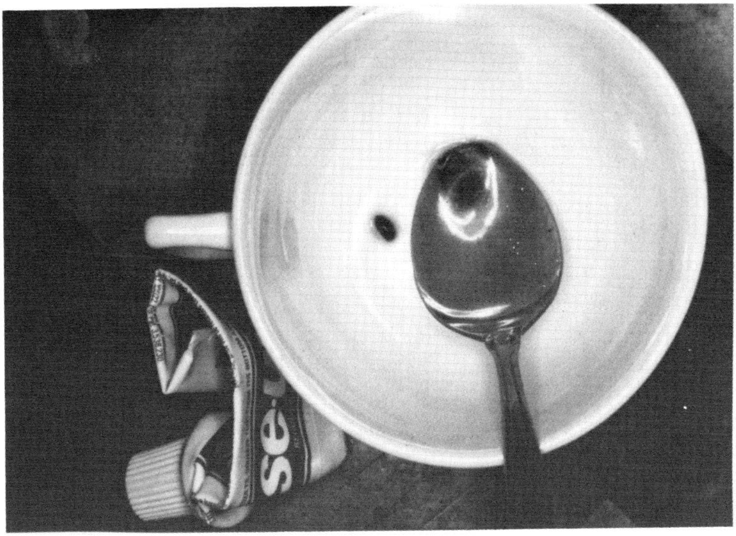

**Figure 11.13.** Mouse droppings in coffee cup could be accidentally ingested. Residence, Hillsgrove, Penn.

population was destroyed by the Black Death in the fourteenth century. Although commensal rats (i.e., *Rattus*) were apparently rare and erratically dispersed both geographically and temporally at the time of the Black Death, *Rattus* has played a major role in other plague epidemics, for example those in India, Italy, England, and the United States (Davis, 1986). Plague persists as a global public health problem because of the continued human contact with infected commensal and wild rodents (Benenson, 1975; Poland, 1986). Plague in wild rodents currently exists in many countries including the western third of the United States. Human plague associated with commensal rodents is more limited though important in some parts of the world, including Vietnam, Burma, and Africa. Murine plague might be expected to appear in areas of the world where it has not been previously recognized when stable ecologic features are disrupted by major developments (e.g., urbanization projects, war) which bring infected wild rodents in close proximity to commensal rats and human activity or dwellings.

### *Tickborne Relapsing Fever*

The diagnosis of relapsing fever is often not considered because the patient may develop clinical illness several days to a week or more after departing from tick-infested areas (Chin, 1986). The disease occurs sporadically or in small outbreaks.

In the western United States and western Canada the tick vector *(Ornithodoros hermsi)* lives in close association with tree squirrels and chipmunks which typically nest in trees or decaying tree stumps (Gelman, 1961). These rodents often move into deserted mountain cabins and cottages during cold weather and carry their infected ticks with them. Once established in a dwelling, the ticks can remain there (without food) for years, remain infective during this period, and pass the infection transovarially to progeny. The danger occurs when vacationers, hunters, and others enter these dwellings and are bitten by infective ticks from rodent nests built in, on, or under the cabins.

In warmer climates, the tick/rodent/human association occurs all year, resulting in a more even distribution of relapsing fever cases over the entire year (Gelman, 1961). Such is the situation with the tick *O. rudis,* the primary vector of endemic tickborne disease in Central and South America. This tick enters human dwellings on rats and, at times, may become responsible for epidemics of the disease.

The control of tickborne relapsing fever in endemic areas depends on the habits of the rodent and human hosts and the tick vector. Preventive measures include elimination of tick populations in dwellings by rodent-proofing and by application of an appropriate residual insecticide (Chin, 1986; Gelman, 1961; Herms and James, 1965).

### *Squirrel Typhus (Epidemic/Fleaborne Typhus)*

Classical epidemic typhus has been one of the great scourges of humankind. Although it has largely disappeared, endemic foci exist in Africa, Central and South America, Eastern Europe, and numerous countries of Asia (Benenson, 1975; Emmons, 1986). The causative agent of epidemic typhus classically has involved only humans and the body louse, with humans being the long-term reservoir. However, flying squirrels have now been recognized as the first extrahuman reservoir of this organism (Bozeman et al., 1975; Sonenshine et al., 1978; Woodman et al., 1977). Human infections have recently been recognized from this source in the eastern United States with fleas as the probable vector (CDC, 1982; McDade et al., 1980). The flying squirrel infests human dwellings (attics or boxed eaves usually) mainly during the colder seasons. Such infestations often go unrecognized because the animal is nocturnal. Flying squirrels have not been implicated in the transmission of other zoonoses to humans. In areas where typhus is known in flying squirrels, they should be denied access to human structures.

### *Rabies*

Rabies is an acute infectious disease of the central nervous system with nearly worldwide distribution (Great Britain, Australia, and some Pacific islands excluded) (Constantine, 1970). All warm-blooded animals are susceptible, but it is most commonly observed in wild and domestic carnivorous mammals. Bat rabies has been reported throughout the contiguous United States and most provinces of Canada; it has been isolated from all of the forty North American bat species that have been adequately sampled (Constantine, 1979). Bat rabies has also been found in many countries of Central and South America, Europe, and Asia. Since 1973, in New York State (with a very active rabies surveillance program) more bats than any other animal have been found to be rabid; nearly all of those confirmed rabid are in the two commensal species, *E. fuscus* and *M. lucifugus*. Commensal bats are also implicated in other parts of the world though general prevalence rates are unknown. It is important to remember, however, that most bats are healthy and should be considered valuable factors in the environment (Fenton, 1983; Greenhall, 1982; Hill and Smith, 1984; Kunz, 1982). Extensive surveys for rabies in asymptomatic bats in the United States usually reveal infection rates of 0.5 percent or less (Constantine, 1970). In fact, the finding of one rabid bat in a colony does not imply that the remaining animals are rabid and the probability of immediately finding others is small (Trimarchi and Debbie, 1977).

The public health impact of bat rabies arises from the many human and companion animal exposures (contacts with bats) each year, difficult decisions regarding postexposure prophylaxis, and mandatory confinement or destruction of unvaccinated pets. When an exposure occurs and the bat escapes, it must be assumed that the bat was rabid and one must proceed with the medical/legal consequences. Probably the most common impact is the psychologic trauma of these bat-contact situations and the chronic anxiety of "living with" the daily threat of rabies from bats roosting in one's residence. The deaths of a Finnish bat researcher (from a rabies-type virus after being bitten by a bat fifty-one days earlier—Lumio et al., 1986) and a young Michigan girl (from rabies after an apparent bat bite several months earlier—CDC, 1983) underscore the importance of preventing direct human contact with bats. Human and companion animal contacts with bats are frequently a result of the commensal habits of bats. Therefore, an important focus of preventive rabies measures is the bat-proofing of buildings where significant risk occurs (e.g., nursery schools, hospitals).

## ARCHITECTURAL INTERVENTION

### General Concept and Case Histories

It is clear that commensal vertebrate pests are globally problematic as a complex form of biologic "pollution," that is, microorganisms, allergens, and deleterious effects. Architecture plays a key role because design features alone may provide exterior harborage and/or allow access to interiors. "Architecture can be the incubator for disease" (Cohen, 1986). Our concern extends to the interrelationship of internal spaces which can serve as harborage and movement routes. Construction errors, poor site management, and inadequate maintenance contribute greatly to infestations. A few examples will illustrate commensal vertebrates' adaptations to favorable architecture.

### *Case 1*

Geis (1976a and b) conducted a methodical study of bird infestations of a wide variety of residence types in the newly built town of Columbia, Maryland. Construction flaws accounted for 45 percent of the infestations and could be directly related to the activities of specific builders at particular times. For example, poor installation of siding resulted in gaps and holes which permitted common starlings to nest in the walls. In fact, building inspectors learned that they could readily detect flaws in construction by merely observing the nesting activities of the birds. The remaining 55 percent of infestations were related to building design features. These included the fitting of circular, widely louvered vents over square holes in attic walls which thereby allowed sparrows to enter and nest in protected cavities in the lower corners of the frame (behind the louvers). The exposed I-beams of a commercial building afforded excellent ledges for pigeon roosting. The resultant accumulation of pigeon droppings became a health concern for the nearby nursery school playground.

### *Case 2*

In 1986, bats were found to be entering a large downtown office building in Albany, New York. Since one of the captured bats proved to be rabid and many workers were at potential risk, further investigation was warranted to determine points of ingress to the concrete, steel, and glass (all windows sealed) high-rise. In one case, it was determined that bats found on the fourteenth floor most probably gained access via the fifteenth-floor fresh air intake system. Bats entering exterior fresh air vents travel short distances in ducts to the air mixing rooms. From these rooms they can escape to the fifteenth-floor interior via a door (opened to direct unfiltered fresh air to the fifteenth-floor machine room) or by entering return air ducts when the fans are periodically shut down (hence no forced air) to conserve energy. The return air ducts lead to various service shafts and plenum areas above drop ceilings. Access to offices is via loose ceiling tiles or directly via a design feature (Figure 11.14). In the other case (the opened door), bats can move to other areas via wide gaps under doors, unused holes in walls (Figure 11.15), floors, and ceilings (Figure 11.16), pipe chases, and so on.

Bats in the basements were found to initially fly into a walled recess at ground level, drop 12 m to enter a large air intake, drop another 7 m to an exterior subbasement air distribution area. From there bats gained entry via the air handling system. Nearby louvered, screened intakes provided entries in two ways: there was a gap between the frame of some screens and the building and an accumulation of leaves, paper, and other debris provided so much resistance to the intake fans that screens had been pulled out of their frames (Figure 11.17). In either case, intruding bats (and various biologic particulates) could next escape from the air handler unit to the subbasement interior via an open door (as noted earlier) or under

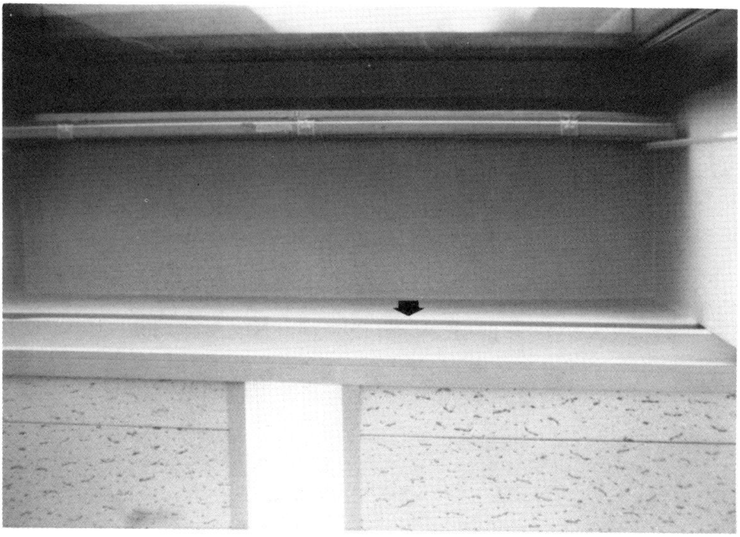

**Figure 11.14.** Design of dropped ceiling provides opening to plenum area near windows throughout much of office complex (fourteenth floor), Albany, N.Y.

the sheet metal walls of the unit which were ill-fitted to the poured cement floor.

Another route from the exterior air distribution area was much more circuitious. Bats were traced more than 115 m through subterranean tunnels, down and up cement shafts, through turning vanes and ducts to finally reach the air handler unit from which escape (as earlier) led into a basement machine room. Movement out of this area could be accomplished as noted with the other bats. Overall, the bats had access to the building interior due to a combination of favorable architecture (air handling system design and construction; interior organization of spaces), inadequate maintenance (unclean intake screens), and human error (opening doors).

### *Case 3*

This third case involves a problem discovered while designing a pest-proofing scheme for a large office building under construction in Baghdad, Iraq (Frantz, 1985). The exterior of the building is clad in marble panels which are individually anchored 3 cm away from the base wall (Figure 11.18). A similar cladding system with a 3-cm panel-wall void is used interiorly and is contiguous with the exterior (Figure 11.19). Horizontal and vertical joints between adjacent panels were open (though specifications called for them to be sealed) and commonly exceeded 0.5 cm (Figure 11.20) as did the expansion joints. Many of the interpanel gaps and occasional breaks were sufficient to allow mice, some rats, and any insects access to the panel-wall void.

**Figure 11.15.** Gaps around conduits pass through wall of office complex (ground floor), Albany, N.Y.

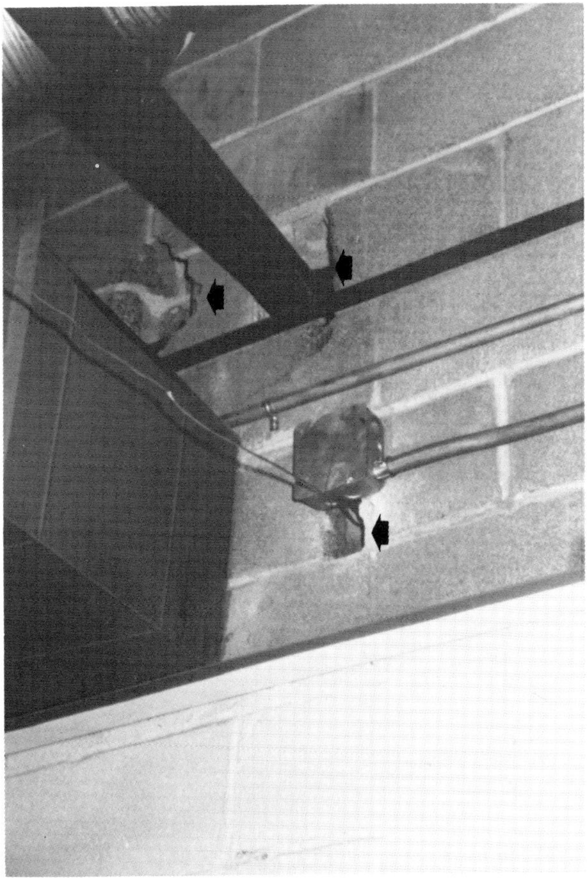

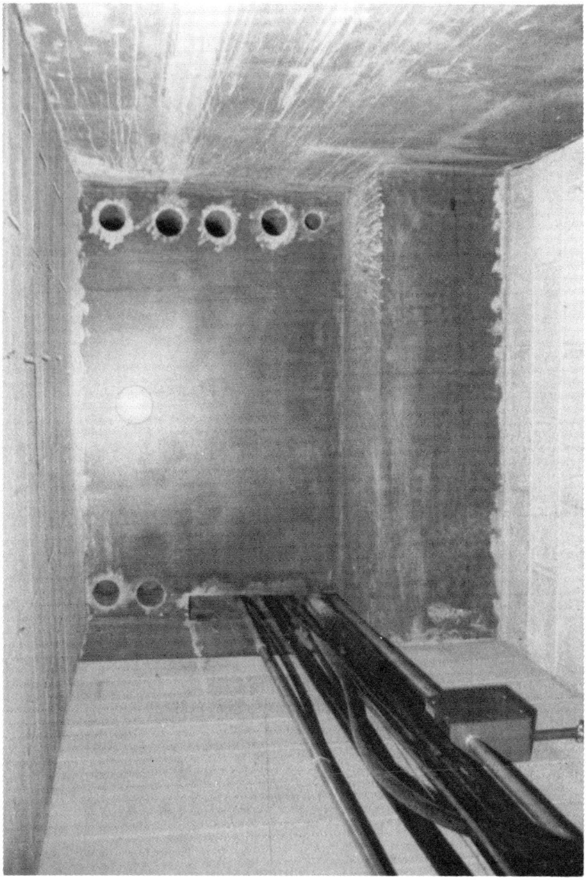

**Figure 11.16.** Unused holes in ceiling (top) of electrical closet; holes and gaps around conduits (bottom) have been filled. Office complex (fifteenth floor), Albany, N.Y.

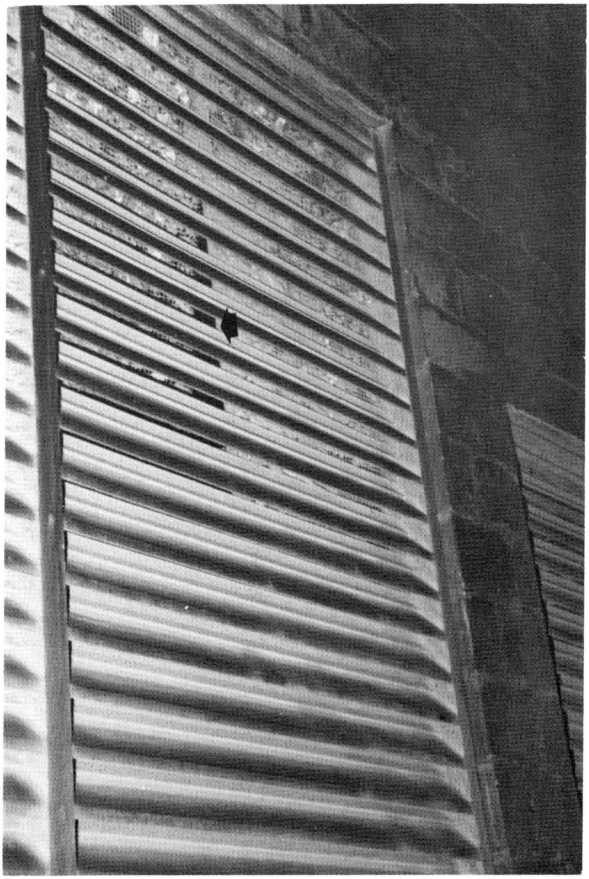

**Figure 11.17.** Leaves, paper, and other debris block air intake screen, resulting in one screen panel being pulled loose from frame. Office complex (subbasement), Albany, N.Y.

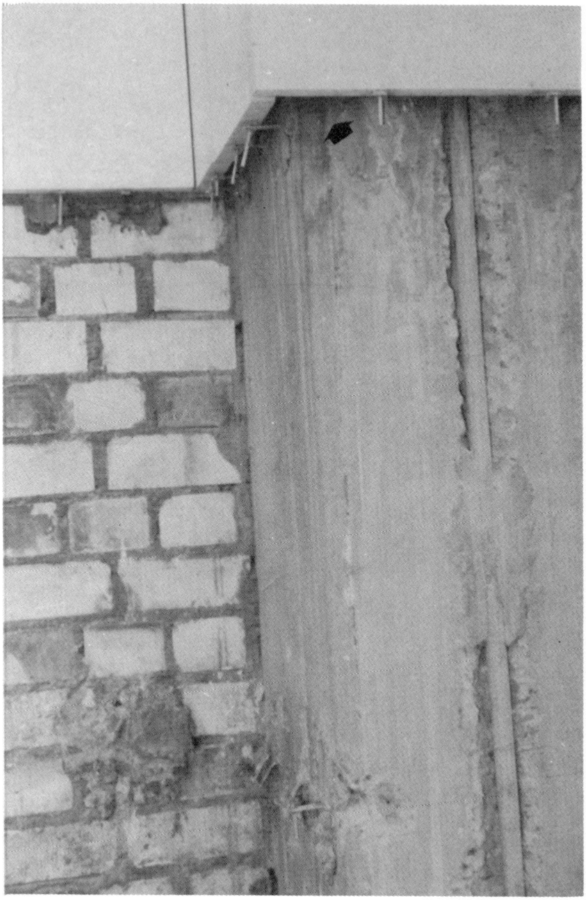

**Figure 11.18.** Marble panels supported by anchor pins provide 3 cm void behind cladding of office complex (ground level), Baghdad, Iraq.

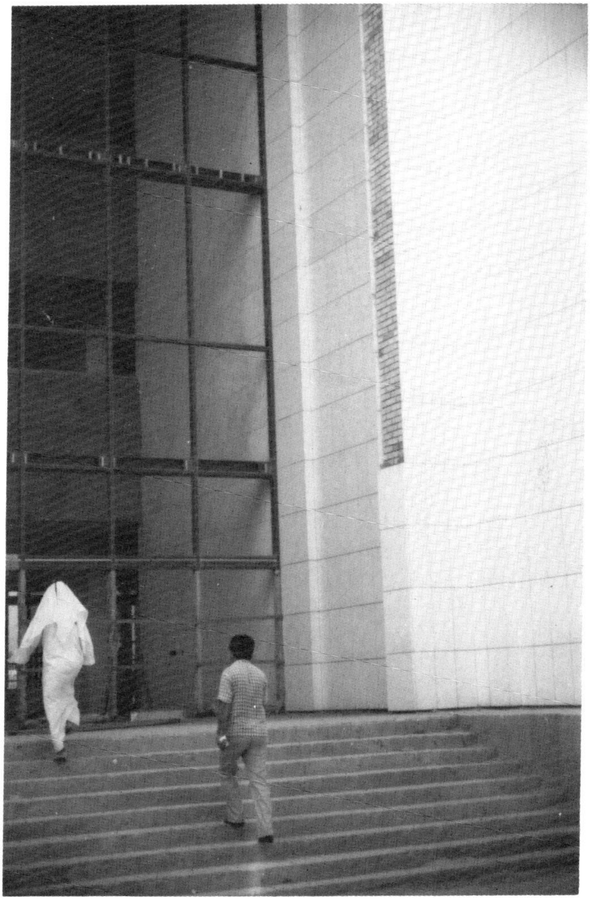

**Figure 11.19.** Marble cladding system is used on exterior and interior walls of office complex (main entrance), Baghdad, Iraq.

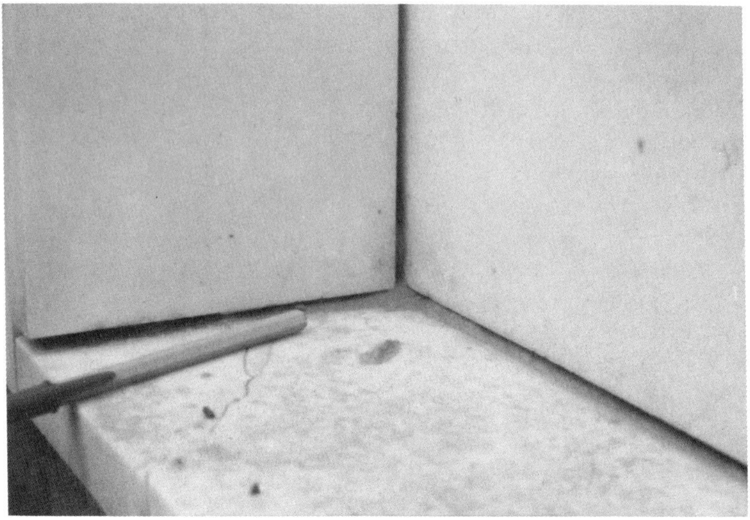

**Figure 11.20.** Gaps between marble cladding panels and at panel-floor junction; corner interpanel gap exceeds 10 mm, sufficient to allow entry of adult house mice. Office complex (main entrance), Baghdad, Iraq.

A major problem was that the panel-wall void was *continuous* between the building exterior and interior. This continuity occurred wherever cladding interfaced with frames of doors and windows (Figure 11.19), at soffits above balcony ceilings, and so on. Although specifications indicated the void would be sealed at the exterior/interior interface, this had not been completed above a height of 2 m (Figure 11.21). Thus, from access holes between exterior cladding panels, mice or rats could move horizontally and vertically within the 3-cm void and eventually pass above an incomplete exterior/interior interface closure. From there, an animal would be free to move about behind the interior cladding, above it to the ceiling plenum (Figure 11.22), and in other ways pass throughout the whole building. In addition to pest infestations, the same basic pathways constituted a serious air handling/energy burden.

## Preventive Design

The objectives of architectural intervention are to prevent pests from infesting a building's exterior shell, from gaining access to the interior, and from freely moving about inside (or using resources therein) if access is achieved. Landscape design is beyond the scope of this chapter, but such designs should be carefully planned so that landscaping neither attracts pest species nor provides easy access to structures (Ebling, 1978; Frantz and Davis, in press; Olkowski and Olkowski, 1984).

**Figure 11.21.** Panel-wall void is filled to only a height of 2 m at exterior/interior interface; provides ready access to building interior for rats, mice and insects. Office complex (ground level), Baghdad, Iraq.

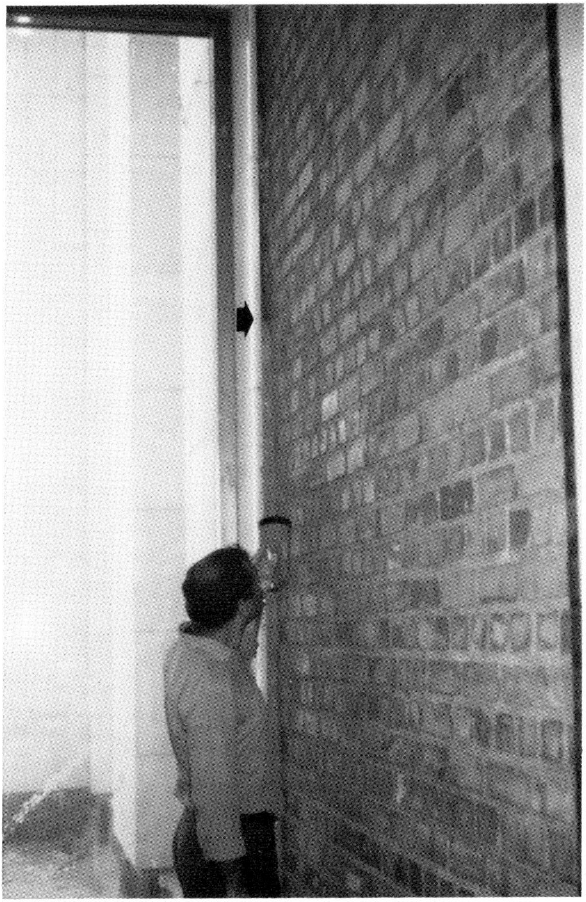

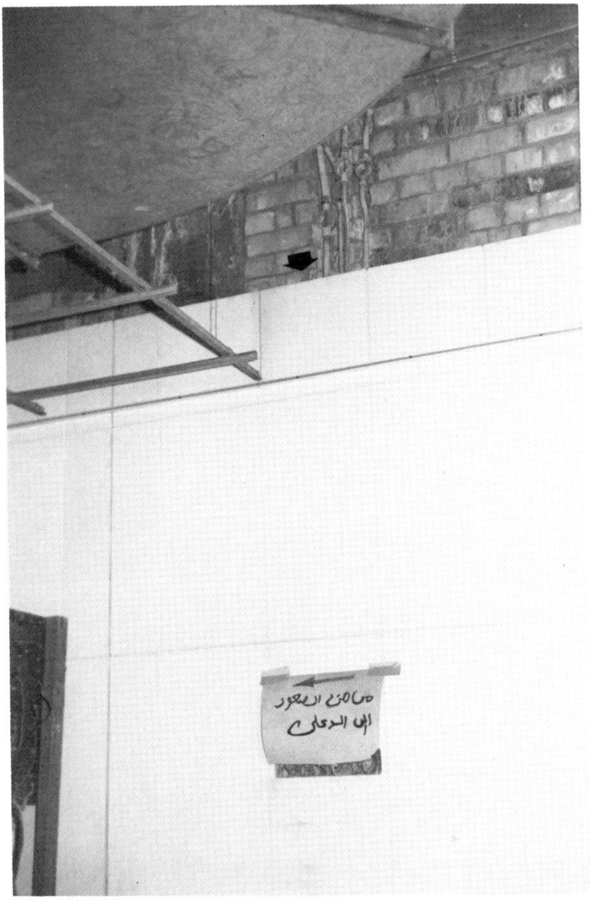

**Figure 11.22.** Panel-wall void is open at top, above false ceiling (see frame), providing vast pest harborage and movement routes. Office complex (level 4), Baghdad, Iraq.

Architectural intervention encompasses the interrelated physical/structural measures that deny commensal vertebrates access to a building's life-support resources. Only general principles and a few newer techniques will be given here. For detailed basic instructions and materials specifications refer to Ebling (1978), Greenhall (1982),

Holsendorf (1937), Imholte (1984), Jenson (1965), Scott and Borom (1977), Silver, Crouch, and Betts (1930), and Vick and Becker (1951). The older references emphasize low technology and inexpensive interventions and may be more applicable to some developing countries or other end-users. A study in Nepal by Blair (1974) provides a synthesis of traditional architectural elements and preventive pest (rodent) measures.

*Pest-proofing* generally relates to designing and building to eliminate or render inaccessible every space that might afford pests harborage (Scott and Borom, 1977). *Stoppage* generally refers to blocking off or removing all passages by which pests are likely to enter or leave existing structures. In practice, the two processes often merge. For example, to prevent birds from roosting on exterior ledges and windowsills, they should be designed with a steep outward pitch (45 degrees minimum) and an extremely smooth surface. If not designed as such, a slanted surface of masonry, wood, or boxed sheet metal can be retrofitted—or an alternative exclusion measure may be more appropriate.

**Figure 11.23.** Bat *(M. lucifugus)* enters gap under fascia which leads into attic of residence, Sloansville, N.Y.

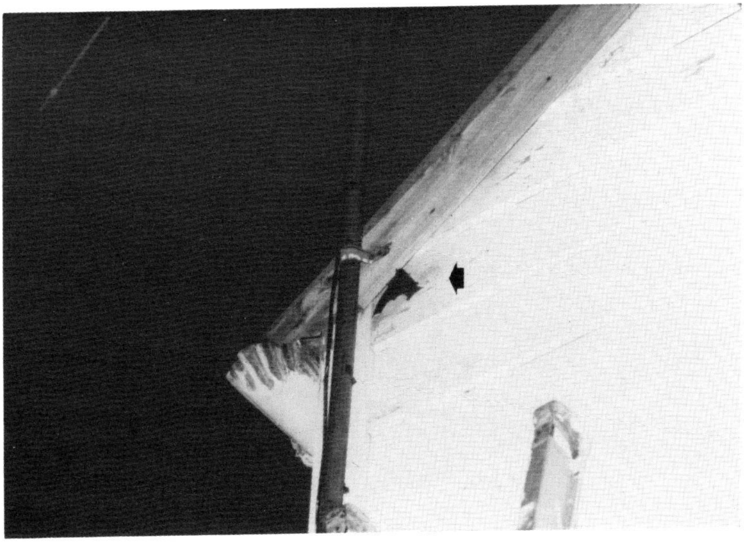

The entire surface of a building is the first structural line of defense against pest intrusion. The walls, floor, and ceiling form a "shell" (for the whole building, for a floor within the building, for a single room, etc.) through which must pass telephone cables, service pipes, air handling ducts, and so forth. Wherever the shell is perforated by a hole 10 mm in diameter or a hole 6 mm × 3.8 cm must be considered a potential entry point, respectively, for adult house mice or little brown bats (Figure 11.23). If cockroaches were the target species, even smaller openings would be of concern (e.g., cracks 1.6 mm wide for the adult German cockroach, *Blattella germanica*).

To be practical, the extent of pest-proofing must be adjusted against tolerable deleterious effects and the economics of excluding the last possible pest. Thorough, detailed inspections and elimination of points of ingress is an ever-changing process. New holes may appear due to construction work, plumbing or electrical changes, deterioration, or direct action by the pests. Systematic inspection programs keep one apprised of structural changes and concomitant responses of commensal vertebrates (Brooks and Rowe, 1979; Frantz and Comings, 1976; Olkowski and Olkowski, 1984).

## Materials and Methods

Many construction materials are impervious (e.g., brick, stone, concrete) to vertebrate pests. Thus, exclusion measures focus largely on doors (Figure 11.24), windows (Figure 11.25), ventilators, chimneys, drains, and gaps relative to construction errors (Figures 11.15, 11.16, 11.21). The same basic concepts of exclusion are applied to the interior of a structure and must include all vertical shafts, horizontal interconnecting subfloor trenches, electrical floor trunking, and gaps around pipes and cables. Interior designers also must take care that decorative moldings, wall and floor coverings, and so on do not simply conceal existing structural gaps that might be utilized by pest species. Maintenance features also must be considered since designs that do not lend themselves to being well maintained often encourage pest situations.

The target species' capabilities determine the opening size to be sealed and the nature of the materials employed. For the pest species under discussion (Tables 11.1 and 11.2), cement mortar (nonshrinking), sheet metal, hardware cloth (5 mm mesh), coarse steel wool

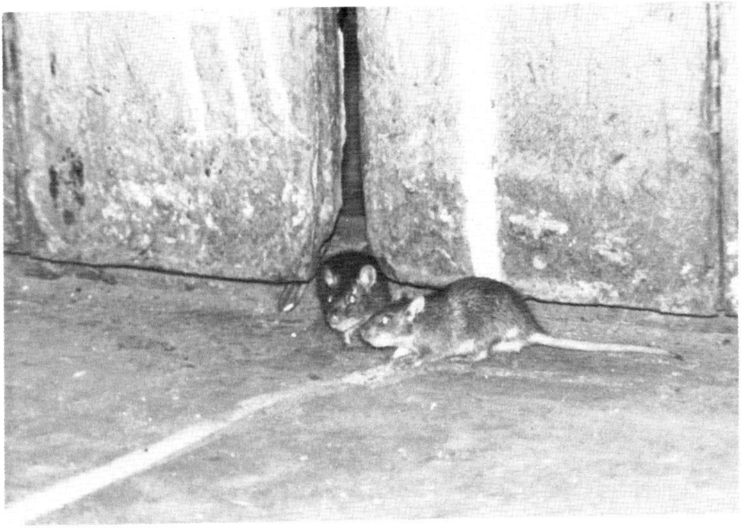

**Figure 11.24.** Two rats *(B. bengalensis)* just inside of rat-gnawed doors, food grain warehouse, Calcutta, India.

**Figure 11.25.** Gaps at bottom of window casing provide rodent entry; note that bird droppings cover much of floor (roost is near ceiling at fifth level). Office complex (lobby) under construction, Baghdad, Iraq.

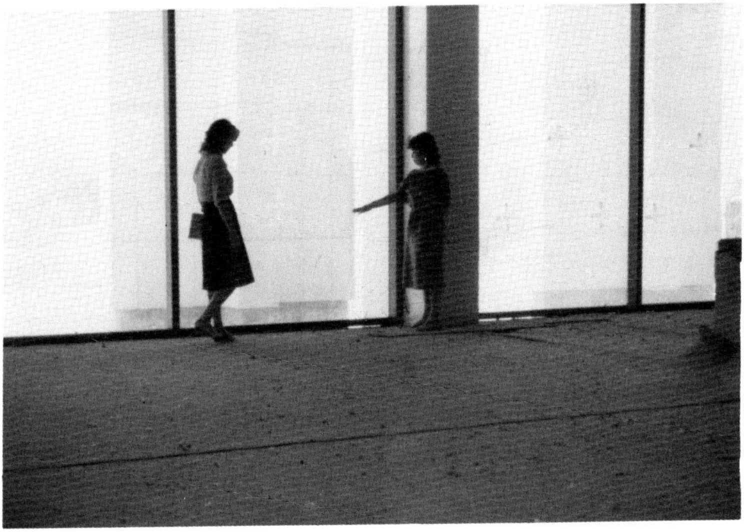

(preferably stainless type) and expanding polyurethane foam sealant are materials of choice. In some developing countries, other materials including scrap metal from biscuit tins, sun-baked mud bricks, plasters of cow dung and clay, tar and pitch have been used (Blair, 1974; Chadurvedi, Patel, and Madsen, 1977; Dias and Dias, 1982; Frantz, 1973; Reddy, 1969). An important point is that it is not always necessary for a material to be totally impervious to an animal so long as it can be very "discouraging." In those situations where commensal vertebrates cannot be excluded from buildings, extreme care should be taken that harborage and/or food are not accessible therein.

### *Polyurethane Foam Sealant*

Polyurethane sealant cures to a woodlike hardness. Though not impervious to rodents or birds, it can discourage them in preventive applications and is excellent for larger openings ($>$7.5 cm) of irregular shape that would be difficult to seal in other ways. Note that foams may provide insect harborage, thus its exposed surfaces must be sealed with epoxy paint. Also, this material is combustible and cannot be used near excessive heat or exposed flame. Silicone (fire-stop) foaming sealants may meet the requirements in high heat areas.

### *Caulking*

Caulking compounds and wood lath are useful for cracks and crevices that may be closed, and screening is used over openings that need to allow ventilation. Numerous caulking products are available (e.g., butyl rubber, siliconized acrylic latex, etc.) depending on the size of the opening, the material to which it must adhere, and how the sealant is to be finished. A prime consideration should be durability; the newer silicone sealants claim to remain flexible for fifty years. Special sealants (e.g., epoxidized polyurethane) may be required for surfaces that could be stained (e.g., light-colored marble and granite) if standard silicone were used. Most of these materials are adequate for small gaps or cracks up to 1 cm wide, and construction-grade silicone sealants are available for gaps of at least 2.5 cm including expansion joints. Larger gaps can be filled with aerosol polyurethane foam or cement if the sealed area or joint need not accommodate movement.

### *Screening*

Insect screening generally should be no coarser than 16 meshes/2.54 cm and can be made of metal or plastic depending on specific application conditions (e.g., subject to mechanical damage, moisture, corrosion) and target species. Where it is necessary to exclude insects as well as rodents and birds, cover the opening with heavy-gauge 5 mm mesh hardware cloth on the exterior and with fine mesh on the interior. The coarse mesh will protect the screening from mechanical damage of animals and people. Since fine screening will reduce the effective opening size and, hence airflow, it may be necessary to increase screen surface area with a box-shaped screen or larger initial opening in order to retain proper ventilation characteristics.

### *Netting*

An effective material for excluding bats and birds is plastic netting, for example Conwed® Birdnetting (Conwed, 1981; Frantz and Trimarchi, 1984; Salmon and Gorenzel, 1981) and ConserVare® Pigeon Control netting (ProSoCo, 1984 and 1985). These nettings are strong, ultraviolet-stabilized, and durable outdoors for many years under most circumstances. Structural-grade Conwed (diagonal hole opening: 1.6 cm) is suitable for bats and birds; it can also be fabricated into checkvalves (Frantz, 1986) to "evict" animals from interior roosts (Figure 11.26). Standard-grade Conwed (diagonal hole opening: 2.4 cm) is suitable for sparrow, starling, and pigeon control; ConserVare (diagonal hole opening: 4.5 cm) probably is best suited to control starlings and pigeons.

Through use of various attachment clips and pins (provided with netting) or sealants, netting can be attached to effectively prevent bird or bat access to open eaves, ventilation shafts or tunnels, ledges, windowsills, ornamental masonry, and statuary. Drop ceilings of netting can be installed in warehouses, stadiums, and pavilions from which it would otherwise be difficult to exclude birds or bats. Where netting must be easily removable for access by maintenance personnel it can be attached with Scotchmate® Dual Lock™ or Velcro® fasteners.

ConserVare netting is available in colors to match masonry or other surfaces; Conwed products are available in black only. In either case, the lightweight, flexible characteristics of the netting allow its

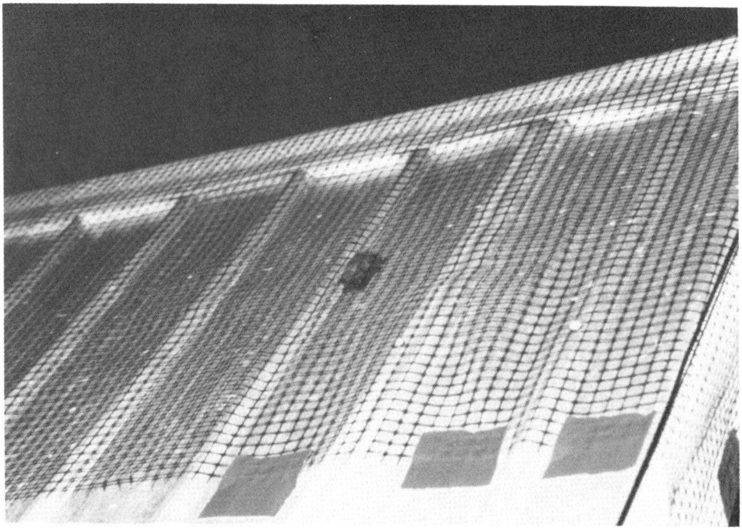

**Figure 11.26.** Bat *(M. lucifugus)* which emerged from under ridge cap, moves down roof to escape from birdnetting "checkvalve"; note that ridge cap design with foam rubber gasket does not exclude bats. Residence, Hadley, N.Y.

installation to be inconspicuous and not detract from architectural or statuary details.

### *Needle Strips/Wires*

Metal strips with projecting needlelike wires (Nixalite, 1985) effectively prevent birds' access to many of the same areas where netting can be used, including ledges, windowsills/frames, louvers, open eaves, cornice returns, and decorative niches associated with doors, windows, frieze work, and so on. It is also useful for preventing birds from resting on *edges* of roofs and gutters, the ridgepole/cap, hardware and *tops* of signs, *tops* of statues and column capitals (Figure 11.27), and on cables. Metal strips with projecting wires can also prevent rodents from climbing posts, cables, and conduits and may be useful in some bat-proofing efforts. Judicious application of needle strips should not conflict with design aesthetics.

A method of keeping birds off narrow pipes or beams is to install a thin wire, centered and tightly stretched, about 2 cm above the surface (Areson, 1984). Piano wire or similarly gauged stainless steel wire works well for this purpose. The wire prevents the bird from sitting comfortably (as do the needle strips) while being too thin to grasp or rest on.

### *Plastic Strips/Automatic Doors/Air Curtains*

Birds and bats (and flying insects) can be excluded from oversized doors and loading dock entrances (Figure 11.28) with strip doors of heavy polyvinyl chloride (PVC) plastic. The overlapping strips part just enough to allow traffic passage then close immediately to reduce the influx of flying pests, dust, and noise; they also prevent an outflow of interior conditioned air. For heavily used doors, it may be most practical to install automatic, rapid-opening (horizontally or vertically) doors. These are made of PVC-coated polyester fabric and meet the same basic requirements as strip doors, but can remain open for several seconds to accommodate traffic.

Somewhat less protective and less energy conserving than the plas-

**Figure 11.27.** Bird roosting on top of capitals can be prevented through installation of needle strips; note droppings defacement of capital. National historic site, New York City.

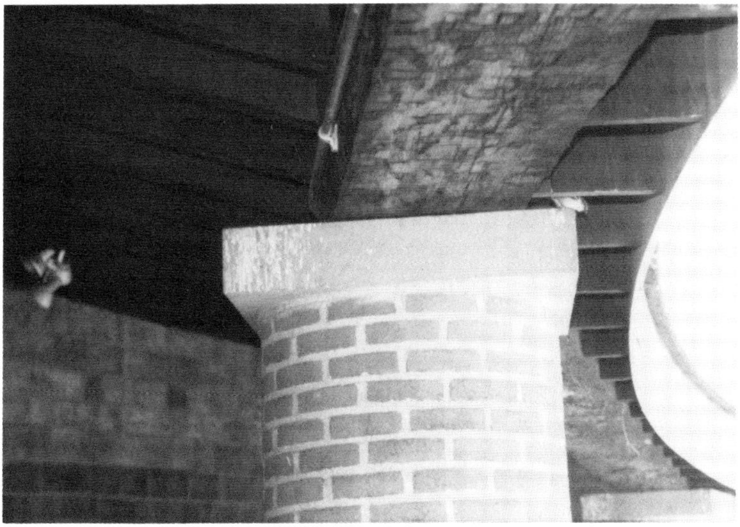

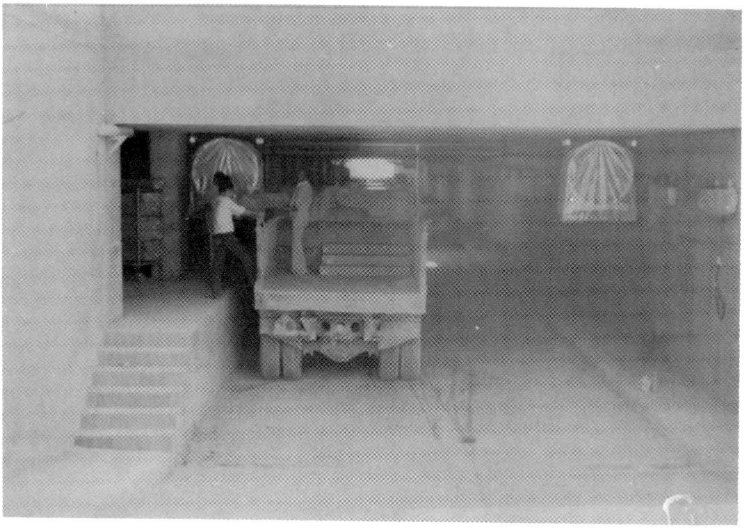

**Figure 11.28.** Most birds, bats, and flying insects can be excluded from large entranceway to loading dock through installation of plastic strip/auto-opening doors or air curtains. Office complex (basement level), Baghdad, Iraq.

tic strips, air curtains can be used at large doors and entrance areas that must be kept fully open. Air curtains (fan-driven) direct a strong and continuous air flow downward and slightly outward from above a doorway (Areson, 1984; Shenker, 1970). This permits full access by people and equipment, but deters bats, birds, and flying insects. If a large entrance area must be kept open for ventilation and has little traffic, an overlapping curtain of birdnetting may be suitable.

## Vulnerable Areas

### *Doors*

For purposes of pest exclusion (as well as energy convervation) all exterior doors must be adequately sealed through use of sheet metal-flashings, built-up thresholds, and/or door bottoms to result in a gap of no more than 5 mm. The remaining gap can be closed with conventional weatherstripping or draft sweeps. Particularly in commercial or multifamily buildings, this treatment should also be applied to interior doors leading to common corridors and those associated with restrooms, and food handling or food storage areas. The latter two areas are at greatest infestation risk for rats and mice (as well as cockroaches and other food storage insect pests) and sealing doors in this way delimits the pests' distribution within a building.

### *Wall/Floor Openings*

Unused openings (or portions thereof) cut into exterior walls for pipes, electrical conduits, air handling ducts, and so on (including gaps around window frames) should be sealed (Figures 11.25 and 11.29). Where necessary, care must be taken to allow for expansion, contraction, or vibration. Ventilator screens must fit tightly into their frames (Figure 11.17) which must fit tightly into the building (Figure 11.30). All exhaust or intake vents and chimneys (from which pests could escape to the interior) should be covered with 1 cm mesh (or finer) hardware cloth (Figure 11.31).

Throughout building interiors a maze of conduits with gaps around them pass through walls (Figures 11.15 and 11.32), floors, and ceilings (Figure 11.16) providing a vast interconnecting system of movement routes for rodents and, to some degree, bats. Ideally, all such openings should be sealed or, at least, those on levels most vulnerable to local pest species. In large commercial and multifamily structures, all openings should be sealed relative to restrooms, food handling or storage areas, and machine/plant rooms. An alternative or companion approach would be to divide up each floor according to bearing walls or other criteria (e.g., at all corridors) and close all openings between the designated areas. This process will make it possible to limit the spread of any infestation that might be introduced from the exterior.

### *Conduit Systems and Subfloor Trenches*

In larger buildings, there may be kilometer upon kilometer of conduits, electrical wireways, and subfloor trenches that could become an endless pest infestation network (Figure 11.33). Access doors and panels to these systems must seal shut to prevent potential pest entry to other areas of a building.

Though subfloor systems must be kept open for maintenance access, it is possible to restrict pest movements therein. For example, at major intersections of electrical trunking systems, all openings

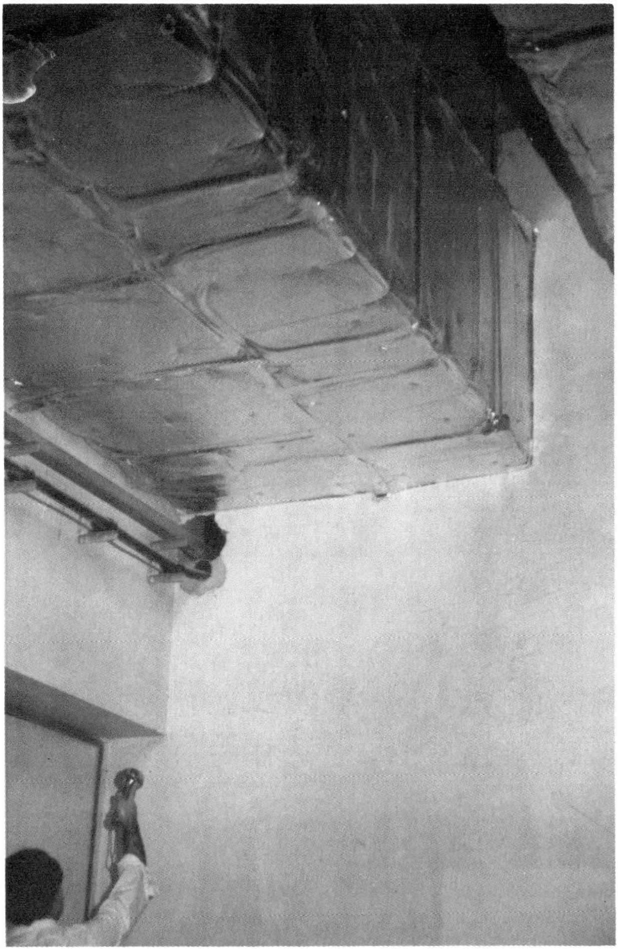

**Figure 11.29.** Conduits and ductwork pass through exterior wall; gaps around conduits will allow pest entry (duct appears well sealed into wall). Office complex (basement loading dock), Baghdad, Iraq.

that lead outward could be sealed (e.g., with removable/alterable polyurethane foam, vermiculite cement, etc.). Service trenches need to be kept open for repair personnel to crawl through; however, major intersections and all openings leading into service shafts (Figure 11.34) could be closed.

**Figure 11.30.** Gap exists between sections of louvered, screened air intake vents; top of service shaft is open to all levels below. Office complex (fifth level [top]), Baghdad, Iraq.

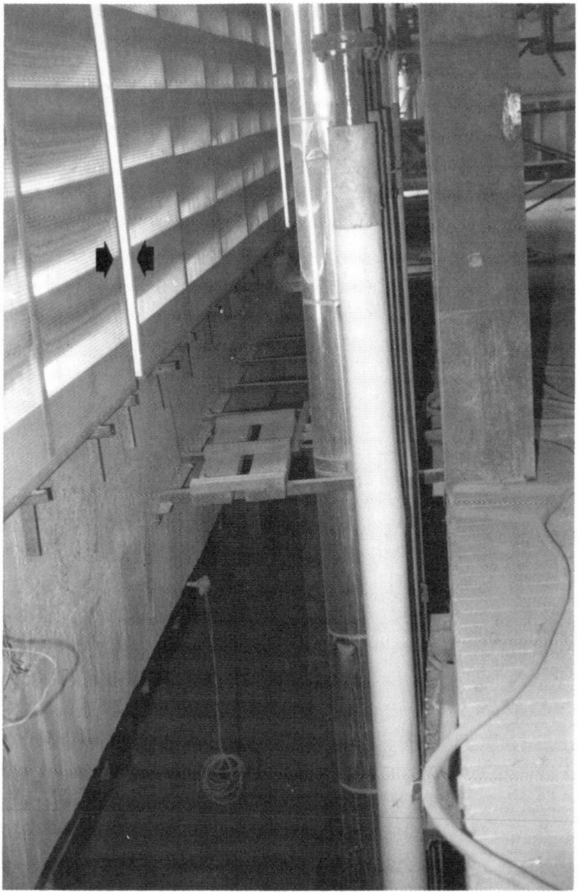

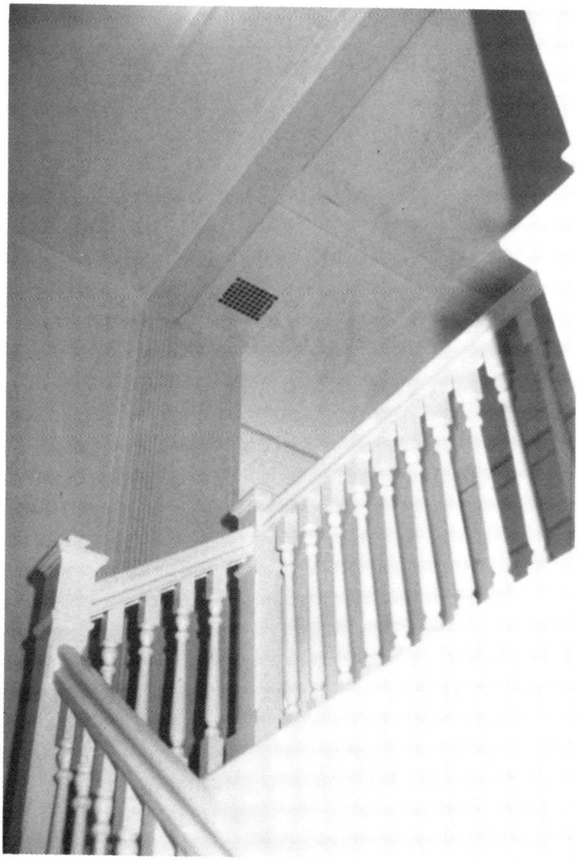

**Figure 11.31.** Ceiling air vent has grillwork openings that allow bat entry from attic; can be batproofed by fitting 10 mm mesh behind grillwork. Residence (third floor), Saratoga Springs, N.Y.

**Figure 11.33.** Subfloor service trench (rear) and electrical trunking junction box (foreground) are interconnected and provide part of pest movement route and harborage throughout building; additional harborage provided by hole in wall at base of electrical panel (rear). Office complex (second-level office), Baghdad, Iraq.

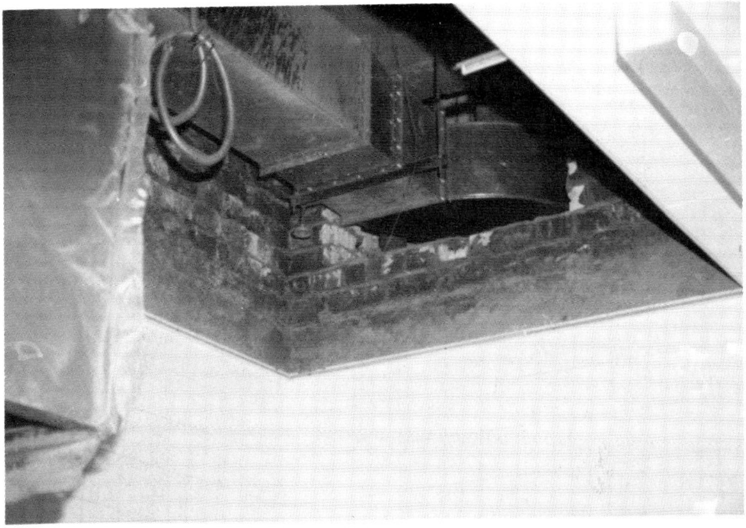

**Figure 11.32.** Large gap around duct passes through wall; it allows pests inter-room access above dropped ceiling of office complex (second-level pantry), Baghdad, Iraq.

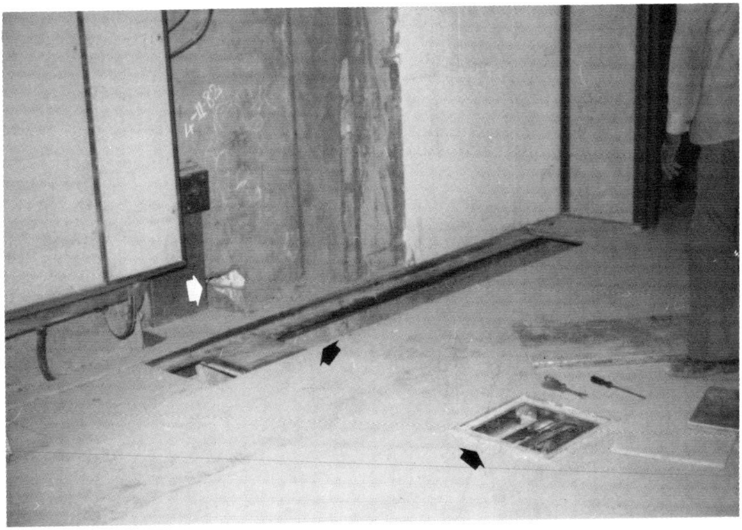

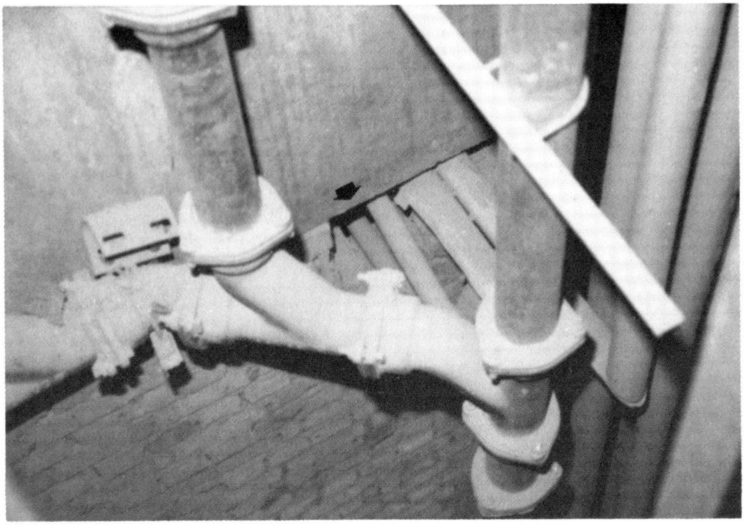

**Figure 11.34.** Plumbing conduits from subfloor service trench connect with interfloor service shaft; sealing the trench/shaft interface will prevent pest movement. Office complex (second level), Baghdad, Iraq.

### *Shafts*

Service shafts of buildings provide vertical connection between most, if not all, levels. Tops of such shafts should be closed to prevent pest access from upper machine rooms (see Figure 11.30) or attics. In large buildings, sealing the shafts at each floor level restricts pest movements as well as reduces fire hazards. Where shafts must be kept open for ventilation, closure with hardware cloth or birdnetting will limit particular pest activities. Water and refuse should not be allowed to accumulate in the bottom of shafts because it may attract pests and/or become a source of microbial pollution.

Elevator shafts are prone to infestation, particularly by rats, mice, and bats. Obviously, in such shafts barriers cannot be applied, except at the top, but other measures can prevent or greatly reduce interfloor access by pests. The elevator car doors should be tight-fitting, using tolerances as close as practical (preferably within 5 mm). In the bottom of shafts, 0.5 m of smooth-surfaced painted cement should be applied as a continuous band to all walls at a height of 1.25–1.75 m. At this height, rats and mice will be unable to jump above it from the floor and unable to climb over its smooth surface. Complete shaft treatment requires the smooth band application just below the door opening at each floor.

### Roofs

Roofs are vulnerable to bats, rats, mice, squirrels, and birds. If the roofing material is impervious (e.g., not thatch, etc.), it is the seams

**Figure 11.35.** Interface of roof, soffit, and house wall with chimney provides bat entry areas; note bat guano and stains on clapboards near chimney of residence, Keeseville, N.Y.

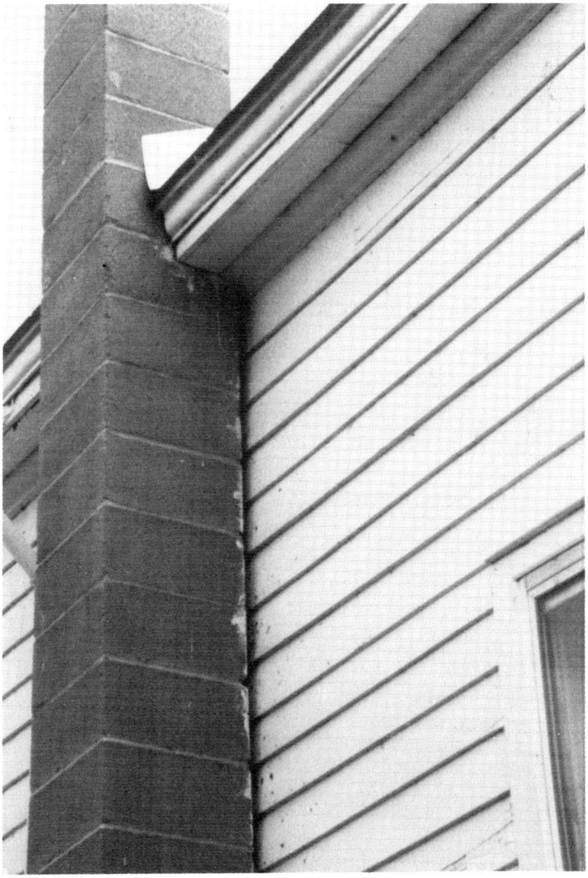

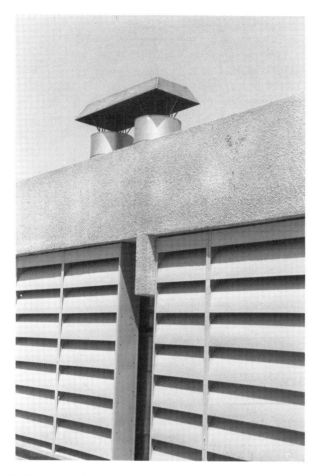

**Figure 11.36.** Covered chimney flue can be pest-proofed to exclude commensal vertebrates with heavy-gauge 1 cm mesh hardware cloth or similar spark arrestor screen (often an integral part of chimney caps); note gap between sections of louvered vent as shown in Figure 11.30.

of that material and its interfaces with vents, chimneys (Figure 11.35), and walls that are potential entry points. Even a slate roof (which commonly has interslate gaps in which bats can hide) does not present as great a problem if it has a "seamless" subroof and sealed ridgepole impervious to bats. A similar argument can be made for tin roofs, in which case the ridge cap must also be bat-proof (Figure 11.26).

As mentioned previously, chimney flues (Figure 11.36) and vents should be pest-proofed with hardware cloth. Self-closing dampers also help to prevent pest access into chimneys and similar devices. Similar protection should be provided to roof equipment, such as air conditioners and cooling towers, to prevent pest access and contamination.

## OVERVIEW

Though our individual tolerance limits may vary, commensal vertebrate pests clearly represent a significant threat to human health and welfare on a global scale. The commensal habits of animals create a potential for human injury, but it is improper architecture that often allows the potential to be realized. Poorly designed architecture permits various species to live in very close proximity to where humans tend to spend most of their time—in buildings. Here, vertebrate pests are often able to exert their deleterious effects and disseminate microorganisms, allergens, and other particulates continuously throughout our living spaces.

It is not suggested that all exterior and interior commensal vertebrate pest infestations are avoidable through proper architectural intervention. However, many potential harborage niches, points of ingress, and movement routes can be systematically "designed out" early in the architectural process. Potential problems need not become active. They can be avoided if building designers (architects, engineers, interior designers, etc.) would carefully consider the habits and capabilities of local pests. The medical, aesthetic, and economic costs of irresponsible design are ubiquitous. Prevention of pest infestations is more efficacious, economical, and safer than waiting for problems to occur and then trying to cure them.

Architectural interventions are largely undramatic actions that require time to manifest themselves, yet the long-term public health benefits are immeasurable. It would pose an interesting challenge to architects if they would recognize biologic imperatives (such as commensal vertebrate pests) and make art of them through environmentally conscious structures.

## ACKNOWLEDGMENTS

I thank the many people who allowed me to study pest problems in their buildings and assisted in this effort. To Christine Tanner and Mary Jane Boulay goes my sincere appreciation for processing the manuscript draft.

## REFERENCES

Areson, C. W. 1984. Structural bird control—an overview. In *Proc. 1st East. Wildl. Damage Control Conf.,* D. J. Decker, ed. Ithaca, N.Y.: Cornell Univ., pp. 333–46.

Azad, A. F. 1986. *Mites of public health importance and their control.* WHO/VBC/86.931. Geneva: World Health Organization.

Bajomi, D., and K. Sasvari. 1986. Results of eight years' examination of the habitats of residual urban Norway rat populations after eradications. In *Proc. 12th vert. pest conf.,* T. P. Salmon, ed. Davis: Univ. California, pp. 66–74.

Barbour, R. W., and W. H. Davis. 1969. *Bats of America.* Lexington: Univ. Kentucky Press.

Benenson, A. S., ed. 1975. *Control of communicable diseases in man.* Washington, D.C. Public Health Assoc.

Blair, K. D. 1974. *The relationship between traditional housing and traditional settlement patterns and urban housing in Nepal.* Washington, D.C.: Fulbright Foundation.

Bozeman, F. M., S. A. Masiello, M. S. Williams, and B. L. Elisberg. 1975. Epidemic typhus rickettsiae isolated from flying squirrels. *Nature* 255:545–47.

Brooks, J. E., and F. P. Rowe. 1979. *Commensal rodent control.* WHO/VBC/79.726. Geneva: World Health Organization.

Bullard, Roger W. 1983. Personal communication.

Bullard, R., and H. Shuyler. 1983. Springing the trap on post-harvest food loss. *Horizons* 2:26–32.

Burge, H. A. 1985. Indoor sources for airborne microbes. In *Indoor air and human health,* R. B. Gammage and S. V. Kaye, ed. Chelsea, Mich.: Lewis Publ., pp. 139–48.

Caslick, J. W., and D. J. Decker. 1981. *Control of wildlife damage in homes and gardens.* Ithaca, N.Y.: Cornell Univ.

Centers for Disease Control (CDC). 1982. Epidemic typhus associated with flying squirrels—United States. *Morbid. Mortal. Weekly Rep.* 31:555, 556, 561.

———. 1983. Human rabies—Michigan. *Morbid. Mortal. Weekly Rep.* 32:159–60.

Chadirji, R. 1986. Architectural education in Iraq: A case study. Presentation made to the Aga Kahn Award for Architecture Seminar, April 1986, Granada, Spain.

Chaturvedi, G. C., M. J. Patel, and C. R. Madsen. 1977. Studies on improved storage systems. In *Proc. All India Rodent Seminar,* Ahmedabad, 1975. Sidhpur, India: Rodent Control Project, 136–38.

Chin, J. 1986. Relapsing fever. In *Maxcy-Rosenau/public health and preventive medicine,* J. M. Last, ed. Norwalk, Conn.: Appleton-Century-Crofts, pp. 359–61.

Cohen, Harold L. 1985. Community intervention for insect and rodent control (CIIRC)—a working paper. Presented at WHO/CIIRC Working Group Meeting, 18–22 August, at State Univ. of New York, Buffalo.

———. 1986. Personal communication.

Constantine, D. G. 1970. Bats in relation to the health, welfare, and economy of man. In *Biology of bats,* vol. 2, W. A. Wimsatt, ed. New York: Academic Press, pp. 319–449.

———. 1979. Bat rabies and bat management. *Bull. Soc. Vector Ecol.* 4:1–9.

Conwed. 1981. *Conwed bird damage control netting applications.* Minneapolis: Conwed Corp.

Cooperative Extension. 1979. *Pesticide applicator training manual; Category 7, industrial, institutional, structural and rodent.* Ithaca, N.Y.: Cornell Univ.

Courtsal, F. R. 1983. Pigeons (rock doves). In *Prevention and control of wildlife damage,* R. M. Timm, ed. Lincoln: Univ. Nebraska, pp. E35–E41.

Davis, D. E. 1986. The scarcity of rats and the Black Death: An ecological history. *J. Interdiscipl. Hist.* 16:455–470.

Davis, D. E., and W. B. Jackson. 1981. Rat control. In *Advances in applied biology,* vol. 6, T. H. Coaker, ed. London: Academic Press, pp. 221–77.

Davis, J. W., R. C. Anderson, L. Karstad, and D. O. Trainer, eds. 1971. *Infectious and parasitic diseases of wild birds.* Ames: Iowa State Univ. Press.

Davis, J. W., L. H. Karstad, and D. O. Trainer, eds. 1970. *Infectious diseases of wild mammals.* Ames: Iowa State Univ. Press.

Deoras, P. J. 1963. Studies on Bombay rats: Frequency of rat population. *Curr. Sci.* 32:163–65.

Diamond, R. C., and D. C. Grimsrud. 1984. *Manual on indoor air quality.* EM-3469 Res. Proj. 2034-3. Berkeley, Calif.: Lawrence Berkeley Laboratory.

Dias, J.C.P., and R. B. Dias. 1982. Housing and the control of vectors of human Chagas' disease in the State of Minas Gerais, Brazil. *PAHO Bull.* 16:117–29.

Dodds, W. Jean. 1987. Conversation with author.

Drummond, D. C. 1973. *The role of population ecology in solving urban rodent problems.* WHO/VBC/SG/73.1 Geneva: World Health Organization.

———. 1974. *Rat control requirements in some large Asian cities.* WHO/VBC/74.487. Geneva: World Health Organization.

Ebling, W. 1978. *Urban entomology.* Rev. ed. Berkeley: Univ. California.

Emmons, R. W. 1986. Rickettsial infections. In *Maxcy-Rosenau/public health and preventive medicine,* J. M. Last, ed. Norwalk, Conn.: Appleton-Century-Crofts, pp. 347–53.

Erz, W. 1966. Ecological principles in the urbanization of birds. *Ostrich. Suppl.* 6:357–63.

Farhang-Azad, A. 1977. Ecology of *Capillaria hepatica* (Bancroft 1893) (Nematoda). 1. Dynamics of infection among Norway rat populations of the Baltimore Zoo, Baltimore, Maryland. *J. Parasitol.* 63:117–22.

Feeley, J. C. 1985. Impact of indoor air pathogens on human health. In *Indoor air and human health,* R. B. Gammage and S. V. Kaye, eds. Chelsea, Mich.: Lewis Publ. pp. 183–87.

Fenton, M. B. 1983. *Just bats.* Toronto: Univ. Toronto Press.

Fitzwater, W. D. 1979. Commensal rodents, Sec. 1. In *Encyclopedia of vertebrate pest control,* vol. 4. Vienna, Va.: National Pest Control Assoc.

———. 1983. House sparrows. In *Prevention and control of wildlife damage,* R. M. Timm, ed. Lincoln: Univ. Nebraska, pp. E43–E51.

Flyger, V., D. L. Leedy, and T. M. Franklin. 1984. Wildlife damage control in eastern cities and suburbs. In *Proc. 1st East. Wildl. Damage Control Conf.,* D. J. Decker, ed. Ithaca, N.Y.: Cornell Univ., pp. 27–32.

Frantz, S. C. 1973. Behavioral ecology of the lesser bandicoot rat, *Bandicota bengalensis* (Gray), in Calcutta, Ph.D. diss., Johns Hopkins University.

———. 1974. Evaluation of rodent infestations in Nepal—A preliminary report. *J. Nepal Med. Assoc.* 12:17–32.

———. 1985. Preventive pest management/Baghdad, Iraq. Consultation report presented to the Architects Collaborative, 21 May, Cambridge, Mass.

———. 1986. Batproofing structures with birdnetting checkvalves. In *Proc.*

*12th Vert. Pest. Conf.*, T. P. Salmon, ed. Davis: Univ. California, pp. 260–68.

Frantz, S. C., and D. E. Davis. In press. Commensal rodent bionomics and integrated pest management. *Ecology and management of food industry pests,* FDA Tech. Bull. No. 4. Washington, D.C.: U.S. Dept. Agriculture.

Frantz, S. C., and J. P. Comings. 1976. Evaluation of urban rodent infestations—an approach in Nepal. In *Proc. 7th Vert. Pest Conf.*, C. C. Siebe, ed. Davis: Univ. California, pp. 279–90.

Frantz, S. C., and C. V. Trimarchi. 1984. Bats in human dwellings: Health concerns and management. In *Proc. 1st East. Wildl. Damage Control Conf.,* D. J. Decker, ed. Ithaca, N.Y.: Cornell Univ., pp. 299–308.

Frishman, A. 1982. Rats and mice. In *A. Mallis/handbook of pest control.* 6th ed., K. Story and D. Moreland, eds. Cleveland: Franzak and Foster, pp. 5–77.

Geis, A. D. 1976a. Bird populations in a new town. *Atlantic Natur.* 31:141–46.

———. 1976b. Effects of building design and quality on nuisance bird problems. In *Proc. 7th Vert. Pest Conf.*, C. C. Siebe, ed. Davis: Univ. California, pp. 51–53.

Gelman, A. C. 1961. The ecology of the relapsing fevers. In *Studies in disease ecology,* J. M. May, ed. New York: Hafner, pp. 113–36, 532, 533.

George, R. B., and R. L. Penn. 1986. Histoplasmosis. In *Fungal diseases of the lung,* G. A. Sarosi and S. F. Davies, eds. New York: Grune and Stratton, pp. 69–85.

Gratz, N. G. 1969. Epidemiology investigations, Item 5.3. In *Proc. FAO/WHO Reg. Train. Seminar on Control of Rodents of Agric. and Public Health Importance.* 8–18 December, Manila, Philippines.

Greenhall, A. M. 1982. *House bat management.* Resource Publ. No. 143. Washington, D.C.: U.S. Dept. Interior.

Hall, E. R., and K. R. Kelson. 1959. *Mammals of North America,* vol. 1. New York: Ronald Press.

Hartlage, J., B. T. Thomas, J. May, and P. Egghorn. 1984. Nuisance bird control in Virginia. In *Proc. 1st East. Wildl. Damage Control Conf.,* D. J. Decker, ed. Ithaca, N.Y.: Cornell Univ., pp. 369–74.

Herms, W. B., and M. T. James. 1965. *Medical entomology.* 5th ed. New York: Macmillan.

Hill, J. E., and J. D. Smith. 1984. *Bats: A natural history.* Austin: Univ. Texas Press.

Holsendorf, B. E. 1937. The rat and ratproof construction of buildings. *Publ. Health Rep.* (suppl.) 131:68.

Hopkins, D. 1974. Status of urban rat control program 1969–1973. In *Proc.*

*National Urban Rat Control Progr. Dir. Meeting,* 30 April–2 May. Atlanta: Center for Disease Control, pp. 3–6.

Imholt, T. J. 1984. Engineering for food safety and sanitation. Crystal, MN: Technical Institute of Food Safety.

Jenson, A. G. 1965. *Proofing of buildings against rats and mice.* Tech. Bull. No. 12. Tolworth, England: Ministry of Agriculture, Fisheries and Food.

Johnsen, A. 1982. Urban habitat use by house sparrows, rock doves, and starlings. M.S. thesis, State University of New York College of Environmental Science and Forestry, Syracuse, NY.

Kellert, S. R. 1976. Perceptions of animals in American society. In *Trans. 41st North Amer. Wildl. Conf.* Washington, D.C.: Wildlife Management Inst., pp. 533–46.

Kimm, P. M. 1986. Laying a solid foundation for urban housing. *Horizons* 5:78–81.

Kundsin, R. B. 1986. Architectural design and microbial pollution. Presentation at N.Y. State Dept. Health, WCL&R, Seminar, 15 May 1986, Albany.

Kunz, T. H., ed. 1982. *Ecology of bats.* New York: Plenum Press.

Last, J. M., ed. 1986. *Maxcy-Rosenau/public health and preventive medicine.* Norwalk, Conn.: Appleton-Century-Crofts.

Lauer, D. M., and D. E. Sonenshine. 1978. Bionomics of the squirrel flea, *Orchopeas howardi* (Siphonaptera: Ceratophyllidae), in laboratory and field colonies of the southern flying squirrel, *Glaucomys volans,* using radiolabeling techniques. *J. Med. Entomol.* 15:1–10.

Leonard, M. A. 1986. Curing 'sick buildings' to protect people inside. *Knickerbocker News* (Albany) 27 October, p. 1B.

Lumio, J., M. Hillbom, R. Roine, L. Ketonen, M. Halha, M. Valle, E. Neuvonen, and J. Lahdevirta. 1986. Human rabies of bat origin in Europe. *Lancet* 1:378.

McCabe, R. A. 1966. Vertebrates as pests: A point of view. In *Scientific aspects of pest control.* Washington: National Academy Press, pp. 115–34.

McDade, J. E., C. C. Shepard, M. A. Redus, V. F. Newhouse, and J. D. Smith. 1980. Evidence of *Rickettsia prowazekii* infections in the United States. *Amer. J. Trop. Med. Hyg.* 29:277–84.

Manski, D. A., L. W. VanDruff, and V. Flyger. 1981. Activities of gray squirrels and people in a downtown Washington, D.C. park: Management implications. In *Trans. 46th North Amer. Wildl. Natur. Resour. Conf.* Washington, D.C.: Wildlife Management Inst., pp. 439–54.

Marsh, R. E., and W. E. Howard, 1982. Vertebrate pests. In *A. Mallis/handbook of pest control.* 6th ed., K. Story and D. Moreland, eds. Cleveland: Franzak and Foster, pp. 791–861.

Miller, J. W. 1975. Much ado about starlings. *Natural History* 84:38–45.

Mix, J. 1986a. Pesticide exposure becomes major concern for industry. *Pest Control* 54:48, 51.

———. 1986b. Survey pinpoints dollars and pests. *Pest Control* 54:22–23.

Monath, T. P., and K. M. Johnson. 1986. Viral infections. In *Maxcy-Rosenau/public health and preventive medicine,* J. M. Last, ed. Norwalk, Conn.: Appleton-Century-Crofts, pp. 323–47.

Moretti, E. R., B. Basso, I. Albesa, A. J. Eraso, and F. O. Kravetz. 1980. Infeccion natual de *Calomys laucha* por *Trypanosoma cruzi. Medicina (Buenos Aires)* 40 (suppl. 1):181–86.

National Pest Control Association (NPCA). 1980. *Tree squirrels, part 1, biology and habits.* Tech. Rel. ESPC 043201A. Vienna, Va.: National Pest Control. Assoc.

National Research Council (NRC). 1980. *Urban pest management.* Washington, D.C.: National Academy Press.

Nixalite. 1985. *How to install Nixalite architectural bird control.* East Moline, Ill.: Nixalite of America.

Nuorteva, P. 1971. The synanthropy of birds as an expression of the ecological cycle disorder caused by urbanization. *Ann. Zool. Fennici* 8:547–53.

O'Donnell, M. A., and L. W. VanDruff, 1984. Wildlife conflicts in an urban area: Occurrence of problems and human attitudes toward wildlife. In *Proc. 1st East. Wildl. Damage Control Conf.,* D. J. Decker, ed. Ithaca, N.Y.: Cornell Univ., pp. 315–23.

Olfert, E. D. 1986. Allergy to laboratory animals. *Lab. Animal* 15:24, 25, 29–31.

Olkowski, W., and H. Olkowski. 1984. *Delivering integrated pest management.* Berkeley, Calif.: Bio-Integral Resource Center (BIRC).

Olsen, O. W. 1974. *Animal parasites.* 3d ed. Baltimore: Univ. Park Press.

Poland, J. 1986. Plague. In *Maxcy-Rosenau/public health and preventive medicine,* J. M. Last, ed. Norwalk, Conn.: Appleton-Century-Crofts, pp. 354–59.

Pratt, H. D., and R. Z. Brown. 1977. *Biological factors in domestic rodent control.* HEW Publ. No. (CDC) 77-81444. Atlanta: Dept. Health, Educ. and Welfare, Public Health Service, CDC.

ProSoCo. 1984. *ConserVare® pigeon control.* Kansas City, Kan.: ProSoCo, Inc.

———. 1985. National building museum opens its doors in revitalized pension building. *ProSoCo News* (Fall 1985):1–6.

Reddy, D. B. 1969. Supplementary information on mechanical proofing against rodents, Item 6.4. In *Proc. FAO/WHO Reg. Train. Seminar on Control of Rodents of Agric. and Public Health Importance.* 8–18 December, Manila, Philippines.

Rennison, B. D. 1981. *Rodent control in Kuwait.* Tolworth, England: Ministry of Agriculture, Fisheries and Food.

Rowe, F. P. 1981. Wild house mouse biology and control. *Symp. Zool. Soc. Lond.* 47:575–89.

Salmon, T. P., and W. P. Gorenzel. 1981. *Cliff swallows: How to live with them.* Coop. Exten. Leaflet 21264. Berkeley, Calif.: Univ. California.

Scott, H. G. 1966. *Rat bite: Epidemiology and control.* Atlanta: Communicable Disease Center, Dept. Health, Educ. and Welfare.

Scott, H. G., and M. R. Borom. 1977. *Rodent-borne disease control through rodent stoppage.* DHEW Publ. No. (CDC) 77-8343. Atlanta: Dept. Health, Educ. and Welfare, Public Health Service, CDC.

Seal, S. C., and R. N. Banerji. 1969. Changing patterns of rodent population in Calcutta and Howrah. In *Indian rodent symposium,* Calcutta, 1966. Johns Hopkins Univ. CMRT, Calcutta, and USAID, New Delhi, pp. 69–83.

Seligmann, J. 1982. Clinical ecology: A shadowy area. *Newsweek* (23 August):45.

Shenker, A. M. 1970. Preventive pest control. *Food Manufact.* (June):1–3.

Silver, J., W. E. Crouch, and M. C. Betts. 1930. *Rat proofing buildings and premises.* Farmers Bull. No. 1638. Washington, D.C.: Dept. Agriculture.

Smith, C.E.G. 1985. Risks from biological research. In *Risk/man-made hazards to man,* M. G. Cooper, ed. Oxford: Clarendon Press, pp. 54–75.

Smith, A., and N. G. Gratz. 1984. *Urban vector and rodent control services.* WHO/VBC/84.4. Geneva: World Health Organization.

Sonenshine, D. E., F. M. Bozeman, M. S. Williams, S. A. Masiello, D. P. Chadwick, N. I. Stocks, D. M. Lauer, and B. L. Elisburg. 1978. Epizootiology of epidemic typhus *(Rickettsia prowazekii)* in flying squirrels. *Amer. J. Trop. Med. Hyg.* 27:339–49.

Squires, S. 1986. The 'sick building' syndrome. *Washington Post,* 2 April.

Sterling, D. A. 1985. Volatile organic compounds in indoor air: An overview of sources, concentrations, and health effects. In *Indoor air and human health,* R. B. Gammage and S. V. Kaye, eds. Chelsea, Mich.: Lewis Publ., pp. 387–402.

Story, K., and D. Moreland, eds. 1982. *A. Mallis/handbook of pest control.* 6th ed. Cleveland: Franzak and Foster.

Tangley, L. 1986. The urban ecologist. *BioScience* 36:68–71.

Traub, R., C. L. Wisseman, Jr., and A. Farhang-Azad. 1978. The ecology of murine typhus—a critical review. *Trop. Dis. Bull* 75:237–317.

Trimarchi, C. V., and J. G. Debbie. 1977. Naturally occurring rabies virus and neutralizing antibody in two species of insectivorous bats of New York State. *J. Wild. Dis.* 13:368–69.

Updike, J. 1977. Rats. From *Tossing and Turning.* New York: Alfred A. Knopf, Inc.

Velimirovic, B. 1969. Rodent borne diseases and their epidemiology, Item 4.1. In *Proc. FAO/WHO Reg. Train. Seminar on Control of Rodents of Agric. and Public Health Importance.* 8–18 December, Manila, Philippines.

Vick, F., and K. Becker. 1951. Ratproofing building techniques (in German). *Schadlingsbekampfung* 43(1–3):1–57.

Weber, W. J. 1982. *Diseases transmitted by rats to man.* Fresno, Calif.: Thomson Public.

Wolcott, R. M., and B. W. Vincent, 1975. *The relationship of solid waste storage practices in the inner city to the incidence of rat infestation and fires.* EPA/530/SW/150. Cincinnati: Environmental Protection Agency.

Woldow, N. 1972. Pigeon and man: A spotty old friendship. *Natural History* 81:26–37.

Woodman, D. R., E. Weiss, G. A. Dasch, and M. Bozeman. 1977. Biological properties of *Rickettsia prowazekii* strains isolated from flying squirrels. *Infect. Immun.* 16(3):853–60.

World Health Organization (WHO). 1974. *Ecology and control of rodents of public health importance.* WHO Tech. Rep. Ser. No. 553. Geneva: World Health Organization.

Zahner, G.E.P., S. V. Kasl, M. White, and J. C. Will. 1985. Psychological consequences of infestation of the dwelling unit. *Am. J. Public Health.* 75:1303–7.

# 12

# Ultraviolet Air Disinfection to Control Tuberculosis in a Shelter for the Homeless

EDWARD A. NARDELL

The most successful application of ultraviolet air disinfection to the control of airborne infection, detailed and referenced by Riley in Chapter 8, was the prevention of measles in day schools in Pennsylvania. The main difference between that trial and subsequent unsuccessful studies was the occurrence of transmission outside of the irradiated areas in the latter situations. Tuberculosis among the homeless within shelters may be another circumstance where transmission occurs predominantly within a limited number of indoor environments, and where air disinfection might be expected to offer some protection, for the homeless as well as the people who staff the shelters. Moreover, because the usual tuberculosis control measures are of limited efficacy among the homeless, primarily due to noncompliance, passive environmental interruption of transmission would be highly desirable.

## TUBERCULOSIS AMONG THE HOMELESS

Because tuberculosis (TB) is associated with poverty, stress, alcoholism, and crowded living conditions, it is not surprising that the disease should be prevalent among the homeless in shelters, especially in shelters frequented by alcoholics and deinstitutionalized mental patients. The largest of Boston's shelters serves this population and has long been associated with a disproportionate number of the city's TB cases (Reilly and McInnis, 1985). In 1971, 41 of Boston's 299 cases were linked to this shelter. In 1973, a shelter-based clinic for TB surveillance and treatment was established; it was staffed by a full-time public health nurse and part-time physicians* and offered on-site chest radiography.

During the first three and a half years after the shelter's relocation to a new, larger facility in 1980, only 2 to 4 new cases per year were associated with the shelter and only 1 skin test conversion in a staff member was detected on routine testing every six months. Late in 1983, however, an unusually large number of tuberculosis cases, many of them drug resistant, began to be diagnosed among the then estimated 6,000 homeless of Boston. Although there are several smaller shelters in Boston, the cases occurred primarily among the male guests of the large shelter under discussion. During the fourteen-month period beginning in January 1984, 16 of the 83 resident and nonresident staff members of the shelter had tuberculin skin test conversions on routine testing. Descriptions of this outbreak and of the TB control efforts that followed have been published (Barry et al., 1986; Drug-resistant tuberculosis among the homeless—Boston, 1985). In addition, the occurrence of exogenous reinfection with TB at the shelter has been documented by Nardell and colleagues (1986). This chapter focuses on the rationale for the use of ultraviolet air disinfection as an adjunct to conventional TB control measures in this shelter setting.

The reasons for the decline in TB in association with the shelter after it moved in 1980, and its subsequent resurgence in 1983, are not entirely clear. The TB surveillance staff, facilities, and the methods employed had not changed, so that better detection was not a likely explanation. Homelessness has been increasing since 1980, resulting in more crowding in shelters and, perhaps, more poverty and stress. Other large cities, such as New York and San Francisco, also have reported more homelessness and more TB among the

*The author served as clinic physician from 1981 to 1986.

homeless (McAdam et al., 1985; Wlodarczyk et al., 1987). In addition, city and state TB case rates are increasing in many areas of the country, a major reversal of the long-standing declining case rates nationally (Tuberculosis provisional data—United States, 1987). Acquired immune deficiency syndrome (AIDS), immigration, and homelessness are believed to account for most of the excess morbidity. The Centers for Disease Control and the American Lung Association considered the homelessness component serious enough to cosponsor a national meeting devoted to sharing observations and strategies for dealing with the problem. Recommendations based on a consensus of the participants at that meeting have been published (Tuberculosis control among homeless populations, 1987).

## DIAGNOSIS AND TREATMENT AMONG THE HOMELESS

The problem of TB among the homeless is of concern, not only because of a high case rate, but because the usual TB control measures are of limited effectiveness in this population. Surveillance cannot depend on self-reporting of symptoms and diagnosis through primary health care providers. Poverty limits access to health care for many homeless persons, but others avoid establishment health care for reasons other than their ability to pay, and are often cared for only when critically ill or injured. Afterward, medical follow-up appointments are often broken. Chronic symptoms such those associated with TB are often endured well beyond the usual threshold for seeking help because they compete for attention with many other acute and chronic socioeconomic and medical problems. Moreover, providers who do see the homeless are often confronted with patients who cannot give accurate histories, and whose life-styles convey a lack of self-concern that evokes little empathy. Special projects aimed at improving health care for the homeless are ameliorating this problem in many cities, including Boston, but much more needs to be done (Barry et al., 1986).

Where available, conventional screening for TB infection by Mantoux skin testing is of limited value among the homeless. Surveys in New York City have shown that as many as half of regular shelter users test positive to the Mantoux test, thereby reducing the test's predictive value in finding current disease, compared to populations where TB infection is less common (McAdam et al., 1985). Moreover, cooperation with skin testing is a major obstacle (Barry et al., 1986). Many of the homeless are fearful of being tested, and those who do consent may not be relocated for reading of the test forty-eight to seventy-two hours later. Screening by chest x-ray usually requires only one encounter, but often means a visit to a clinic or hospital, which may be resisted by the homeless. Having chest x-rays available at the shelter avoids that hurdle, but the results obtained may be nonspecific. Bronchitis, emphysema, bacterial pneumonias, chest trauma, and lung cancer are common among the homeless and may produce symptoms and radiographic findings indistinguishable from TB. Even among high incidence populations, routine, periodic chest x-ray screening for TB is no longer recommended, based on cost-effectiveness considerations (Chest x-ray screening examinations, 1983). Screening by sputum smear and culture is more specific and may be more sensitive, but like chest x-rays, has its greatest yield among those with chronic symptoms that increase the probability of TB. Ongoing screening at the shelter has intensified since 1983, employing a combination of skin tests, x-rays, and sputum examinations, guided by the suspicions of an experienced public health nurse who sees many of the guests regularly and is in the best position to detect changes in their well-being. Although the goal of screening is primarily the detection of current TB disease, some of those found to be infected have been candidates for an attempt at preventive therapy.

Containment of TB disease, once diagnosed, presents additional problems. Drug treatment is often incomplete because of noncompliance. Drug-resistant disease, which results from erratic drug ingestion, may require therapy for as long as two years, further expanding the opportunities for noncompliance. Alcoholism and other chronic diseases further complicate treatment. Patients who fail to comply with daily treatment receive twice-weekly, supervised therapy; if this fails, they may require hospitalization for the entire duration of treatment in order to assure completion and to interrupt transmission, sometimes under the restraint of public health laws. Yet, despite all of these efforts, incomplete therapy, leading to reactivation and transmission, remains the most important source of new cases in shelters, as demonstrated by the data that follow.

**Table 12.1** Phage Type and Drug-Resistance Pattern of Organisms among Forty-two Homeless Men with Tuberculosis*

| Phage Type | Drug Resistance | | | | | | Total |
|---|---|---|---|---|---|---|---|
| | Isoniazid and Streptomycin | Isoniazid, Streptomycin, and Ethambutol | Isoniazid | Streptomycin | Ethambutol | No Resistance | |
| 8 (7, 9, 12, 13, 14, 15) | 22 | 1 | | | 1 | 1 | 25 |
| 7 (7, 9, 12, 14) | | | 1 | | | | 1 |
| 2 (9, 13, 14, 15) | | | | | | 1 | 1 |
| 2 (7, 12, 13, 15) | | | | | | 1 | 1 |
| 1 (13, 14) | | | | | | 2 | 2 |
| 1 | | | | | | 2 | 2 |
| Not determined or not viable | 5 | | | 1 | | 4 | 10 |
| Total | 27 | 1 | 1 | 1 | 1 | 11 | 42 |

*From* Nardell, E., et al., 1986. Reproduced with the permission of the authors and publisher.

*In seven patients, TB was diagnosed on clinical grounds, without bacteriologic confirmation.

## EVIDENCE FOR TRANSMISSION WITHIN THE SHELTER

As indicated in Table 12.1, of the first forty-two cases among the homeless, twenty-two were due to organisms resistant to both isoniazid and streptomycin, and of the same phage type, indicating a common origin for nearly half of the cases. The probable source case for the twenty-two linked cases was known ten years earlier to have had isoniazid and streptomycin resistance. This man had not complied with previous courses of therapy. He was again diagnosed with reactivation TB, with the same resistance pattern, in January 1983, eleven months before the first of the twenty-two cases presented. Isoniazid and streptomycin resistance has been seen on occasion among the homeless in the past, and in isolated cases with no direct homeless connection; the pattern was found in only 1.9 percent of 1,035 cultures processed at the state mycobacteriology laboratory from 1981 through 1983. Combined with the specificity of the phage type, it can be confidently stated that the twenty-two cases were the result of recent transmission associated with the large shelter in Boston. This finding contradicts the widely held view that TB among the homeless results predominantly from the episodic reactivation of old infections, known to be prevalent among long-term shelter users. A reactivation pathogenesis would necessitate a sequence of events highly unlikely in this transient population: a common source for at least twenty-two infections at some time in the past, followed by independent reactivations over a relatively short period, all in association with one shelter and occurring almost nowhere else in the area.

The observation that TB disease resulted from new infection as well as reactivation has implications for public health interventions. If reactivation of old disease was primarily the problem, rather than ongoing transmission, prevention, however difficult, would rely heavily on isoniazid prophylaxis of those already infected who do not yet have disease. However, if transmission and new infection are important components of the pathogenesis, the strategies should be diagnosis and treatment of active cases to render them noninfectious, preventive therapy for those newly infected, and air disinfection to prevent further transmission. Another strategy for shelter planners would be to build many smaller shelters rather than fewer larger ones where widespread transmission is more likely to occur. Before we describe the ultraviolet air disinfection within the large Boston shelter, one more consideration regarding the mode of transmission deserves mention.

## EXOGENOUS REINFECTION AND THE POSSIBILITY OF ACCELERATED EPIDEMIC TRANSMISSION WITHIN THE SHELTER

The twenty-two linked cases associated with the shelter were remarkable not only for their drug resistance and for the recent transmission indicated by the bacteriologic markers, but for the high frequency of extensive, cavitary, lung disease; the type usually associated with reactivation disease and with contagiousness. Yet, as explained earlier, the markers precluded reactivation as the pathogenic mechanism for these cases. An alternative explanation for the cavitation was that some of those recently infected had been previously infected and were, therefore, already hypersensitive to tuberculoproteins and prone to lung cavitation on reinfection with the resistant strain. Exogenous reinfection was proven in four of the twenty-two cases where convincing evidence of previous infection or disease was obtained from the review of old records and chest x-rays (Nardell et al., 1986). An additional three cases of reinfection have subsequently been identified; other cases, in which reinfection is suspected, remain unproven due to the lack of reliable past medical data. All seven proven reinfection cases had advanced cavitary lung disease, positive sputum smears, and, therefore, a high likelihood of having been contagious. In contrast, four other bacteriologically linked cases, known to be Mantoux-negative just before the outbreak, had disease typical of primary TB, without cavitation or smear positivity (Table 12.2). These cases were not likely to have been contagious. Unlike measles and some other rapidly spreading viral illnesses, most new TB infections never progress to clinical disease, and those that do develop symptomatic primary disease are usually not highly contagious. Based on these seven cases, however, and other observations in the literature, we have theorized that exogenous reinfection may have been associated with a propensity for prompt lung cavitation

**Table 12.2** Previous Tuberculosis Histories of Eight Patients with Bacteriologically Linked Tuberculosis

| Patient No. | Age | Time in Shelters | Prior TB History* | Current Disease | Diagnosis Date | Sputum Smear |
|---|---|---|---|---|---|---|
| Known previous infection | | | | | | |
| 1 | 34 | 11 yr | Positive PPD 1973<br>Abnormal x-rays†<br>Treated | Cavitary | 12/29/83 | ++++ |
| 2 | 53 | 6 yr | Positive PPD 1980<br>Abnormal x-rays†<br>Treated | Cavitary | 07/05/84 | ++++ |
| 3 | 55 | 6 yr | Positive PPD 1979<br>Abnormal x-rays† | Cavitary | 10/31/84 | ++++ |
| 4 | 68 | 8 yr | Positive TB culture 1978<br>Sensitive to all drugs<br>Treated | Cavitary | 10/01/85 | +++ |
| Negative Mantoux before outbreak | | | | | | |
| 5 | 57 | 5 yr | Negative PPD 12/83<br>Negative x-ray | Lung infiltrate | 03/14/84 | Negative |
| 6 | 29 | 3–4 mo | Negative PPD 1/84<br>No x-rays | Pleural effusion | 05/01/84 | Negative |
| 7 | 25 | 1 yr | Negative PPD 2/83<br>No x-rays | Lung infiltrate | 07/06/84 | Negative |
| 8 | 26 | 1 yr | Negative PPD 12/83<br>No x-rays | Adenopathy, lung nodule | 08/13/84 | + |

*From* Nardell, E., et al., 1986. Reproduced with the permission of the authors and publisher.

*PPD denotes the test for reaction to purified protein derivative of tuberculin.

†X-ray abnormalities were consistent with mycobacterial disease.

and an acceleration of the usual pattern of epidemic transmission (Grange, 1986; Nardell et al., 1986).

Unknown local and systemic host factors might also explain the disease progression observed in this population. But even if reinfection itself did not accelerate transmission, its occurrence strongly indicates heavy air contamination. The demonstration of transmission and of reinfection within the shelter amplifies the need for air disinfection, in addition to good surveillance and treatment, if TB control among the homeless is to be achieved.

## ULTRAVIOLET AIR DISINFECTION

The shelter facility was remodeled for its current use in 1980. It consists of several large, joined buildings. It sleeps 350 persons on beds in three upper floors, with a public dining area and the medical clinic, including x-ray facilities, on the main floor. However, on cold winter nights, until the recent opening of another building nearby, the shelter allowed as many as 350 additional homeless people to sleep on the benches and floors of the first-floor lobby areas. Under crowded conditions, inadequate ventilation may have contributed to the airborne transmission of TB infection.

Fresh air ventilation in the dormitory areas was probably adequate, as estimated by ambient $CO_2$ measurements taken in the early morning hours. In the first-floor lobby areas, however, ventilation, which would have been adequate for normal occupancy, was suboptimal for the large numbers of people sleeping and eating in that space. Increasing ventilation to meet peak requirements would not be a practical solution. Moreover, mathematic modeling of indoor TB transmission indicates that when the number of tuberculin bacilli generated is large, as postulated at the shelter, increasing ventilation is relatively ineffective in reducing transmission. At the levels needed to offer significant protection, increased ventilation would be expensive, noisy, and uncomfortably drafty. Further modeling predicts that ultraviolet air disinfection would offer more than twice the protection achievable by optimal levels of ventilation (Nardell et al., 1987).

Ultraviolet air disinfection is being employed in this shelter as a way to help reduce TB transmission without requiring active participation by guests or staff. However, as indicated previously, air disinfection would be predicted to help protect the homeless from TB only if their main source of exposure was at the shelter. The evidence, so far, suggests that this may be true. As a rule, shelter guests are required to leave the building after breakfast. During the day, the homeless are generally outside or in relatively large public buildings. Although the homeless frequent several soup kitchens and smaller shelters in Boston, none of these places has been associated with TB at rates approaching that of the large shelter.

The ultraviolet light installation was planned and executed in two stages. The large public areas were well suited to overhead irradiation because of their high ceilings. This was especially true of one large lobby (Figure 12.1). These areas were considered to have high priority due to crowding during the winter months when the shelter case rate soared. The ultraviolet dosage was based on one 30-watt fixture per 200 sq ft of floor space (see Riley, Chapter 8). Twenty-three fixtures were required for the ground floor, most of which were the long, hanging type operating at 29 watts. In addition, two special circular units and three wall-mounted fixtures were best suited to certain structural requirements. The installation considerations out-

**Figure 12.1.** Ultraviolet light installation in lobby of homeless shelter. (Photo by E. A. Nardell.)

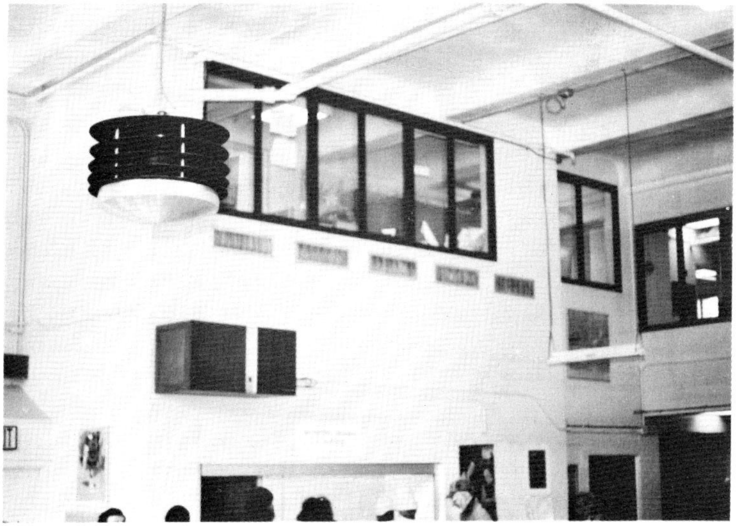

lined by Riley were closely followed (see Appendix, Chapter 8). After installation, the lights were checked for the possibility of eye irritation, and metered for both safety and effective output before routine use. Fixtures were adjusted to expose room occupants to no more than 0.2 $\mu W/cm^2$ of ultraviolet intensity. Excess reflection was reduced by moving fixtures or by using low-reflecting paint (aerosolized stove black).

The second phase was to irradiate the dormitory areas on the remaining three floors, wherever ceiling height was adequate. In all, forty-seven fixtures were required, all of the long, hanging type. The same dosage calculations and installation procedures were used. However, competitive bids for the contract resulted in considerable savings over the initial installation, without compromising quality. A grant from the American Lung Association of Boston helped defray the cost. The grant was given with the understanding that the entire installation would be completed and that an attempt to study the efficacy of the intervention would follow. That study is now under way. Although this installation was not inexpensive, its total cost was less than the cost of three months' in-patient care for one homeless TB case—when transmission was not prevented.

## EFFICACY OF ULTRAVIOLET AIR DISINFECTION

Studying the effect of ultraviolet air disinfection on tuberculosis transmission with a shelter for the homeless is replete with even more problems than studying ultraviolet disinfection's effectiveness on measles transmission in schools. Observing TB case rates in parallel populations at equal risk for TB infection, with and without air disinfection, is not possible. Symptomatic cases reflect only a fraction of those infected; furthermore, these cases present episodically and vary widely in infectiousness. As indicated previously, surveillance among the homeless is difficult at best. A failure to reduce the number of cases may mean that the ultraviolet lights are ineffective, but it could also reflect a simultaneous increase in cases due to other factors. Tuberculosis infection acquired outside the irradiated areas, for example, as in the measles trials, would reduce apparent efficacy. Similarly, a reduction in cases may reflect other factors, such as more effective treatment or less crowding due to the availability of additional shelters.

We have chosen to monitor skin test conversions among the staff, relative to the cases among the guests, as an indicator of transmission within the shelter. New TB cases have continued to be diagnosed at a rate of about twenty per year over the period of installation and since completion of the project in February 1987. While bacteriologic markers link most of the recent cases to those that first presented in 1983, it has not been possible to determine whether transmission occurred before or after air disinfection began. However, whereas sixteen of eighty-three resident and nonresident shelter staff had PPD conversions over the fourteen-month period beginning January 1984, only nine more have occurred through 1986 and none through 1987.

Assuming efficacy can be demonstrated in the field situation, other problems remain to be solved. Does it make sense to calculate dosage by room floor area in shelters where room occupancy varies widely? Would it be more appropriate to base dosage on occupancy, similar to fresh air ventilation standards? Riley (Chapter 8) has suggested one 30-watt fixture for each six to seven room occupants. How does room height effect the calculation? Theoretically, a higher space above the lights provides a larger irradiation chamber which should improve efficacy. Is there a role for ultraviolet light in ductwork under some circumstances? These and other questions may be answered in years to come. The current problem of TB in shelters for the homeless, and the absence of good solutions for its control, led to the use of ultraviolet air disinfection based on what is known today. At least one other public health program arrived at the same idea independently and also uses ultraviolet lights in its shelters (Stead, 1986). The ultimate solutions to homelessness and its ramifications may be socioeconomic, political, and moral. In the meantime, renewed interest in ultraviolet light air disinfection may help alleviate TB transmission among the homeless, and should result in new knowledge to better guide its application.

## REFERENCES

Barry, M. A., C. Wall, L. Shirley et al. 1986. Tuberculosis screening in Boston's homeless shelters. *Public Health Rep.* 101:487–94.

Chest x-ray screening examinations. 1983. U.S. Department of Health and Human Services, Rockville, Md. (HHS) Publication (FDA) 83-8204.

Drug-resistant tuberculosis among the homeless—Boston. 1985. *Morbidity and Mortality Weekly Report (MMWR)* 34:429–31.

Grange, J. M. 1986. Environmental mycobacteria and BCG vaccination. *Tubercle* 67:1–4.

McAdam, J., P. W. Brickner, R. Glickman, D. Edwards, B. Fallon, P. Yanowitch. 1985. Tuberculosis in the SRO/homeless population. In P. W. Brickner, L. K. Scharer, B. Conanan, A. Elvy, and M. Savarese, eds. *Health care of homeless people.* New York: Springer, pp. 155–75.

Nardell, E., B. McInnis, B. Thomas, and S. Weidhaas. 1986. Exogenous reinfection with tuberculosis in a shelter for the homeless. *N. Engl. J. Med.* 315:1570–75.

Nardell, E., S. Weidhaas, J. Keegan, L. Cheney, L. Mofenson, and J. Greenspan. 1987. Tuberculosis transmission in a tight office building: The theoretical limits of protection achievable by increased ventilation. *Am. Rev. Resp. Dis.* (suppl.) 135:A33.

Reilly, E., and B. N. McInnis, 1985. Boston, Massachusetts: The Pine Street Inn Nurses' Clinic and Tuberculosis Program. In P. W. Brickner, L. K. Scharer, B. Conanan, A. Elvy, and M. Savarese, eds., *Health care of homeless people.* New York: Springer, pp. 291–99.

Stead, W. 1986. Personal communication.

Tuberculosis control among homeless populations. 1987. *MMWR* 36:257–60.

Tuberculosis provisional data—United States, 1986. 1987. *MMWR* 36:254–55.

Wlodarczyk, D., G. Schecter, and P. Hopewell. 1987. Screening for tuberculosis in shelters for the homeless in San Francisco. *Am. Rev. Resp. Dis.* 135 (suppl.):A31.

# Index